FIRST AID FOR THE®

Medicine Clerkship

Third Edition

MATTHEW S. KAUFMAN, MD

Assistant Professor
Albert Einstein College of Medicine
Department of Hematology
North Shore–Long Island Jewish Medical Center
New Hyde Park, New York

LATHA G. STEAD, MD, MS, FACEP

Chief, Division of Clinical Research
Professor of Emergency Medicine
University of Florida College of Medicine at Gainesville
Adjunct Professor of Emergency Medicine
Mayo Clinic, College of Medicine
Rochester, Minnesota
Editor-in-Chief, *International Journal of Emergency Medicine*

ARTHUR RUSOVICI, MD

Cardiology Fellow
Division of Cardiology
University of Medicine and Dentistry of New Jersey
Newark, New Jersey
Formerly Chief Medical Resident
Department of Internal Medicine
North Shore–Long Island Jewish Medical Center
New Hyde Park, New York

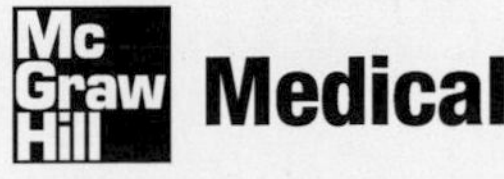

Medical

New York / Chicago / San Francisco / Lisbon / London / Madrid / Mexico City
Milan / New Delhi / San Juan / Seoul / Singapore / Sydney / Toronto

The McGraw-Hill Companies

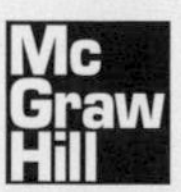

FIRST AID FOR THE® MEDICINE CLERKSHIP, THIRD EDITION
International Edition 2010

NOTICE

Medicine is an ever-changing science. As new research and clinical experience broaden our knowledge, changes in treatment and drug therapy are required. The authors and the publisher of this work have checked with sources believed to be reliable in their efforts to provide information that is complete and generally in accord with the standards accepted at the time of publication. However, in view of the possibility of human error or changes in medical sciences, neither the authors nor the publisher nor any other party who has been involved in the preparation or publication of this work warrants that the information contained herein is in every respect accurate or complete, and they disclaim all responsibility for any errors or omissions or for the results obtained from use of the information contained in this work. Readers are encouraged to confirm the information contained herein with other sources. For example and in particular, readers are advised to check the product information sheet included in the package of each drug they plan to administer to be certain that the information contained in this work is accurate and that changes have not been made in the recommended dose or in the contraindications for administration. The recommendation is of particular importance in connection with new or infrequently used drugs.

10 09 08 07 06 05 04 03 02
20 15 14 13 12 11
CTP COS

Library of Congress Cataloging-in-Publication Data
Kaufman, Matthew S.
First aid for the medicine clerkship / Matthew S. Kaufman, Latha G. Stead, Arthur Rusovici. -- 3rd ed.
p. ; cm.
Other title: Medicine clerkship
Rev. ed. of: First aid for the medicine clerkship / series editors, Latha G. Stead, S. Matthew Stead, Matthew S. Kaufman ; supervising editor and contributing author, Samy I. McFarlane. 2nd ed. 2005.
Includes index.
ISBN-13: 978-0-07-163382-6
ISBN-10: 0-07-163382-0 1. Clinical clerkship. I. Stead, Latha G. II. Rusovici, Arthur . III. Title. IV. Title: Medicine clerkship.
[DNLM: 1. Clinical Clerkship--Handbooks. 2. Career Choice--Handbooks. 3. Fellowships and Scholarships--Handbooks. 4. First Aid--Handbooks. W 49 K21f 2010]
R839.F57 2010
610.71'1--dc22

2010011625

When ordering this title, use ISBN 978-007-108301-0 or MHID 007-108301-4

Printed in Singapore

DEDICATION

To my mother, Madeleine, and stepfather, Costas, for their love and support. — MK

To my parents, Ganti and Prabha Rao, for giving me the peace and encouragement to excel, always. — LS

I would like to dedicate this book to my family. Mom, Dad, Tommy, and Grandma, I love you dearly and I thank you for the lessons, the care, and the support you have all given me. — AR

CONTENTS

PREFACE

In the 2010 edition of *First Aid for the® Medicine Clerkship*, a complete and thorough revision has been done to make the book an even more effective tool to ace both the clerkship and the shelf exam. These changes have been made carefully according to valuable feedback from extensive student and faculty reviews.

In addition to stylistic updates, the following changes have been made:

- An overhaul of topic organization with additions to some and reductions of others to emphasize the most relevant information.
- Update of information according to newer guidelines and data.
- The addition of minicases which provide classic exam scenarios.
- Additional exam tips to point out the favorite tested facts.

We are grateful to all of the student and faculty contributors who made this edition the best yet and we welcome additional feedback for the continued improvement of *First Aid for the® Medicine Clerkship*. (See How to Contribute, p. ix.)

New Hyde Park, New York Matthew Kaufman
Rochester, New York Latha Stead

HOW TO CONTRIBUTE

We are grateful for and welcome any updates, corrections, and study hints. Contributors will receive compensation and credit at the discretion of the authors. Also let us know about material in this edition that you feel is low yield and should be deleted.

The preferred way to submit entries, suggestions, or corrections is via e-mail:

Mattkaufman1@gmail.com; Latha.Stead@gmail.com; firstaidclerkships@gmail.com; Catherine_Johnson@mcgraw-hill.com.

NOTE TO CONTRIBUTORS

All contributions become property of the authors and are subject to editing and reviewing. Please verify all data and spellings carefully. In the event that similar or duplicate entries are received, only the first entry received will be used. Include a reference to a standard textbook to facilitate verification of the fact. Please follow the style, punctuation, and format of this edition if possible.

CONTRIBUTORS

Jian Li Campian, MD, PhD
Resident
North Shore–LIJ Health System
Long Island Jewish Medical Center
New Hyde Park, New York
Endocrinology

Bella Fradlis, MD
Medical Student
Department of Medicine
Columbia University Medical Center
New York–Presbyterian Hospital
New York, New York
Dermatology

Abhishek Jaiswal, MBBS
Resident, Department of Internal Medicine
Long Island Jewish Medical Center
New Hyde Park, New York
Gastroenterology
Health Maintenance and Evidence Based Medicine

Tim Johnson, MD
Internal Medicine
Emergency Medicine
Critical Care
Long Island Jewish Medical Center
New Hyde Park, New York
Neurology

Pralay K. Sarkar, MD, MRCP(UK)
Attending Physician
Hospitalist Division, Department of Internal Medicine
Long Island Jewish Medical
New Hyde Park, New York
Pulmonary Diseases

Peter Bryan Schrier, MD
Resident
Internal Medicine
Long Island Jewish Medical Center
New Hyde Park, New York
Nephrology and Acid-Base Disorders

Bilal K. Siddiqui, MD
Resident
Long Island Jewish Medical Center
New Hyde Park, New York
Hematology-Oncology

Avneet Singh, MD, MRCP(UK)
Resident
Internal Medicine Residency Program
Long Island Jewish Medical Center
New Hyde Park, New York
Cardiology
Rheumatology

Joshua N. Vernatter, MD
Resident
Long Island Jewish Medical Center
New Hyde Park, New York
Infectious Disease

FACULTY EDITOR

Samy I. McFarlane, MD, MPH, MBA, FACP
Professor of Medicine
Division of Endocrinology
Medical Director of Clinical Research
College of Medicine
State University of New York–Dowstate Medical Center
Kings County Hospital
Brooklyn, New York

STUDENT REVIEWERS

Jean C. Ancelet
Medical Student
LSUHSC New Orleans School of Medicine

Mary M. Bonar
Medical Student
Ohio University College of Osteopathic Medicine

Kenneth Marc Fomberstein
Class of 2010
Albert Einstein College of Medicine

Dmitriy Kedrin
Medical Student
Albert Einstein College of Medicine

Eileen Kisilis
Medical Student
Albert Einstein College of Medicine

Vibhuti Kowluru
Medical Student
Albert Einstein College of Medicine

Christy Nolan
Medical Student
Lake Erie College of Medicine

Brian Park
Medical Student
Albert Einstein College of Medicine

Sharon Rose
Medical Student
Albert Einstein College of Medicine

Matthew Saybolt
Medical Student
UMDNJ Robert Wood Johnson Medical School

David Scoville
Medical Student
Kansas University Medical Center

SECTION I

How to Succeed in the Medicine Clerkship

HOW TO BEHAVE ON THE WARDS

Be on Time

Most medical ward teams begin rounding between 7 and 8 AM. If you are expected to "pre-round," you should give yourself at least 10 minutes per patient that you are following to see the patient and learn about the events that occurred overnight. Like all working professionals, you will face occasional obstacles to punctuality, but make sure this is occasional. When you first start a rotation, try to show up at least 15 minutes early until you get the routine figured out. If the morning vitals are not yet recorded, take them yourself. Also, look at the chart to update yourself on any developments.

Dress in a Professional Manner

Even if the resident wears scrubs and the attending wears stiletto heels, you must dress in a professional, conservative manner. Wear a *short* white coat over your clothes unless discouraged (as in pediatrics).

- **Men** should wear long pants, with cuffs covering the ankle, a long collared shirt, and a tie. No jeans, no sneakers, no short-sleeved shirts.
- **Women** should wear long pants or knee-length skirt and a blouse or dressy sweater. No jeans, no sneakers, no heels greater than 1½ inches, no open-toed shoes.
- **Both men and women** may wear scrubs occasionally, during overnight call or in the operating room. Do not make this your uniform.

Act in a Pleasant Manner

The medical rotation is often difficult, stressful, and tiring. Smooth out your experience by being nice to be around. Smile a lot and learn everyone's name. Don't be afraid to ask how your resident's weekend was. If you do not understand or disagree with a treatment plan or diagnosis, do not "challenge." Instead, say, "I'm sorry, I don't quite understand, could you please explain. . ." Show kindness and compassion toward your patients. Never participate in callous talk about patients.

Be Aware of the Hierarchy

The way in which this will affect you will vary from hospital to hospital and team to team, but it is always present to some degree. In general, address your questions regarding ward functioning to interns or residents. Address your medical questions to attendings; make an effort to be somewhat informed on your subject prior to asking attendings medical questions. It's always good to make your residents look good on rounds (. . . "Dr. Smith was nice enough to teach me about . . ."). Make sure the resident knows new patient developments ASAP.

Address Patients and Staff in a Respectful Way

Address patients as Sir, Ma'am, or Mr., Mrs., or Miss. Try not to address patients as "honey," "sweetie," and the like. Although you may feel these names are friendly, patients will think you have forgotten their name, that you are being inappropriately familiar, or both. Address all physicians as "doctor," unless told otherwise.

Show Initiative

Often, residents are busy with work and neglect their teaching responsibilities. Read up on your patient's condition, find an article, and offer to summarize in a few minutes what you learned. Give a copy of the article to your resident. This kind of initiative goes a long way in evaluations.

Take Responsibility for Your Patients

Know everything there is to know about your patients: their history, test results, details about their medical problem, and prognosis. Keep your intern or resident informed of new developments that they might not be aware of, and ask them for any updates you might not be aware of. Assist the team in developing a plan; speak to radiology, consultants, and family. Never give bad news to patients or family members without the assistance of your supervising resident or attending.

Respect Patients' Rights

1. All patients have the right to have their personal medical information kept private. This means do not discuss the patient's information with family members without that patient's consent, and do not discuss any patient in hallways, elevators, or cafeterias.
2. All patients have the right to refuse treatment. This means they can refuse treatment by a specific individual (you, the medical student) or of a specific type (no nasogastric tube). Patients can even refuse lifesaving treatment. The only exceptions to this rule are if the patient is deemed to not have the capacity to make decisions or understand situations, in which case a health care proxy should be sought, or if the patient is suicidal or homicidal.
3. All patients should be informed of the right to seek advance directives on admission. Often, this is done by the admissions staff, in a booklet. If your patient is chronically ill or has a life-threatening illness, address the subject of advance directives with the assistance of your attending.

Volunteer

Be self-propelled, self-motivated. Volunteer to help with a procedure or a difficult task. Volunteer to give a 20-minute talk on a topic of your choice. Volunteer to take additional patients. Volunteer to stay late. If the answer is "You don't have to," do it anyway.

Be a Team Player

Help other medical students with their tasks; teach them information you have learned. Support your supervising intern or resident whenever possible. Never steal the spotlight, steal a procedure, or make a fellow medical student look bad. Making other people look good always helps you, too.

Be Honest

If you don't understand, don't know, or didn't do it, make sure you always say that. Never say or document information that is false (a common example: "bowel sounds normal" when you did not listen). This can get you into serious trouble.

Keep Patient Information Handy

Use a clipboard, notebook, or index cards to keep patient information, including a miniature history and physical, and lab and test results, at hand. The first day of the rotation, learn the computer system so that you can get lab and test results on your own. Know all of these results *before* your resident does; don't ask him or her what a test showed, tell them!

Present Patient Information in an Organized Manner

Here is a template for the "bullet" presentation:

> "This is a [age]-year-old [gender] with a history of [major history such as HTN, DM, coronary artery disease, CA, etc.] who presented on [date] with [major symptoms, such as cough, fever, and chills] and was found to have [working diagnosis]. [Tests done] showed [results]. Yesterday, the patient [state important changes, new plan, new tests, new medications]. This morning the patient feels [state the patient's words], and the physical exam is significant for [state major findings]. Plan is [state plan].

The newly admitted patient generally deserves a longer presentation following the complete history and physical format.

Some patients have extensive histories. The whole history should be present in the admission note, but in ward presentation, it is often too much to absorb. In these cases, it will be very much appreciated by your team if you can generate a **good summary** that maintains an accurate picture of the patient. This usually takes some thought, but it's worth it.

Document Information in an Organized Manner

A complete medical student initial History and Physical is neat, legible, organized, and usually two to three pages long. Major topics should include: chief complaint, history of present illness, medical history, surgical history, medications, allergies, sexual history, smoking and alcohol history, occupation, travel, review of systems, vital signs, physical exam, lab results, test results, assessment or problem list, and plan.

HOW TO ORGANIZE YOUR LEARNING

The main advantage to doing the medical clerkship is that you get to see patients. The patient is the key to learning medicine, and the source of most satisfaction and frustration on the wards. Plan your learning before the rotation starts as follows.

Make a List of Core Material to Learn

This list should reflect common symptoms, illnesses, and areas in which you have particular interest, or in which you feel particularly weak. Do not try to learn every possible topic. The Committee of Directors in Internal Medicine (*www.im.org/cdim/*) publishes a list of core content, on which this book is based. The CDIM emphasizes:

Symptoms and Lab Tests
- Abdominal pain
- Altered mental status
- Anemia
- Back pain
- Chest pain
- Cough
- Dysuria
- Fluid, electrolyte, and acid-base disorders

Common Illnesses
- Chronic obstructive pulmonary disease (COPD)
- Congestive heart failure
- Depression
- Diabetes mellitus
- Dyslipidemia
- Human immunodeficiency virus (HIV) infection
- Hypertension
- Smoking cessation
- Substance abuse
- Common cancers

We Also Recommend
- Adult vaccinations
- Domestic violence
- Dysrhythmias
- Nutritional disorders

Select Your Study Material

We recommend:

- This review book, *First Aid for the Clinical Clerkship in Medicine*
- A major medicine textbook such as *Harrison's Principles of Internal Medicine* (costs about $135)
- A full-text online journal database, such as www.mdconsult.com (subscription is $99/year for students)
- A small pocket reference book to look up lab values, clinical pathways, and the like, such as *Maxwell Quick Medical Reference* (costs $7)
- A small book to look up drugs, such as *Pocket Pharmacopoeia* (Tarascon Publishers, $9.95)

Make a Schedule to Learn the Illness-Based Topics

This schedule should reflect the rotation you are doing. For example, for the time you are going to be rotating in a clinic or office, make a schedule to study smoking cessation, dyslipidemia, depression, and diabetes. First, read this review book on each topic, then read the major textbook, taking notes. Make sure to include all chosen topics in your schedule, but leave room at least 2 weeks before the clerkship exam for review.

As You See Patients, Note Their Major Symptoms and Diagnosis for Review

Your reading on the symptom-based topics above should be done with a specific patient in mind. For example, if a patient comes to the office with cough, fever, and night sweats and is thought to have tuberculosis, read about chronic and acute cough, postnasal drip, asthma, gastroesophageal reflux disease (GERD), pneumonia, and tuberculosis in this review book that night.

Prepare a Talk on a Topic

You may be asked to give a small talk once or twice during your rotation. If not, you should volunteer! Feel free to choose a topic that is on your list; however, realize that this may be considered dull by the people who hear the lecture. The ideal topic is slightly uncommon but not rare, for example, cardiomyopathy. To prepare a talk on a topic, read about it in a major textbook and a review article not more than 2 years old, and then search online or in the library for recent developments or changes in treatment.

HOW TO PREPARE FOR THE CLINICAL CLERKSHIP EXAM

If you have read about your core illnesses and core symptoms, you will know a great deal about medicine. To study for the clerkship exam, we recommend:

2–3 weeks before exam: Read this entire review book, taking notes.
10 days before exam: Read the notes you took during the rotation on your core content list and the corresponding review book sections.
5 days before exam: Read this entire review book, concentrating on lists and mnemonics.
2 days before exam: Exercise, eat well, skim the book, and go to bed early.
1 day before exam: Exercise, eat well, review your notes and the mnemonics, and go to bed on time. Do not have any caffeine after 2 PM.

Other helpful studying strategies include:

Study with Friends

Group studying can be very helpful. Other people may point out areas that you have not studied enough and may help you focus on the goal. If you tend to get distracted by other people in the room, limit this to less than half of your study time.

Study in a Bright Room

Find the room in your house or in your library that has the best, brightest light. This will help prevent you from falling asleep. If you don't have a bright light, get a halogen desk lamp or a light that simulates sunlight (not a tanning lamp).

Eat Light, Balanced Meals

Make sure your meals are balanced, with lean protein, fruits and vegetables, and fiber. A high-sugar, high-carbohydrate meal will give you an initial burst of energy for 1–2 hours, but then you'll drop.

Take Practice Exams

The point of practice exams is not so much the content that is contained in the questions, but the training of sitting still for 3 hours and trying to pick the best answer for each and every question.

Tips for Answering Questions

All questions are intended to have one best answer. When answering questions, follow these guidelines:

Read the answers first. For all questions longer than two sentences, reading the answers first can help you sift through the question for the key information.

Look for the words "EXCEPT, MOST, LEAST, NOT, BEST, WORST, TRUE, FALSE, CORRECT, INCORRECT, ALWAYS, and NEVER." If you find one of these words, circle or underline it for later comparison with the answer.

Evaluate each answer as being either true or false. Example:

Which of the following is *least* likely to be associated with pulmonary embolism?

A. Tachycardia **T**
B. Tachypnea **T**
C. Chest pain? **F not always**
D. Deep venous thrombosis? **T not always**
E. Back pain? **F aortic dissection**

By comparing the question, noting LEAST, to the answers, "E" is the best answer.

As the Boy Scouts say, "BE PREPARED."

POCKET CARDS FOR THE WARDS

The "cards" on the following page contain information that is often helpful in family practice. We advise that you make a copy of these cards, cut them out, and carry them in your coat pocket.

History

CC:	complaint (pt's words)
HPI:	- age, race, sex - chronological description of illness, include relevant PMH - include dates, times, sx, prior occurrences & treatment - sx description: location, duration, frequency, timing, quality, radiation, aggravating or relieving factors, & associated sx
PMH:	illnesses not mentioned in HPI
PSH:	surgeries not mentioned in HPI
OBH:	ob/gyn Hx in women (if not in HPI)
Psy:	psychiatric Hx, if present
All:	drugs (foods, insects, pollen, etc.), transfusion rxns, describe rxn
Med:	current medications, home remedies, vitamins
FH:	ages, health, causes of death, HTN, HD, DM, CA, arthritis, hereditary diseases, Sx similar to pt's
SH:	occupations (past & present), home situation, lifestyle, sexual practices, religion
Trv:	country of origin, travel history
Tox:	- toxic habits (tobacco, alcohol, illicit drugs) - CAGE: Cut down/Annoyed/Guilty/Eye-opener

ROS:

Gen:	fever, weight change, appetite, sleep, night sweats
Skin:	rash, itch, growths, color change, hair loss/growth
Head:	headaches, trauma
Eyes:	acuity, spots, flashes, diplopia, pain
Ears:	acuity, tinnitus, vertigo, infection, discharge
Nose:	bleed, sinusitis, congestion, rhinorrhea, acuity
Mouth:	lesions, sore throat, teeth/gums, bruxism, TMJ
Neck:	pain, stiffness, swollen glands
Lung:	cough, wheeze, sputum (color), SOB, pleuritic pain, emphysema, bronchitis, TB, last CXR
Heart:	CP, palpitations, HTN, edema, orthopnea, murmurs
GI:	pain, N/V, diarrhea/constipation, bleeding, abd girth
GU:	pain, dysuria/frequency/urgency, nocturia, discharge, masses, STDs, sexual dysfunction/libido
Gyn:	menarche/menopause, hot flashes, contraception LMP, meno/metrorrhagia, dyspareunia
Breast:	pain, lumps, discharge, self-exam
Musc:	cramps, bone pain, joint pain/swelling, arthritis, gout
Vasc:	varicose, DVTs, claudication/rest pain, Raynaud's
Endo:	heat/cold intolerance, polydipsia/uria, polyphagia
Heme:	anemia, excess bleeding, easy bruising
Neuro:	seizures, syncope, weakness/paralysis, paresthesias, tics, tremors, memory deficits, blackouts
Psych:	anxiety/tension, depression/suicide, insomnia, concentration, mood swings, paranoia, voices

Physical

VS:	T, HR, RR, BP (upright vs recumbent, R arm vs leg), O_2 sat pain
Gen:	appearance, distress/anxiety, obese/wasted, apparent age
Skin:	texture, color, turgor, temp, lesions, rashes, scars, hair texture/distribution, cyanosis, edema
Hands:	deformities, arthritic nodes, nail pitting/stippling, capillary refill, clubbing
LN:	axillary, cervical, postauricular, supraclavicular, inguinal (mobility, size, texture)
H/N :	size, symmetry, trauma (palpate), neck ROM, thyroid, carotid pulses/bruits, JVD
Eyes:	pupils, EOMs, alignment, acuity, visual fields, conjunctiva/sclera, fundi, nystagmus, strabismus
Ears:	location/symmetry, auditory acuity, TMs, discharge
Nose:	discharge, congestion, frontal/maxillary sinus tenderness
Mouth:	pharynx (erythema, exudate), uvula, tonsils, palate, gums, lips, tongue
Back:	alignment, spinal/CV tenderness, ROM
Chest:	symmetry, retractions, air entry, breath sounds, percussion
CVS:	PMI, thrills, heart sounds, murmurs, rhythm, peripheral pulses
Murm:	grade (I - VI), timing (midsystolic, diastolic, etc), quality (rumbling, click, vibratory, etc.) location (e.g. lower left sternal border), radiation (axilla, neck, back, etc.), accentuating maneuvers (squatting, Valsalva, etc.)
Breast:	symmetry, dimples, masses, pain, nipple shape/discharge
Abd:	bowel sounds/bruits, distention, tenderness, rebound, guarding, rigidity, liver borders (palpation, percussion, scratch test), hepatojugular reflux, Murphy's, spleen, masses, aorta (AAA), percussion (tympany), shifting dullness/fluid wave
Rectal:	sphincter tone, prostate, mass, hemorrhoid/fissure/abscess, guaiac
♂ GU:	lesions, meatal discharge, pain, scrotal veins/mass/swelling, (transilluminate) inguinal/femoral masses (reducible)
♀ GU:	lesions, discharges, odors, swelling, pelvic if indicated
Neuro:	strength (0-5), tone, DTRs (0-4+, 2+ N), Babinski, FTN/HTS, rapidly alternating movements, gait, sensory (light touch, pin prick, vibration, joint position), Romberg, mini MS if indicated
CN:	I - smell, II/III/IV/VI - EOMs/visual fields/pupils/acuity, V - bite (masseter, temporalis)/facial sensation, VII - facial expression, VIII - hearing, IX/X - gag/swallow/uvula midline, XI - turn head/shrug shoulders, XII - stick out tongue

Laboratory Values

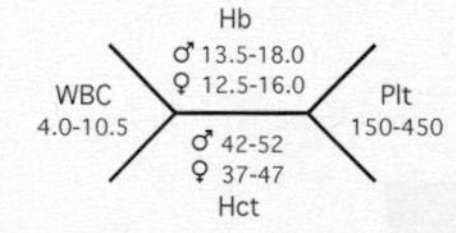

57-67N / 23-33L / 3-7M / 1-3E / 0-1B

neutrophils: 54-62 segs, ≤5 bands
absolute 1.5-6.6

Na^+	Cl^-	BUN	Glu
135-145	98-106	7-18	70-115
3.5-5.1	22-29	0.6-1.2	
K^+	HCO_3^-	Cr	

Ca^{2+}	total 8.4-10.2, ionized 4.6-5.3
Mg^{2+}	1.3-2.1
PO_4^{2-}	♂ 2.3-3.7, ♀ 2.8-4.1, >60y 2.7-4.5

Fe	♂ 65-175, ♀ 50-170
TIBC	250-450
Fe sat	♂ 20-50, ♀ 15-50
Ferritin	♂ 20-250, ♀ 10-120

ABG:

pH	$PaCO_2$	PaO_2	HCO_3^-	O_2 Sat	B.E.
7.35-7.45	35-45	80-100	20-28	>95	±2

VBG:

pH	$PvCO_2$	PvO_2	HCO_3^-	O_2 Sat	B.E.
7.32-7.42	45-50	37-43	22-30	60-80	±2

Urinalysis:

Color	yellow
Clarity	clear
Spec. grav.	1.001-1.035
pH	4.6-8.0

Negative: Bilirubin, Ketones, Blood, Glucose, Protein, Nitrites, Leukocyte esterase

CSF:

Opening pressure:	70-180
WBC	5-10
RBC	0
Protein	15-45
Glucose	45-80

Cardiac enzymes:

CK	♂ 38-174, ♀ 26-140
CK-MB	<5
Troponin I	I <0.6, T <0.1
Myoglobin	serum <90, urine <2

RBC	♂ 4.7-6.0, ♀ 4.2-5.4
Retic	0.5-1.5
MCV	78-100
MCH	27-31
MCHC	31-37
RDW	11.5-14.0

Haptoglobin	40-270
Bilirubin	total <1.0, direct <0.6
AST (SGOT)	♂ 15-45, ♀ 5-30
ALT (SGPT)	♂ 10-40, ♀ 5-35
LD	50-150
PT	11-15
aPTT	20-35
Bleeding Time	2-7
Thrombin Time	6.3-11.1
FDP	<10
D-dimers	<200
GGT	♂ 9-50, ♀ 8-40
CPK	♂ 38-174, ♀ 26-140
ESR	♂ <15, ♀ <20
CRP	<0.8
Alk Phos	♂ 38-126, ♀ 70-230
Protein	total 6.0-8.0 albumin 3.5-5.5
Amylase	25-125
Lipase	10-140, >60y 18-180
C peptide	0.7-1.9
HbA_{1c}	4.0-6.7

Tot Chol	<200
LDL	<130
HDL	♂ >29, ♀ >35
Trig	♂ 40-160, ♀ 35-135

TFTs:

T4	5.0-12.0
FreeT4	0.8-2.3
T3	100-200
TBG	15-34
TSH	<10

Serum drug levels:

	peak	trough
Gentamicin	5-10	<2
Tobramycin	5-10	<2
Amikacin	15-25	<5
Vancomycin	30-40	5-10
	therapeutic	**toxic**
Lidocaine	1.5-5.0	>7
Theophylline	10-20	>20
Digoxin	0.1-2.0	>2.4
Phenobarbital	15-40	>50
Phenytoin	10-20	>20
Carbemazepine	8-12	>15
Valproic acid	50-100	>200

Formulae

Anion Gap:
$(Na^+) - (HCO_3^- + Cl^-)$

Osmolality:
$(2 \times Na^+) + (Glu / 18) + (BUN / 2.8)$

Creatinine Clearance:
$$\frac{(\text{urine Cr}) \times (\text{urine volume [mL]})}{(\text{serum Cr}) \times (\text{time [min]})}$$
$$\frac{(140 - \text{age}) \times (\text{weight [Kg]}) \times (0.85 \text{ for } ♀)}{72 \times (\text{serum Cr})}$$

Fractional Excretion of Sodium:
$$\frac{(\text{urine } Na^+) \times (\text{serum Cr})}{(\text{serum } Na^+) \times (\text{urine Cr})}$$
$$\frac{\left(\frac{\text{urine } Na^+}{\text{serum } Na^+}\right)}{\left(\frac{\text{urine Cr}}{\text{serum Cr}}\right)}$$

Maintenance Fluids:

100 mL/d/kg for 1st 10 kg *plus*
50 mL/d/kg for 2nd 10 kg *plus*
20 mL/d/kg for remaining weight

4 mL/hr/kg for 1st 10 kg *plus*
2 mL/hr/kg for 2nd 10 kg *plus*
1 mL/hr/kg for remaining weight

Body Water Deficit [Liters]:
$$\frac{0.6 \times (\text{weight [kg]}) \times (Na^+ - 140)}{140}$$

Unit Conversions:

1 in = 2.54 cm	1 cm = 0.394 in
1 ft = 0.305 m	1 m = 3.28 ft
1 mi = 1.61 km	1 km = 0.621 mi
1 ft ≈ 30 cm	
1 fl oz = 29.6 mL	1 mL = 0.0338 fl oz
1 qt = 0.946 L	1 L = 1.06 qt
1 gal = 3.79 L	1 L = 0.264 gal
1 tsp = 5 mL	1 tbs = 15 mL
	1cc = 1 mL
1 oz = 28.4 g	1 g = 0.0353 oz
1 lb = 0.454 kg	1 kg = 2.20 lb
70 kg = 154 lb	

$°F = (1.8 \times °C) + 32$ $\quad °C = \frac{(°F - 32)}{1.8}$

Aa Gradient:
$$(713 \times FIO_2) - \frac{PaCO_2}{0.8} - PaO_2$$

ABG Rule:
$\Delta\ 10\ PaCO_2 = \Delta\ 0.08\ pH$

Corrected Total Ca^{2+}:
$Ca^{2+} + 3.6 - (0.8 \times \text{albumin})$

Corrected Na^+:
$$Na^+ + \left(\frac{Glu}{62.5}\right) - 1.6$$

Regular Insulin Sliding Scale (RISS):
$\left(\frac{Glu}{25}\right)$ - 6 units, for $200 \le Glu \le 450$

Mean Arterial Pressure (MAP):
$$\frac{\text{systolic} + 2(\text{diastolic})}{3}$$

Body Surface Area:
$$\frac{\sqrt{\text{height [cm]} \times \text{weight [kg]}}}{60}$$

Body Mass Index:
$$\frac{\text{weight [kg]}}{(\text{height [m]})^2}$$

Normal Weights (lbs) for ♂ and ♀:

Height	Age 19-34	Age ≤ 35
5'0"	97-128	108-138
5'1"	101-132	111-143
5'2"	104-137	115-148
5'3"	107-141	119-152
5'4"	111-146	122-157
5'5"	114-150	126-162
5'6"	118-156	130-167
5'7"	121-160	134-172
5'8"	125-164	138-178
5'9"	129-169	142-183
5'10"	132-174	146-188
5'11"	136-179	151-194
6'0"	140-184	155-199
6'1"	144-189	159-205
6'2"	148-195	164-210

SECTION II

High-Yield Facts in Internal Medicine

HIGH-YIELD FACTS IN

Cardiology

COMMON CAUSES OF CHEST PAIN

- **Myocardial infarction (MI)/angina:** Chest heaviness, pressure, or pain, typically radiating to left arm, shoulder, or jaw. *Diaphoresis is a key symptom also.* Shortness of breath is another. Often described as "An elephant sitting on my chest."
- **Pericarditis:** Chest pain radiating to shoulder, neck, or back, worse with deep breathing or cough (pleuritic), relieved by sitting up and leaning forward.
- **Aortic dissection:** Severe chest pain radiating to the back, can be associated with unequal pulses or unequal blood pressure in right and left arms.
- **Thoracic abscess or mass:** Often sharp, localized pain, can be pleuritic.
- **Pulmonary embolism:** Often pleuritic. Frequently associated with tachypnea and tachycardia.
- **Pneumonia:** Pleuritic, frequently associated with cough, sputum, and hypoxia if severe.
- **GERD/esophageal spasm/tear:** Burning pain, midline, substernal, may be associated with dysphagia. Pain made worse with lying flat, certain foods, also bitter taste in mouth known as "water brash." May be similar to pain of MI.
- **Costochondritis/musculoskeletal:** Sharp, localized pain with ***reproducible tenderness*** (touch chest wall and feel the pain); often exacerbated by exercise (second or third costochondral junction inflammation, aka Tietze's syndrome).
- **Other causes:** Peptic ulcer disease, biliary disease, herpes zoster, anxiety, pneumothorax, pleuritis (infection, systemic lupus erythematosus [SLE]), pulmonary embolus.

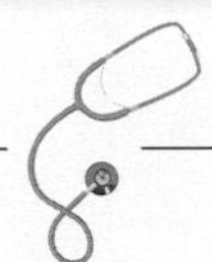

Myocardial infarction can be *silent*, with no symptoms or atypical symptoms in diabetics (due to neuropathy) or heart transplant (denervated heart).

CARDIOLOGY

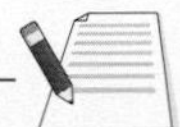

Criteria for **family history** of coronary artery disease:
MI before age 40 in men
MI before age 55 in women

RISK FACTORS FOR CORONARY ARTERY DISEASE

Modifiable
- Smoking
- Hypercholesterolemia
- Hypertension
- Obesity (central)
- Diabetes mellitus
- Physical inactivity
- Metabolic syndrome

Nonmodifiable
- Age
- Male sex/ postmenopausal female
- Family history

A 55 year-old male with HTN complains of claudication. Further questioning reveals increasing shortness of breath with exertion. Coronary artery disease should be suspected and stress testing should be performed.

CARDIAC TESTING

Stress Tests

A stress test is a noninvasive test to assess for possible coronary artery disease (CAD) or risk of MI. There are different types.

- Indications for stress test:
  - Symptoms consistent with angina (to rule out, or in CAD).
  - Post MI (to evaluate risk of having another; poor exercise tolerance correlates with higher mortality).

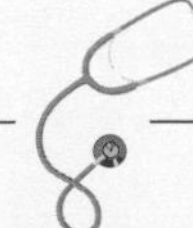

The *normal* maximum heart rate is estimated as: [220 – patient's age].

- **Exercise stress test:** Patients are asked to walk on a treadmill at ↑ levels of difficulty to reach a heart rate that is 85% of predicted maximum for age. Patients should not be taking meds that prevent heart rate from rising (beta blockers or digoxin).
- **Pharmacologic stress test: Agents** such as dobutamine may be administered IV to stimulate myocardial function (and cause cardiac exertion) in a patient who cannot exercise.
- Electrocardiographic (ECG) monitoring during the procedure detects changes.
- A test is considered positive for CAD if the patient develops:
  - ECG changes (ST elevation or depression).
  - ↓ blood pressure.
  - Failure to exercise more than 2 minutes due to cardiac symptoms.

Stress Myocardial Perfusion Imaging

This is similar to other stress tests except imaging allows the visualization of the amount of blood perfusion in the myocardium. "Defects" indicate that the blood is not getting to a part of the myocardial tissue (fixed defects = infarct, reversible = inducible ischemia). Thallium or technetium is typically used.

Echocardiography

- Echocardiography, or ultrasound of the heart, provides a picture of the heart and can evaluate its function. It is used to evaluate many different types of heart disease, from valvular defects to the strength of the heart muscle (described as ejection fraction). It can demonstrate a myocardial infarction (either acute or old) by showing a defect in movement of one of the walls (called "wall motion abnormality").
- In transthoracic echocardiography (TTE) the probe is placed on the chest wall. Transesophageal echo requires the probe to be placed into the esophagus (TEE); it is used for more precise imaging of valves and aorta.
- For specific uses of echocardiography, see Table 2.1-1.

Cardiac Catheterization

- Cardiac catheterization is used for diagnosis and treatment of many different types of heart disease. In left heart catheterization, a wire is inserted through a vessel (usually the radial or femoral artery) and threaded up to the coronary vessels. Dye is injected into the coronary vessels (angiogram), and stenosis (narrowing) or blockage can be visualized. The dye also allows visualization of heart function. These are *diagnostic*. Cardiac catheterizations can include therapeutic *intervention*, such as angioplasty or stenting (see below). A right heart catheterization is the same as above but through a vein.
- For other uses of cardiac catheterization, see Table 2.1-2.

TABLE 2.1-1. Uses of Echocardiography

DISORDER	USE OF ECHO
Myocardial infarction	Assess wall motion abnormalities, or new valve abnormalities induced by the MI.
Heart failure	Assess ventricular function, ejection fraction.
Heart murmur	Identify and evaluate valvular disease.
Pericardial effusion	Assess volume of effusion and tamponade.
Aortic dissection	Identify presence of tear (especially TEE).
Pulmonary embolism	Identify saddle emboli or evidence of ↑ right-sided heart pressure caused by the PE.
Patent foramen ovale	Assess bubbles traversing PFO (air administered through peripheral IV).
Endocarditis	Identify vegetation, abscess (sensitivity TEE > TTE).
Congenital heart disease	Identify coarctation of the aorta, pulmonary stenosis, tetralogy of Fallot, ventricular septal defect (VSD), atrial septal defect (ASD).

TABLE 2.1-2. Uses of Cardiac Catheterization

DISORDER	THERAPY
Myocardial infarction and unstable angina	Coronary artery angiography (visualize the blockage); also can intervene with balloon dilatation of stenoses, stent placement (percutaneous transluminal coronary angioplasty [PTCA]), or laser techniques.
Valvular heart disease	"Balloon valvuloplasty": Dilatation of valves with a balloon. This can be used for mitral stenosis, pulmonary stenosis, aortic stenosis.
Dysrhythmias	When a patient has an arrhythmia, the cause can be located and removed. This is called "electrophysiologic mapping" and radiofrequency ablation.
Myocardial disease	Biopsy of myocardium for cardiomyopathies.
Congenital heart disease	Can diagnose valvular disorder and correct in some cases (ASDs, VSDs, PFOs).
Pericardial disease	Simultaneous left and right heart catheterization will measure heart pressures and diagnose a pericardial abnormality such as restriction.

ANGINA

Typically left-sided chest pain caused by temporary myocardial ischemia.

- **Stable angina:** A chronic, episodic, predictable, pain syndrome due to temporary myocardial ischemia. Pattern of pain is similar to that of acute MI, but resolves with rest or medication. Doesn't change (ie, it's stable). **Treatment:** Beta blocker (reduces myocardial oxygen demand); aspirin; nitroglycerin.
- **Unstable angina** (further discussed in next section; a type of acute coronary syndrome). Defined as (1) new onset of anginal pain, (2) anginal pain that accelerates or changes in pattern location or severity, (3) anginal pain at rest. **Treatment:** See Acute Coronary Syndromes section.
- **Prinzmetal's angina (variant angina):** Angina due to coronary vasospasm, not linked to exertion. Distinguished from unstable angina by chronic, intermittent nature. Pain usually occurs at a specific hour in the early morning. Coronary vessels are normal (no stenosis or plaques). ECG may show transient ST elevations. **Treatment:** Calcium channel blockers and nitrates to reduce vasospasm.

A 62-year-old smoker presents complaining of three episodes of severe chest heaviness this morning. Each episode lasted 3–5 minutes, but he has no pain now. He has never had this type of pain before. *Think: Unstable angina.*

A middle-aged woman comes to the ER with severe chest pain and ST elevations on ECG. She is rushed for a cardiac catherization, which shows no obstruction in her coronary arteries. What is it? *Variant angina (aka Prinzmetal's angina/vasospasm).*

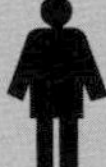

A 62-year-old man presents with frequent episodes of dull chest pain on and off for 8 months. He says the pain wakes him from sleep. *Think: Prinzmetal's angina.*

ACUTE CORONARY SYNDROMES (ACS)

- Acute coronary syndromes (ACS) refers to unstable angina (chest pain in which an MI can happen at any second) or an actual MI. On a physiologic level, this is due to an imbalance of myocardial oxygen supply and demand. The most common cause of ↓ oxygen supply is narrowing of coronary artery by thrombus or plaque that has become unstable.
- **Ischemia** is reversible insult to the tissue by oxygen deprivation.

- **Infarction** is when the damage is permanent (as in MI). When there is tissue damage (infarction), there is enzyme leakage (eg, creatinine phosphokinase [CPK] and troponin see below).
- **ACS events are classified according to the changes on ECG:** (1) **non-ST-elevation** (includes non-ST elevation myocardial infarction or unstable angina) or (2) **ST-elevation** (includes ST-elevation MI [STIMI]).

Serum Markers for MI

- Myoglobin: Elevated within 1 hour of MI; peak 6 hours; nonspecific.
- Creatinine phosphokinase (CPK): Elevated within 4–8 hours; peak 18–24 hours of MI; total is nonspecific but CK MB is specific. CK MB isoenzyme is the subgroup of CPK specific for myocardial tissue damage. The extent of elevation correlates with the amount of cardiac damage.
- Troponin T or I: Very sensitive and specific markers for cardiac muscle injury. Elevated within 3 hours and can stay elevated for more than a week. Renal insufficiency can → high levels that can be mistaken for cardiac damage. Troponin may also be slightly chronically elevated in CHF.
- "Serial enzymes": Consists of cardiac biomarkers followed every 6–8 hours for a 24-hour period. This is standard practice for patients presenting to the hospital for chest pain and when you want to rule out or in an MI.

Enzyme	Onset (hrs)	Peak (hrs)	Duration
Myoglobin	1–4	6–8	24 hrs
Troponin T/I	3–12	18–24	7–10 days
Creatinine kinase (total and CK MB)	3–12	18–24	3–4 days
Lactate dehydrogenase	6–12	24–48	6–8 days

A 47-year-old man presents to the ER with left-sided chest pain at rest. He is a chronic smoker with family history of diabetes and hypertension. On examination, he is found to have stable vitals. ECG showed new ST flattening in II, III, and AVF. ASA, Plavix and nitrate were administered and patient still complained of pain. **Next step:** Start heparin drip and send patient for cardiac catheterization.

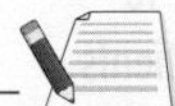

Patients presenting with ACS should be given MONA + beta blocker (unless contraindicated):

Oxygen
Nitrate
Aspirin
Morphine

Note: Morphine should be the last medication given. It may mask angina and should only be given when a diagnosis of ACS is certain and the patient still has severe pain.

What Do You Do With a Patient Suspected of ACS?

- **Detailed history and physical:**
  - **Typical symptoms for any anginal/MI:** Left-sided/substernal chest pressure with radiation to the left shoulder, arm, or jaw. Patient may characterize this by putting a closed fist over the chest (Levine`s sign), shortness of breath, diaphoresis, nausea or vomiting.

- **Specific situations:**
  - **Syncope or cardiac arrest** (arrhythmia can result from the ischemic insult).
  - **Unstable angina** is associated with ↑ frequency and/or severity of symptoms, symptoms at rest or new onset of symptoms
  - **Atypical presentation:** No symptoms or just one. Presentation may be atypical in diabetics (they may have a neuropathy that blunts the sensation of pain; many diabetics have "silent MIs" where the MI has no symptoms). Women may also have atypical symptoms.
- **Initial tests:** (1) ECG, and (2) cardiac enzymes.

Initial Treatment for All ACS

- Patients should also be placed on a cardiac monitor (telemetry) because during ischemia they are at high risk for arrhythmias.
- Beta blockers ↓ cardiac oxygen demand and have been shown to ↓ mortality.
- Antiplatelet and anticoagulation: Aspirin (chewable preferred). Clopidogrel is an alternative for those with true aspirin allergy.
  - *Note:* Morphine helps with pain control but does not affect outcome.
- Other possible additions:
  - Either unfractionated heparin or low-molecular-weight heparin can be used. The rationale behind using both aspirin and heparin is that they act at different sites.
  - GP IIb/IIIa inhibitors have shown to be beneficial for high-risk patients.
  - *Note:* Thrombolytics are not used in unstable angina or non-ST-elevation MI because 60–80% of the time the infarcted artery is not occluded.
- **MONA + beta blocker for all ACS patients, but additional treatment depending on type of ACS.** ACS is divided into two major types:
  1. **ST-elevation MI (STEMI):** This is the most dangerous type of ACS. (This group also includes those with a new left bundle branch block [LBBB] on ECG).
     - **Treatment:** These patients need aggressive treatment in addition to MONA + beta blocker. They need urgent opening of blockage (revascularization). This can be done with (1) thrombolytics (medicines that break up clots) and/or (2) cardiac catheterization and stent (percutaneous transluminal coronary angioplasty [PTCA]) (see section on cardiac catheterization above). Cardiac catheterization is generally considered superior to thrombolytics in STEMI. **Thrombolytics:** Examples include streptokinase, urokinase, anistreplase, alteplase, and reteplase. Contraindications are risks of bleeding, particularly in the brain: prior intracranial hemorrhage, stroke within 1 year, brain tumor, active internal bleeding, or suspected aortic dissection.
  2. **Unstable angina** and **non-ST-elevation MI (NSTEMI):** These two have similar pathogenesis. Non-ST-elevation MI differs from unstable angina in that the lack of oxygen is severe enough to cause myocardial damage and enzyme leakage (unlike unstable angina, where there is no enzyme leakage).
     - **Treatment:** MONA + beta blocker as described above. Can treat with invasive treatment (cardiac catheterization) or conservatively (medications). Ongoing chest pain and signs of cardiac dysfunction would prompt intervention.

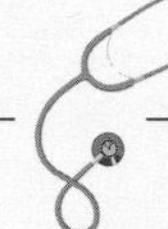

Heparin does not dissolve already-present clots; rather, it prevents future ones from forming.

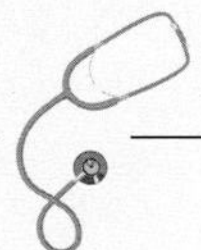

What is a TIMI score?
Scoring system used to evaluate risks of patients with NSTEMI and determine if early invasive management (ie, cardiac cath) is warranted. Each item is worth a point:

- Age > 65
- ≥ 3 CAD risk factors
- Prior coronary stenosis > 50%
- ST changes on ECG
- ≥ 2 anginal episodes in 24 hours
- Use of aspirin in prior week
- Positive serum markers

TIMI > 4: Patient should get invasive management.

- Cocaine can cause MI without a clot, rather vasospasm, or simply drug-induced heart strain in which the oxygen supply cannot keep up (do urine drug screen if suspicious).
- **Inferior wall MI—a special case:** Inferior wall MI (ECG changes in II, III, and aVF) affects the right ventricle. Therefore, there is a *major danger of dropping preload.* Treatment must maintain preload with aggressive fluids and *avoid nitrates* (will drop preload).

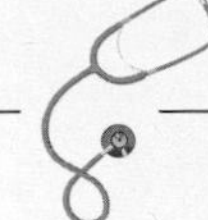

Cardiac output = stroke volume × heart rate.

Typical ECG Findings in MI

Location of ECG abnormalities tells which vessel in the heart is infected.

- **Inferior wall MI:** ST elevation in II, III, aVF (cor pulmonale: ST *depression* in II, III, aVF) (see Figure 2.1-1).
- **Anteroseptal MI:** ST elevation in V_1, V_2, V_3 (see Figure 2.1-2).
- **Lateral wall MI:** ST elevation in V_5, V_6, I, aVL.
- **Posterior wall MI:** Tall ST elevation in II, III, AVF, tall R with ST depression in V1, V2, and ST elevation in V4R.

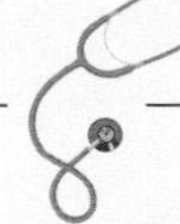

Causes of ST elevation:
- MI
- Pericarditis
- Left ventricular (LV) aneurysm
- Early repolarization (young people)

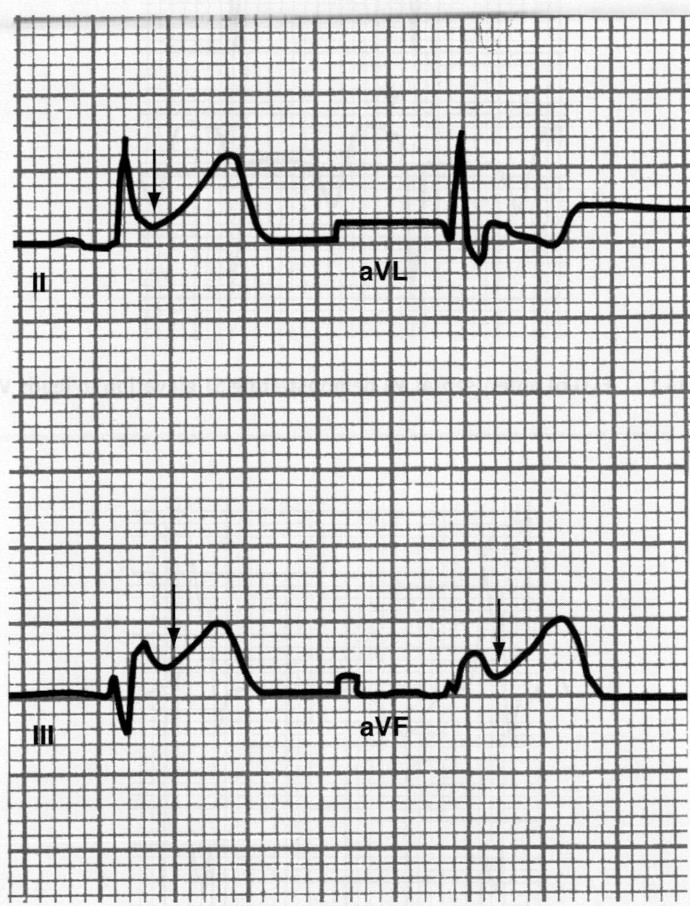

FIGURE 2.1-1. ECG of inferior wall MI demonstrating ST elevation in leads II, III, and aVF.

CARDIOLOGY

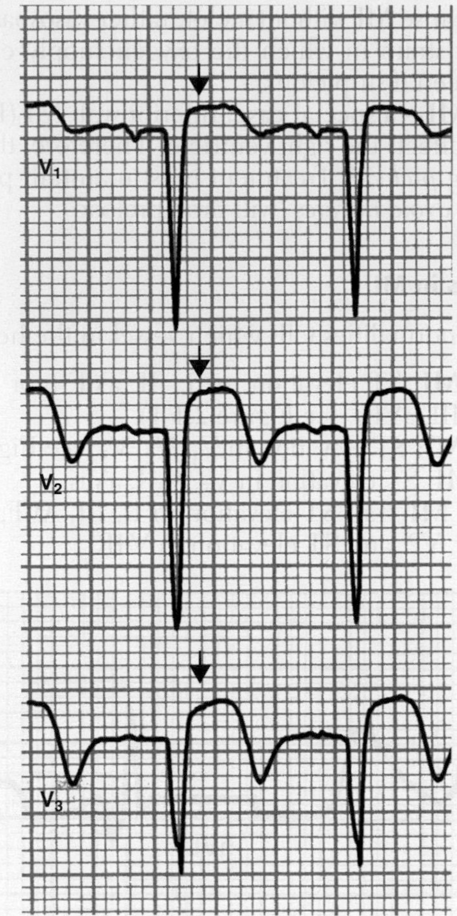

FIGURE 2.1-2. ECG of anteroseptal MI demonstrating ST elevation in leads V_1, V_2, and V_3.

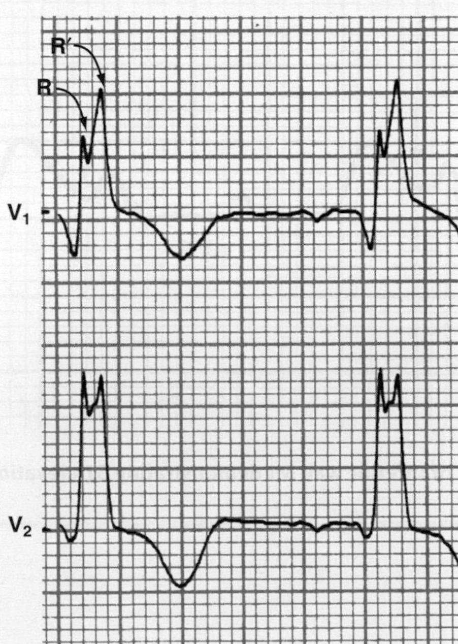

FIGURE 2.1-3. Right bundle branch block.

Medications at Discharge for Patients with ACS

- Aspirin indefinitely.
- Beta blocker indefinitely.
- Angiotensin-converting enzyme (ACE) inhibitor indefinitely; can particularly help patients with resulting low cardiac function (congestive heart failure [CHF]).
- Statin (hydroxymethylglutaryl coenzyme A [HMG CoA] reductase inhibitor) to maintain LDL < 70.
- Clopidogrel (Plavix) if a stent was placed.

Secondary Prevention of MI

- Smoking cessation
- Diabetes control
- Hypertension control
- Control of hyperlipidemia

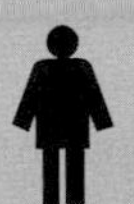

A 65-year-old woman with a history of CAD and drug-eluting stent (DES) placed 6 months ago presents with acute crushing chest pain. She says that she had stopped taking her Plavix 1 week ago for a dental procedure. *Think: Acute in-stent thrombosis.*

Next step: ECG (may show ST elevation; send for urgent cardiac catheterization).

Post-MI patient upon discharge: aspirin, beta blocker, angiotensin-converting enzyme (ACE) inhibitor, and statin (and Plavix if a stent was placed).

Postinfarction Complications

- **Ruptures** (usually occur within 4–5 days of a large MI). These can be in the free wall of the heart, the intraventricular septum, or the papillary muscle, which causes acute mitral regurgitation.
- **Arrhythmias:** Ventricular tachycardia (usually within 48 hours, when the myocardium reperfuses), bradycardia (usually from inferior wall MI), atrioventricular block (can be from anterior wall or inferior wall MI).
- **Dressler's syndrome:** Usually occurs 1 or 2 weeks after cardiac injury (MI or cardiac surgery). It is associated with fever, pericarditis, and sometimes pericardial or pleural effusions; likely a hypersensitivity process. Treat with nonsteroidal anti-inflammatory drugs (NSAIDs) and steroids.

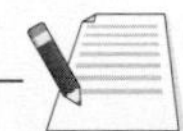

A patient presents with a known history of CHF with a low EF. What is the most likely cause of death? Arrhythmia.

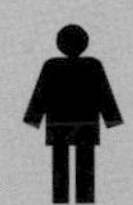

A 58-year-old man who was discharged from the hospital after an MI 2 weeks ago presents with fever, chest pain, and generalized malaise. ECG shows diffuse ST-T wave changes. *Think: Dressler's syndrome.* Treat with NSAIDs.

HEART FAILURE

Congestive heart failure (CHF) is the failure of the heart to pump blood effectively to the tissues. Left heart failure (LHF) causes pulmonary venous congestion (blood flow back-up into the lungs) and compromised systemic circulation. Right heart failure (RHF) causes systemic venous congestion.

Most Common Causes of Right- and Left-Sided Heart Failure

Right Heart Failure	Left Heart Failure
CAD (MI that has damaged the right ventricle)	CAD (MI that has damaged the left ventricle)
2° to LHF (then further "backup" of blood)	Hypertension
Pulmonary hypertension (right ventricle has to push against a higher pressure and gets hypertrophied and damaged)	Mitral and aortic valve disease
Endocarditis damaging triscuspid valve	Endocarditis
Ventricular septal defect (VSD)	Dilated cardiomyopathy

Decompensated Heart Failure

Refers to the worsening or exacerbation of an underlying CHF. It can be precipitated by:

- Ischemia (most common).
- Noncompliance with meds (eg, skipped diuretic).
- Dysrhythmias.
- Other noncardiac causes (pulmonary embolism, EtOH, thyrotoxicosis, wet beriberi, viruses).

SIGNS AND SYMPTOMS OF HEART FAILURE

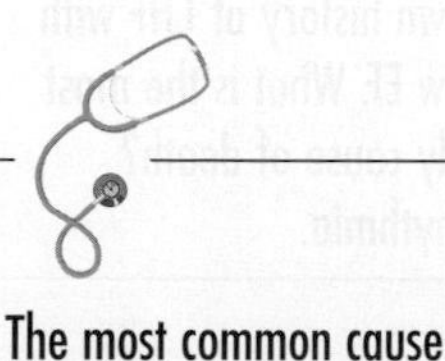

The most common cause of right heart failure is left heart failure.

Left Heart Failure

- Symptoms:
  - Shortness of breath (SOB).
  - Orthopnea.
  - Paroxysmal nocturnal dyspnea (PND)—SOB when lying down.
  - Dyspnea on exertion (DOE).
  - Cough.
  - Diaphoresis.
  - Nocturia.
- Signs:
  - Rales.
  - S3 gallop.
  - Tachycardia.
  - Peripheral edema.

Right Heart Failure

- Symptoms:
  - RUQ pain (due to hepatic congestion).
  - SOB.
  - Abdominal swelling (ascites).
  - Weight gain (fluid retention).

- **Signs:**
  - Hepatomegaly.
  - Hepatojugular reflex.
  - Jugular venous distention (JVD).
  - Ascites.
  - Cirrhosis.
  - Abnormal LFTs (congestive hepatopathy).
  - Peripheral edema.
  - Cyanosis.

DIAGNOSIS

- Chest x-ray can show enlargement of cardiac silhouette, pulmonary vascular congestion with redistribution to upper lobes, and effusion.
- Echocardiogram can show ↓ cardiac function.
- Brain natriuretic peptide (BNP) is elevated in CHF.

TREATMENT

- **Nonpharmacologic**: Sodium and water restriction, exercise, education, and avoidance of alcohol.
- **Pharmacologic:**
  - First-line therapy:
    - **ACE inhibitors:** ↓ afterload; ↓ symptoms, mortality, incidence of heart failure symptoms, and hospitalization.
    - **Diuretics:** Use in NHYA class II–IV for fluid retention. Helps to reduce preload. Thiazides and loop diuretics (furosemide) are examples.
    - **Beta blockers:** For NYHA class II–III (↓ symptoms, improve survival).
    - **Digoxin:** Add for NYHA class III–IV (for symptomatic relief only; **does not** improve survival but reduces hospitalization).
    - **Spironolactone (potassium-sparing diuretics):** Low dose, use in New York Heart Association (NYHA) class III–IV. ↓ mortality. Monitor potassium closely. Concomitant use of ACE inhibitors can make potassium go very high, so monitor closely.
    - **Epleronone:** Similar to spironolactone, but fewer side effects (namely gynecomastia).
  - Second-line therapy:
    - **Angiotensin receptor blockers (ARBs):** If ACE inhibitors are not well tolerated (eg, cough).
    - **Nitrate-hydralazine combination:** Improve symptoms and survival. High rate of intolerance and lower effect on mortality make this therapy a second line to ACE inhibitors.
    - **Cardiac resynchronization therapy:** Reserved for patients who are in Class III HF despite maximal therapy. Essentially a pacemaker that times the contractions of atria and ventricles for maximum efficiency.

Acute Cardiogenic Pulmonary Edema

- **Acute pulmonary edema (APE)** is caused by rapid decompensation of LV function due to dysrhythmias (atrial fibrillation, ventricular tachycardia [VT], supraventricular tachycardia [SVT]), MI, ↑ sodium intake, noncompliance with medications (ie, diuretics), drugs, infection (less common).

Diastolic Dysfunction
CHF that may have a normal ejection fraction; the problem occurs during filling (diastole) due to cardiac wall stiffness.

- Accounts for 40–60% of heart failure.
- Signs/symptoms of heart failure with normal ejection fraction (> 50%).
- More common in women.
- Associated with hypertension, left ventricular hypertrophy (LVH), dilated cardiomyopathy, and ischemia.
- Treat the hypertension, use diuretics for congestion and edema, and control rate if atrial fibrillation.

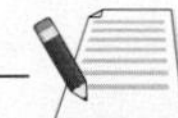

New York Heart Association Functional Classification of Heart Failure
Class I: No limitation
Class II: Slight limitations (symptoms at ordinary efforts)
Class III: Marked limitation (comfortable at rest, symptoms at minimal efforts)
Class IV: Symptomatic at rest

In pregnancy there is ↑ cardiac output, ↓ vascular resistance, and ↑ plasma volume. These cause ↑ shortness of breath! And the plasma volume ↑ causes a drop in hemoglobin (dilutes blood!).

- First-line therapy: NOMAD
  - Nitroglycerin
  - Oxygen
  - Morphine
  - Aspirin
  - Diuretic
- Other therapy: MDDN
  - Milrinone ↑ inotropy with vasodilation.
  - Dobutamine ↑ inotropy without vasoconstriction.
  - Dopamine ↑ inotropy with vasoconstriction.
  - Nesiritide is basic natriuretic peptide—causes smooth muscle to relax and diuresis.

Paroxysmal Nocturnal Dyspnea (PND)

A brief episode of breathlessness that awakens patient from sleep. Also called cardiac asthma.

Etiology

Due to ↑ volume load on the heart when lying in the horizontal position or sudden ↓ in myocardial contractility, which results in pulmonary edema, impairing the exchange of oxygen.

Diagnosis

Distinguished from true asthma by improvement with sitting upright, walking a few steps, and lack of improvement with bronchodilators.

Treatment

Nitroglycerin, oxygen, diuretic (NOD).

CARDIOMYOPATHIES

Dilated Cardiomyopathy

Left or right ventricular enlargement with loss of contractile function resulting in congestive heart failure, dysrhythmias, or thrombus formation.

Etiology

ITEMM:

- Infectious: Viral myocarditis (one-third improve, one-third stay the same, one-third get worse).
- Toxic: Reversible—prolonged EtOH abuse.
- Endocrine: Reversible—thyroid disease (hypo or hyper). Irreversible—acromegaly, pheochromocytoma.
- Metabolic: Reversible—hypocalcemia, hypophosphatemia, thiamine deficiency (wet beriberi), selenium deficiency. Irreversible—genetic: 20% of cases have positive family histories; pregnancy (postpartum cardiomyopathy, 1–9 months after delivery—similar prognosis as viral); neuromuscular; idiopathic.
- Mechanical: Dysrhythmias (tachycardia induced cardiomyopathy); valvular disease.

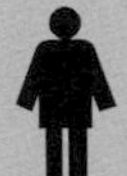

A 26-year-old man presents with SOB, PND, orthopnea, and pleuritic chest pain for 1 week. He had an upper respiratory infection (URI) 1 week prior to onset of symptoms. *Think: Viral myocarditis.*

Next step: ECG shows diffuse ST-segment elevation and PR-segment depression. Treat with NSAIDs and steroids if severe.

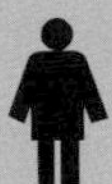

A known alcoholic presents with orthopnea and swelling of legs, but no ascites. *Think: Alcohol-induced cardiomyopathy.*

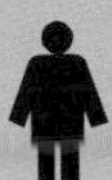

A patient with multiple myeloma has SOB and a chest x-ray showing pulmonary edema. An echo shows a "speckled" appearance. Diagnosis? Cardiac amyloidosis. Type of cardiomyopathy? Restrictive.

Signs and Symptoms

- Symptoms of heart failure.
- Angina due to ↑ O_2 demands of enlarged ventricles.
- Sudden death from arrhythmias.

Diagnosis

Echocardiography shows dilated ventricles/atria, regurgitant valves, low ejection fraction.

Treatment

- Address any reversible causes (eg, discontinue toxic agent).
- Supportive care—medical management of heart failure (ACE inhibitors and diuretics reduce mortality).
- Anticoagulation with Coumadin (with severe LV dysfunction, even if no evidence of thrombus).
- Implanted automatic defibrillator for patients with life-threatening dysrhythmias or EF < 30% despite maximal therapy at 3 months.
- Heart transplant.

Stress-Induced Cardiomyopathy (Takotsubo Cardiomyopathy)

Etiology

- Rare form of cardiomyopathy that is precipitated by emotional and physical stress. More commonly seen in female patients in postmenopausal age group.
- It may happen in situations with sudden sympathetic surge (eg, subjects undergoing dobutamine stress test).
- Pathophysiology thought to be combination of sympathetic overactivation, coronary microcirculation dysregulation, and hormonal effects.

Symptoms

Chest pain and/or SOB.

Management

- Supportive care with cardiac monitoring, serial echocardiograms, treatment of heart failure, and arrhythmias.
- Beta blockers have important role in management as sympathetic stimulation seems to play a central role.

Prognosis

Usually good, with recovery within 1–3 months.

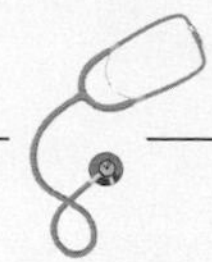

Restrictive cardiomyopathy is often difficult to distinguish from constrictive pericarditis—biopsy can usually confirm.

Restrictive Cardiomyopathy

Scarring and infiltration of the myocardium causing ↓ right or LV filling.

Etiology

Amyloidosis; endomyocardial fibrosis; hemochromatosis; sarcoidosis; carcinoid heart disease; congenital (Gaucher's, Hurler's, glycogen storage disease).

Signs and Symptoms

- Signs of LHF/RHF; RHF usually predominates.
- Exercise intolerance is a common presenting symptom.

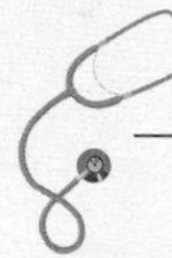

Hypertrophic cardiomyopathy used to be called idiopathic hypertrophic subaortic stenosis, or IHSS. Don't get this confused with ventricular hypertrophy.

Diagnosis

- Endomyocardial biopsy may detect eosinophilic infiltration or myocardial fibrosis or amyloid.
- Echocardiography—normal-sized ventricles, large atria, thickened ventricular walls, mitral/tricuspid regurgitation; typically has a speckled appearance if amyloid is cause. *Ejection fraction is normal or ↑.*
- **Other findings:**
  - **Auscultation:** S3 and/or S4 gallop murmurs, occasional mitral or tricuspid regurgitation.
  - **ECG:** Low voltages, conduction abnormalities, nonspecific ST segment/T wave changes, left bundle branch block.
  - **CXR:** Normal cardiac silhouette or enlarged atria, pulmonary venous congestion.

In HCM, symptoms prior to 30 years of age correlate with ↑ risk of sudden death, but severity of symptoms (whenever they occur) does not correlate with risk of death.

Treatment

Treat underlying cause; treat the resulting heart failure; heart transplant if candidate.

Hypertrophic Cardiomyopathy (HCM)

Hypertrophy of the interventricular septum narrows the LV outflow tract. High-velocity systolic flow draws the anterior leaflet of the mitral valve into the tract (via the Bernoulli effect) causing a dynamic LV outflow tract obstruction. **Put simply,** thick intraventricular septum obstructs blood flow out of the heart and can cause sudden death by arrhythmia.

Etiology

~ 50% idiopathic, ~ 50% familial (autosomal dominant, with variable penetrance).

Clinical Sequelae

These are the young patients with sudden death!!

- Conditions that ↓ the LV end-diastolic volume ↑ the obstruction and make it worse (and make murmur more pronounced (eg, inotropic drugs, afterload reduction, Valsalva).
- Outflow obstruction can result in left atrial dilatation, atrial fibrillation, CHF, right heart failure.
- May have angina for reasons poorly understood, also syncope, or arrhythmias.
- **Sudden death due to arrhythmia.**
- **Diagnosis:** Echocardiography: Septal hypertrophy and LVH.
- **Other findings:** The murmur changes with position—systolic ejection murmur heard best along the left sternal border, ↓ with ↑ LV blood volume (squatting), ↑ with ↑ blood velocities (exercise), and ↓ LV end-diastolic volume (Valsalva) and standing. Paradoxical splitting of S2.
- **Treatment: Counseling** and **screening** should be offered to immediate family members. Patient should refrain from vigorous exercise. Beta blockers reduce heart rate, ↑ LV filling time and ↓ inotropy; calcium channel blockers are considered second-line agents. Septal myomectomy (not always effective); implantable cardioverter defibrillator (ICD) for primary prevention as well as secondary prevention; avoid anything that ↓ preload (nitrates, diuretics, volume depletion) as this will worsen obstruction by allowing LV collapse.

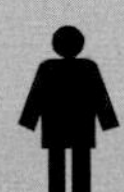

A 25-year-old man becomes severely dyspneic and collapses while running laps. His father died suddenly at an early age. *Think: Hypertrophic cardiomyopathy.*

Very few murmurs ↓ with squatting (HCM does).

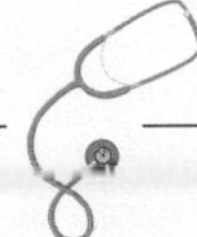

Causes of paradoxical splitting of S2:

- Hypertrophic cardiomyopathy
- Aortic stenosis
- LBBB (left bundle branch block)

Splitting of S2:
Normal physiologic: Aortic before pulmonic valve closure. Split widened by inspiration as increasingly negative intrathoracic pressure augments right heart filling, resulting in longer ventricular emptying times.
Paradoxical: Pulmonic before aortic valve due to a delay in aortic valve closure. Inspiration still delays pulmonic closure but now brings it closer to aortic closure, *paradoxically* narrowing the split.

MYOCARDITIS

Inflammation of the myocardium.

Etiology

- **Viral:** Coxsackie A or B, echovirus, HIV, cytomegalovirus (CMV), influenza, Epstein–Barr (EBV), hepatitis B virus (HBV), adenovirus.
- **Bacterial:** Group A beta-hemolytic strep (rheumatic fever), *Corynebacterium, meningococcus, Borrelia burgdorferi* (Lyme), *Mycoplasma pneumoniae.*
- **Parasitic:** *Trypanosoma cruzi* (Chagas'), *Toxoplasma, Trichinella, Echinococcus.*

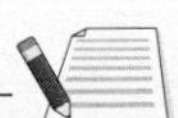

Coxsackie B is the most common viral cause of myocarditis.

- **Systemic disease:** Kawasaki's, systemic lupus erythematosus (SLE), sarcoidosis, inflammatory conditions.
- **Drugs:** Cocaine, ephedra.
- Idiopathic.

Signs and Symptoms

- Spectrum of disease ranges from asymptomatic to fulminant cardiac failure and death.
- Findings may include: chest pain, fever, recent upper respiratory infection, fatigue, signs of CHF.

Diagnosis

- Myocardial biopsy.
- Echocardiography shows hypokinetic wall movement, dilated ventricles/atria and sometimes pericardial effusion.
- **Other findings:**
  - **Auscultation:** S3/S4, mitral or tricuspid regurgitation, friction rub (if pericardium involved.
  - **ECG:** Nonspecific changes, low voltage, dysrhythmias.
  - **Labs:** Leukocytosis, elevated ESR, elevated cardiac enzymes (slower rise and fall than acute MI, troponin I is most sensitive).

Treatment

- Primarily supportive.
- Limit activity.
- Treat CHF and dysrhythmias.
- Address etiology if known/applicable (eg, antivirals, antibiotics, diphtheria—antitoxin, discontinue drug use); intravenous immunoglobulin G (IVIG) may be of benefit.

PERICARDITIS

Inflammation of the pericardium.

Etiology

- **Viral:** Recent viral URI, though a definitive cause is not known.
- **Bacterial:** Tuberculosis (TB), streptococci, staphylococci (rheumatic fever causes pancarditis).
- **Metastases:** 1° tumors usually breast, lung, or melanoma.
- **Immediate post MI:** Pericarditis occurs within 24 hours of a *transmural* infarction due to direct pericardial irritation from injured myocardium.
- **Dressler's syndrome:** Pericarditis occurring 1 week to months after an MI due to an autoimmune response to infarcted myocardium.
- Uremia.
- Rheumatologic condition (SLE, scleroderma).
- Drug reaction.
- Myxedema.
- Trauma.

Signs and Symptoms

Chest pain, often pleuritic, radiating to left shoulder; often relieved by leaning forward; does not respond to nitroglycerin.

DIAGNOSIS

- **Auscultation:** Pericardial friction rub on expiration, pathognomonic but variably present.
- **ECG:** *Diffuse* ST elevations and PR depressions (no discreet pattern of infarction) (see Figure 2.1-4).

TREATMENT

- Address **underlying cause** if known/applicable (eg, hemodialysis for uremia).
- **NSAIDs** to relieve pain and reduce inflammation (aspirin, indomethacin, ibuprofen).
- **Steroids** for intractable cases (eg, Dressler's), generally not used < 10 days post MI.

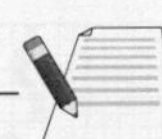

Always suspect a patient with lupus (or any rheumatologic condition) who presents with shortness of breath of having cardiac tamponade. These patients get pericardial effusions. JVD would be a tip off. **Next step:** Give IV fluid to ↑ preload, then immediately do a pericardiocentesis.

PERICARDIAL TAMPONADE

Tamponade is the physiologic result of rapid accumulation of fluid within the relatively inelastic pericardial sac. Pericardial tamponade impairs cardiac filling and reduces cardiac output.

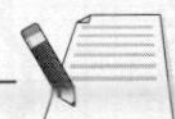

Pulsus paradoxus is a transient fall in measured blood pressure > 10 mm Hg associated with inspiration (due to reduced stroke volume during inspiration).

ETIOLOGY

- Pericarditis.
- Trauma (accidental or iatrogenic).
- Ruptured ventricular wall (post MI).
- Aortic dissection with rupture into pericardium.
- Malignancy.

SIGNS AND SYMPTOMS

In addition to dyspnea and tachycardia:

- **Beck's triad:** (1) Hypotension, (2) muffled heart sounds, (3) JVD.
- **Pulsus paradoxus:** Systolic blood pressure ↓ by > 10 mm Hg with inspiration.
- **Narrow pulse pressure:** Only a small difference between systolic and diastolic blood pressure.

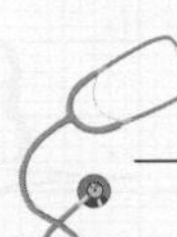

Tamponade physiology: During inspiration, venous return to the right atrium ↑ because of greater negative pressure. In tamponade, the transiently enlarged right atrium bulges leftward, reducing left ventricular volume and output, causing BP to fall with inspiration. Pericardiocentesis yielding *clotted* blood probably came from the right ventricle, not the pericardial sac. Fluid in the pericardium usually is not entirely blood (ie, usually other fluid, too) and therefore won't clot.

DIAGNOSIS

- Echocardiogram will show large pericardial effusion and ↓ filling.
- **Other findings:**
  - ECG: May show low voltage or electrical alternans.
  - CXR: Enlarged cardiac silhouette.
  - Auscultation: Distant heart sounds.

TREATMENT

- Immediate pericardiocentesis (aspirate fluid from pericardial sac) for unstable patients.
- Infuse fluids to expand volume.
- Pericardial window (surgery) for stable patients and recurrent effusions.

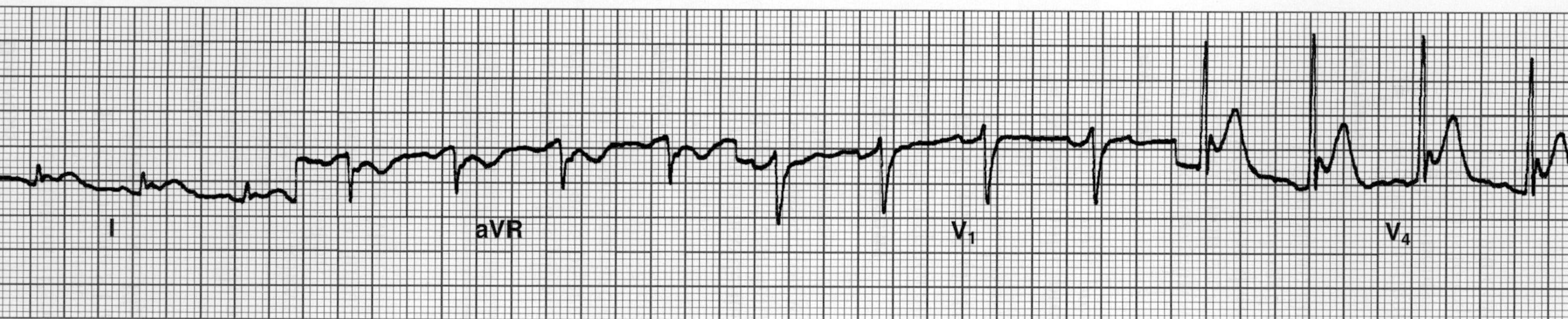

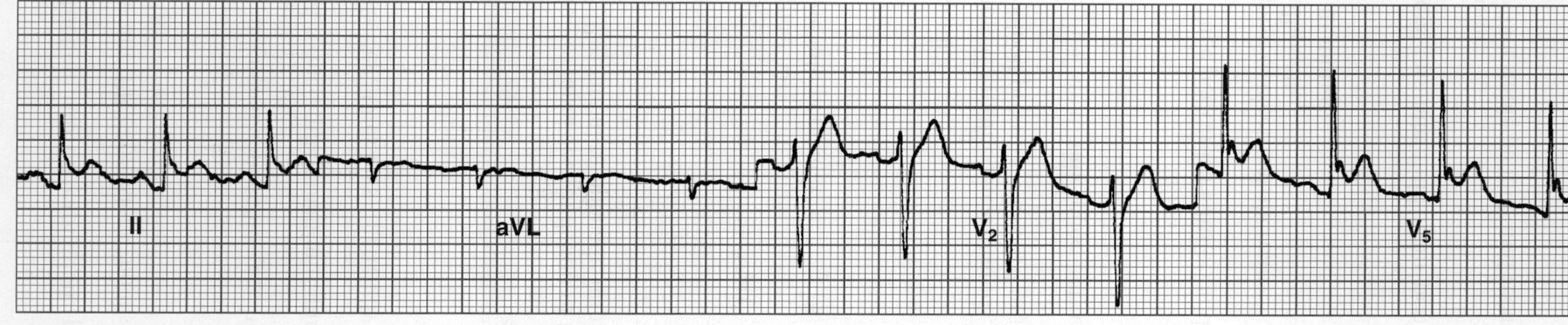

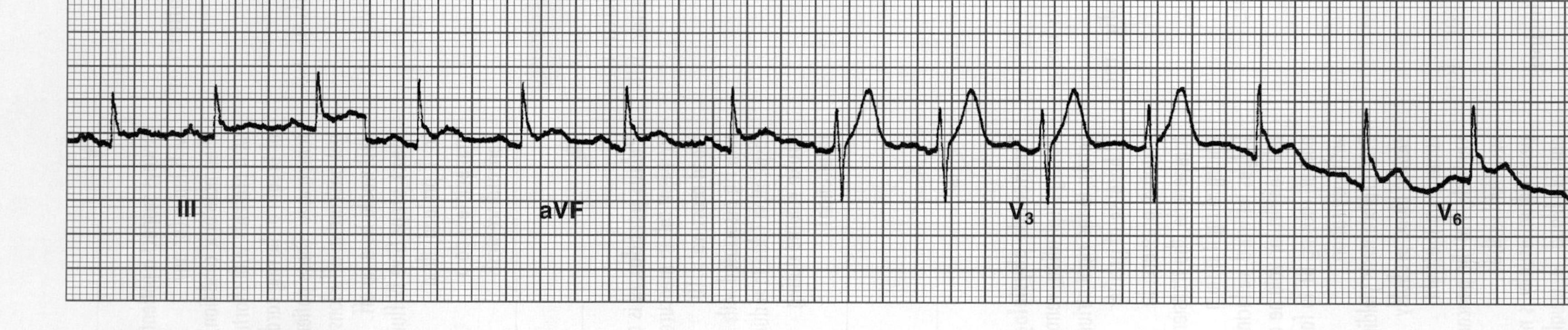

FIGURE 2.1-4. Pericarditis.

Note diffuse ST segment elevation and PR depression.

CONSTRICTIVE PERICARDITIS

Granulation and scarring of the pericardium secondary to acute pericarditis. Cardiac output is diminished.

SIGNS AND SYMPTOMS

- Dyspnea.
- Fatigue.
- Tachycardia.
- JVD with patient upright.
- Kussmaul's sign: Paradoxic rise in JVD during inspiration.
- LV failure.
- Peripheral edema.

DIAGNOSIS

- Echocardiogram will show *normal left ventricular function* and may show pericardial thickening.
- **Other findings:**
  - Auscultation may demonstrate distant heart sounds. Pericardial "knock" may be heard.
  - CXR may show pericardial calcification.
  - ECG may show low voltage, T wave flattening or inversion in V_1 and V_2, notched P waves.

TREATMENT

Pericardiectomy.

VALVULAR HEART DISEASE (VHD)

Mitral Stenosis

ETIOLOGY

Rheumatic heart disease (most common), congenital (rare).

EPIDEMIOLOGY

Most cases occur in women.

SIGNS AND SYMPTOMS

These are due to resulting decompensation of cardiac function; from the left atrium backing up into the lungs and then the right heart: symptoms of CHF and right-sided failure (dyspnea on exertion, rales, cough). See Table 2.1-3 for classic signs and symptoms of valvular diseases.

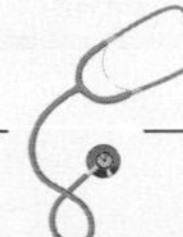

Any disorder that causes dilation of the atria can → atrial fibrillation. Also any disorder that causes dilation can → thrombus in the ventricle and emboli.

DIAGNOSIS

- Echocardiography demonstrates diseased valve.
- **Other findings:**
  - Murmur is mid-diastolic with opening snap, low-pitched rumble best heard over left sternal border between 2nd and 4th interspace (see Figure 2.1-5).

CARDIOLOGY

TABLE 2.1-3. Classic Signs and Symptoms of Valvular Diseases

	Etiology	Symptoms	Signs/Murmur
Mitral stenosis	■ Rheumatic heart disease ■ Congenital ■ Degenerative	■ Right heart failure ■ SOB (orthopnea, PND) ■ Cough/hemoptysis ■ Atrial fibrillation	■ Loud S2/tapping apex ■ Opening snap followed by mid-diastolic rumbling murmur
Mitral regurgitation	■ Rheumatic heart disease ■ Papillary muscle rupture (post MI) ■ Physiologic ■ Dilated cardiomyopathy ■ Ischemia ■ Endocarditis	■ SOB, orthopnea, PND ■ Pulmonary edema ■ Right heart failure	■ Holosystolic murmur best heard at the apex with radiation to the axilla
Aortic stenosis	■ Congenital ■ Degenerative ■ Bicuspid valve ■ Rheumatic heart disease	■ SOB ■ Chest pain ■ Syncope	■ Systolic ejection murmur, crescendo/decrescendo, radiating to the carotids ■ Low-volume pulse, slow rising (pulsus parvus et tardus)
Aortic regurgitation	■ Rheumatic heart disease ■ Congenital bicuspid valve ■ Endocarditis ■ 2° aortic root dilatation (eg, syphilis, ankylosing spondylitis)	■ SOB, orthopnea, PND	■ Early diastolic decrescendo murmur best heard at left 3rd/4th intercostal space
Tricuspid regurgitation	■ Endocarditis ■ 2° left heart failure ■ Pulmonary hypertension ■ Carcinoid	■ Pedal edema ■ Ascites ■ Fatigue	■ Holosystolic murmur left sternal border, ↑ by inspiration (Carvallo`s sign) ■ Hepatomegaly (may be pulsatile)
Tricuspid stenosis	■ Rheumatic heart disease ■ Congenital ■ Carcinoid	■ Fatigue ■ Abdominal discomfort (2° hepatomegaly) ■ Pedal edema	■ Diastolic murmur left sternal edge ■ Hepatomegaly ■ Icterus, edema

- CXR may show straight left heart border due to enlarged left atrium and Kerley B lines from pulmonary effusion.

TREATMENT

- Surgical repair or balloon valvuloplasty in symptomatic patients with severe stenosis.
- Endocarditis prophylaxis.
- Treat for heart failure (diuretics, digitalis) and dysrhythmias as needed.

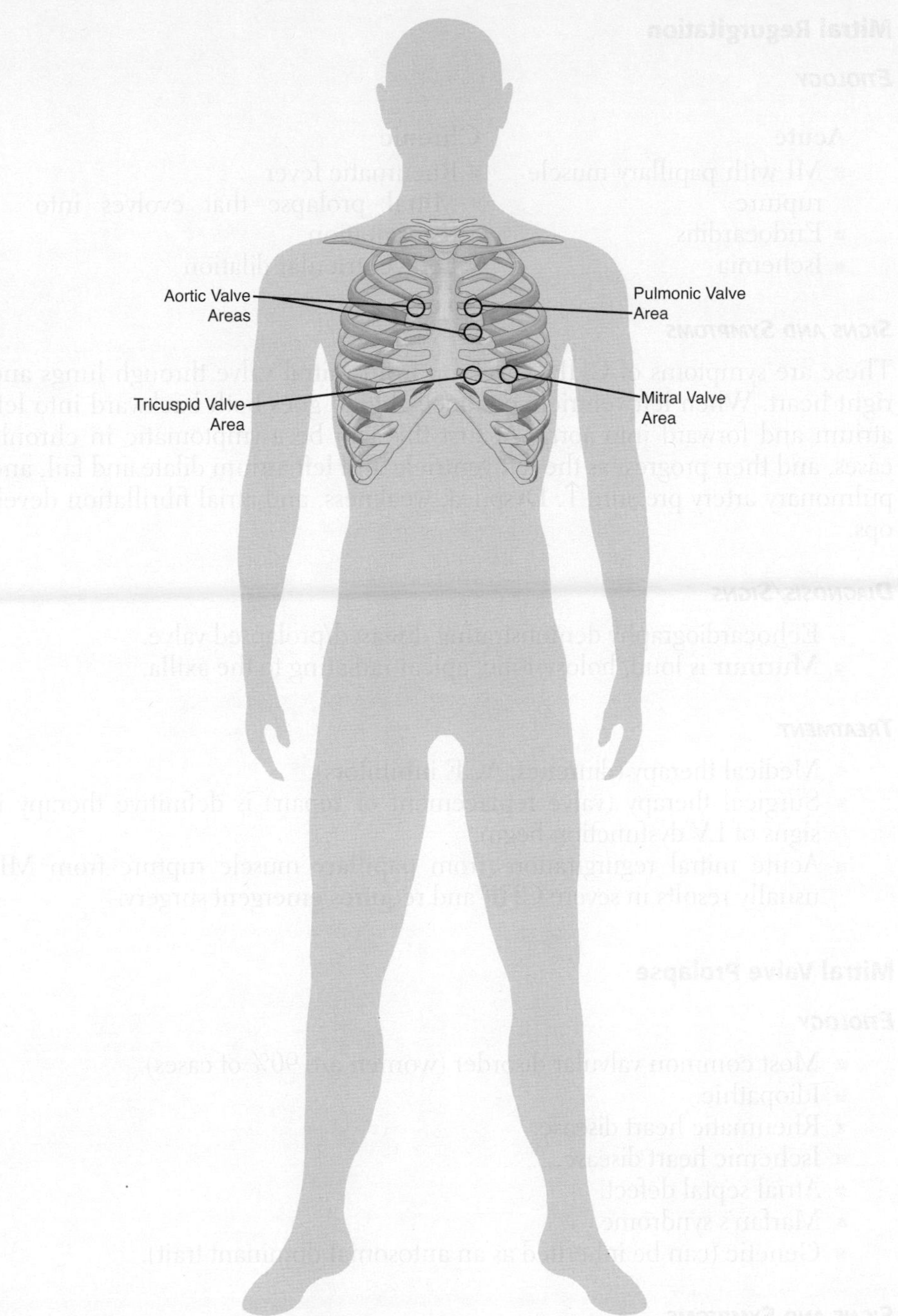

FIGURE 2.1-5. Cardiac auscultation sites.

(Reproduced, with permission, from DeGowin RL. *DeGowin & DeGowin's Diagnostic Examination,* 6th ed. New York: McGraw-Hill, 1994: 359.)

Mitral Regurgitation

Etiology

Acute
- MI with papillary muscle rupture
- Endocarditis
- Ischemia

Chronic
- Rheumatic fever
- Mitral prolapse that evolves into regurgitation
- Left ventricular dilation

Signs and Symptoms

These are symptoms of CHF—back up from mitral valve through lungs and right heart. When left ventricle contracts, blood goes both backward into left atrium and forward into aorta. At first this can be asymptomatic in chronic cases, and then progress as the left ventricle and left atrium dilate and fail, and pulmonary artery pressure ↑. Dyspnea, weakness, and atrial fibrillation develops.

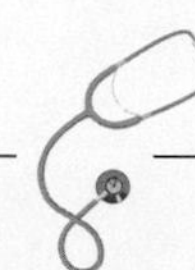

Patient with mitral regurgitation has a good prognosis if LV function is preserved.

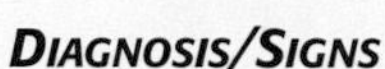

Diagnosis/Signs

- Echocardiography demonstrating diseased/prolapsed valve.
- **Murmur** is loud, holosystolic, apical radiating to the axilla.

Treatment

- Medical therapy (diuretics, ACE inhibitors).
- Surgical therapy (valve replacement or repair) is definitive therapy if signs of LV dysfunction begin.
- Acute mitral regurgitation (from papillary muscle rupture from MI) usually results in severe CHF and requires emergent surgery.

Mitral Valve Prolapse

Etiology

- Most common valvular disorder (women are 90% of cases).
- Idiopathic.
- Rheumatic heart disease.
- Ischemic heart disease.
- Atrial septal defect.
- Marfan's syndrome.
- Genetic (can be inherited as an autosomal dominant trait).

Signs and Symptoms

Mostly asymptomatic, but can rarely have chest pain and shortness of breath.

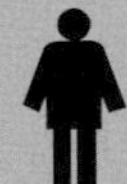

A young woman presents with atypical chest pain and mid-systolic click. *Think: Mitral valve prolapse.*

DIAGNOSIS/SIGNS

- Echocardiography.
- **Murmur:**
  - ***Mid-systolic click*** (that's what you get on exams); followed by late systolic, high-pitched murmur (*if mild regurgitation is present also*).
  - Best heard at apex.
  - Wide splitting of S2.

TREATMENT

None.

Aortic Stenosis (AS)

ETIOLOGY

Degenerative calcific (calcification) disease (idiopathic, older population); also bicuspid aortic valve (most common *congenital* valve abnormality) can result in aortic stenosis around age 40.

SYMPTOMS

Classic triad: (1) angina, (2) syncope, (3) CHF.

PATHOPHYSIOLOGY

- **Asymptomatic** early in course.
- Then develop **angina and syncope**, particularly during exercise. Exertion increases heart rate, which results in less filling time and decreased flow across the stenotic valve. Syncope results from decreased blood flow to the brain. Angina results from subendocardial ischemia as a result of LVH.
- With longstanding severe aortic stenosis, the left ventricle ultimately fails and CHF develops.

PROGNOSIS

- Mean survival for patients with AS correlates with symptoms:
  - Angina: 5 years
  - Syncope: 2–3 years
  - Heart failure: 1–2 years
- **Murmur:** Loud systolic ejection murmur, crescendo–decrescendo, medium pitched loudest at second right intercostal space, radiates to carotids.

DIAGNOSIS

- Echocardiography.
- **Other possible findings:**
  - Narrow pulse pressure.
  - Paradoxical splitting of S2.
  - Calcification of aortic valve may be seen on CXR.
  - Carotid pulse is "parvus and tardus" (weak and slow).

TREATMENT

- Avoid strenuous activity.
- Valvuloplasty produces only temporary improvement as rate of restenosis is very high.
- Valve replacement is definitive therapy.

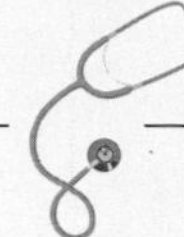

Conditions with narrow pulse pressure (small difference between systolic and diastolic blood pressure):

- Aortic stenosis
- Cardiac tamponade
- Heart failure
- Hypovolemia
- Shock/Anaphylaxis

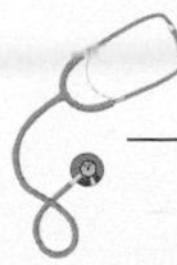

Left ventricular strain pattern is ST segment depression and T wave inversion in I, aVL, and left precordial leads.

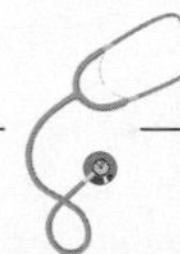

When to go for valve replacement surgery?

- Persistent symptoms
- Aortic orifice < 0.7 cm^2
- Gradient > 70 mm Hg across valve

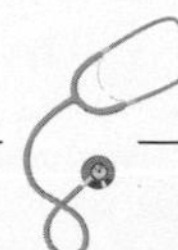

Acute valvular disorders (eg, acute MR or AR) result in severe decompensation into CHF due to the absence of hemodynamic compensation. Emergent surgery is required.

Aortic Regurgitation

Etiology

- Can be caused by a dilation of the aortic root causing the valve not to work, or a problem with the aortic valve itself.
- **Causes of aortic root dilatation:** Idiopathic, Marfan's, collagen vascular disease.
- **Causes of aortic valve problem:** Rheumatic heart disease, endocarditis, syphilis, Marfan's, Ehlers-Danlos syndrome, Turner's syndrome, trauma.

Diagnosis

- Echocardiography.
- **Murmur:**
  - High-pitched, blowing, decrescendo diastolic murmur best heard over second right interspace or third left interspace, accentuated by leaning forward.
  - **Austin Flint murmur:** Observed in severe regurgitation, low-pitched diastolic rumble due to regurgitated blood striking the anterior mitral leaflet (similar sound to mitral stenosis).
- **Other findings:**
  - Hyperdynamic, down and laterally displaced point of maximum impulse (PMI) due to LV enlargement.
  - ECG shows LVH (see Figure 2.1-6).
  - Wide pulse pressure.

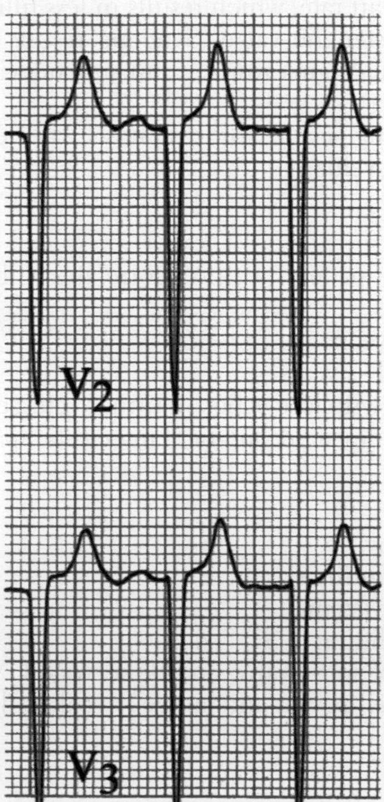

FIGURE 2.1-6. Left ventricular hypertrophy.

SIGNS AND SYMPTOMS

- Dyspnea, orthopnea, PND.
- Angina (due to reduced diastolic coronary blood flow due to low pressure in aortic root).
- LV failure.
- **Other signs with fancy names:**
  - Bounding "Corrigan" pulse, "pistol shot" femorals, pulsus bisferiens (dicrotic pulse with two palpable waves in systole).
  - **Duroziez sign:** Presence of diastolic femoral bruit when femoral artery is compressed enough to hear a systolic bruit.
  - **Hill's sign:** Systolic pressure in the legs > 20 mm Hg higher than in the arms.
  - **Quincke's sign:** Alternating blushing and blanching of the fingernails when gentle pressure is applied.
  - **De Musset's sign:** Bobbing of head with heartbeat.

Acute valvular disorders (eg, acute MR or AR) result in severe decompensation into CHF due to the absence of hemodynamic compensation. Emergent surgery is required.

Conditions with wide pulse pressure:
- **Aortic regurgitation**
- **Hyperthyroidism**
- **Anemia**
- **Wet beriberi**
- **Hypertrophic subaortic stenosis**
- **Hypertension**

TREATMENT

- Treat LV failure.
- Endocarditis prophylaxis.
- Valve replacement is necessary for severe cases and is the only definitive treatment.

Tricuspid Stenosis

ETIOLOGY

- Rheumatic heart disease, congenital, carcinoid.
- Rare.

SIGNS AND SYMPTOMS

Right-sided heart failure (peripheral edema, JVD, hepatomegaly, ascites, jaundice).

DIAGNOSIS

- Echocardiography demonstrates diseased valve.
- **Murmur** is diastolic, rumbling, low pitched accentuated with inspiration. Best heard over left sternal border between fourth and fifth interspace.

TREATMENT

Surgical repair.

Tricuspid Regurgitation

ETIOLOGY

- ↑ pulmonary artery pressure (eg, from left-sided failure or mitral regurgitation/stenosis).
- Right ventricular dilation stretching the outflow tract (eg, from right heart failure, infarction, or tricuspid regurgitation itself).
- Right papillary muscle rupture from infarction.
- Tricuspid valvular lesions (eg, from rheumatic heart disease or bacterial endocarditis).

Signs and Symptoms

Signs of right heart failure: Prominent JVD, pulsatile liver.

Diagnosis

- Echocardiography.
- **Murmur:** Holosystolic, blowing, medium-pitched murmur heard best along the left sternal border in the fifth interspace, accentuated with inspiration.
- **Other findings:**
  - ECG shows right ventricular enlargement.
  - Atrial fibrillation is common.

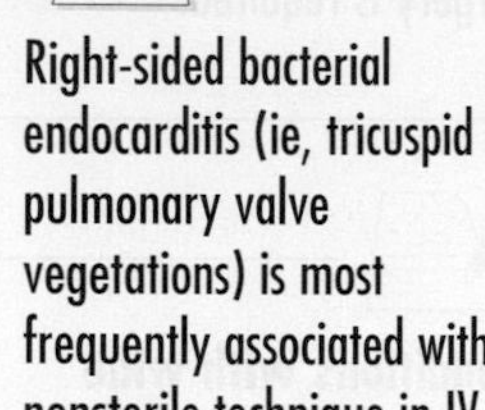

Right-sided bacterial endocarditis (ie, tricuspid or pulmonary valve vegetations) is most frequently associated with nonsterile technique in IV drug abusers.

Treatment

- Treat left heart failure, if applicable.
- Diuresis to reduce volume load.
- Endocarditis prophylaxis.
- Surgical repair.

DYSRHYTHMIAS

Ventricular Fibrillation and Pulseless Ventricular Tachycardia

- **Ventricular fibrillation** (see Figure 2.1-7) is disorganized electrical activity of the ventricular myocardium. Because the myocardium depolarizes in an irregular, disorganized fashion, regular myocardial contraction does not occur (looks like a "bag of worms").
- **Pulseless ventricular tachycardia:** Organized rapid contraction of myocardium, with insufficient filling time and lack of forward flow resulting in loss of pulse. It may degenerate into ventricular fibrillation. Both of these conditions are medical emergencies and require immediate cardioversion (shocking) and IV administration of amiodarone or lidocaine.

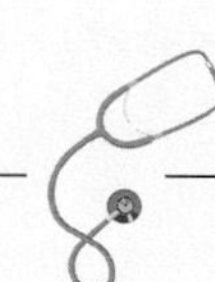

Ventricular fibrillation usually occurs after ventricular tachycardia.

Etiology

- Can be caused by many things, but MI is the most common.
- Prolonged QT syndrome.
- Torsades de pointes.
- Wolff-Parkinson-White (WPW) with atrial fibrillaton and rapid ventricular response.
- Drugs (usually antidysrhythmic drugs!).

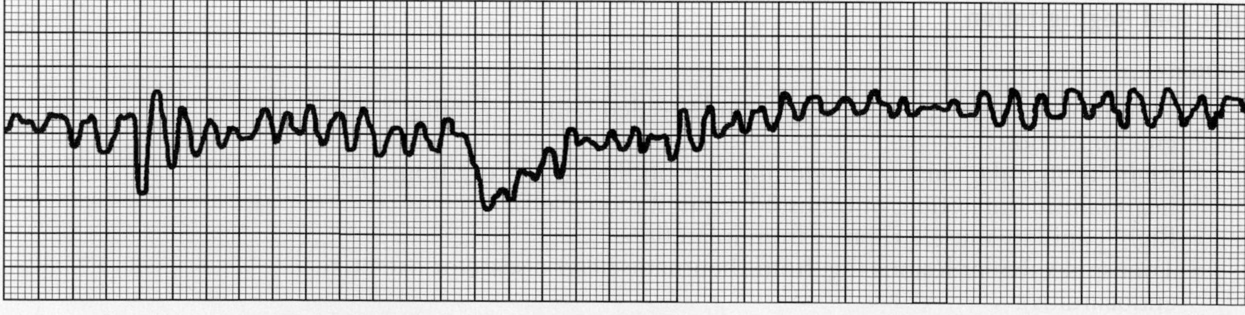

FIGURE 2.1-7. Ventricular fibrillation.

SIGNS AND SYMPTOMS

Ventricular fibrillation is not compatible with life. A patient with V-fib lasting more than 5–6 seconds will lose consciousness.

TREATMENT

- Emergent electrical cardioversion (shocking).
- Medications: Amiodarone/lidocaine as per ACLS protocol.
- **For prevention:**
  - Implanted cardioverter/defibrillator (ICD) in patients who have underlying conditions that predispose to VT/VF or survivors of cardiac arrest 2° to VT/VF (this does not prevent the rhythm, but treats it if it comes about).
  - Electrophysiologic testing and radiofrequency ablation for accessory bypass tracts, AV nodal re-entrant SVT, and others (basically you find the abnormal electrical tract in the myocardium and ablate it).

> ***Etiology of Torsades–***
>
> ***POINTES***
>
> **P**henothiazines
> **O**ther meds (tricyclic antidepressants)
> **I**ntracranial bleed
> **N**o known cause (idiopathic)
> **T**ype I antidysrhythmics (quinidine and procainamide)
> **E**lectrolyte abnormalities (low K^+ or Mg^+)
> **S**yndrome of prolonged QT

CARDIOLOGY

Torsades de Pointes

Wide-complex arrhythmia with rotating axis and prolonged QT (see Figure 2.1-8). Emergency—usually degenerates into ventricular fibrillation!

TREATMENT

- Magnesium IV
- Overdrive pacing
- Beta blockers for prolonged QT syndrome

Atrial Fibrillation

Disorganized electrical activity of the atrial myocardium, causing ineffective atrial contractions.

ETIOLOGY

Seen often in patients with dilated atria, related to heart failure or valvular disease.

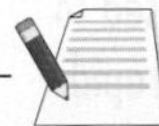

> Rapid atrial fibrillation with a low blood pressure and symptoms. **Next step:** Cardioversion (key is that the patient is unstable).

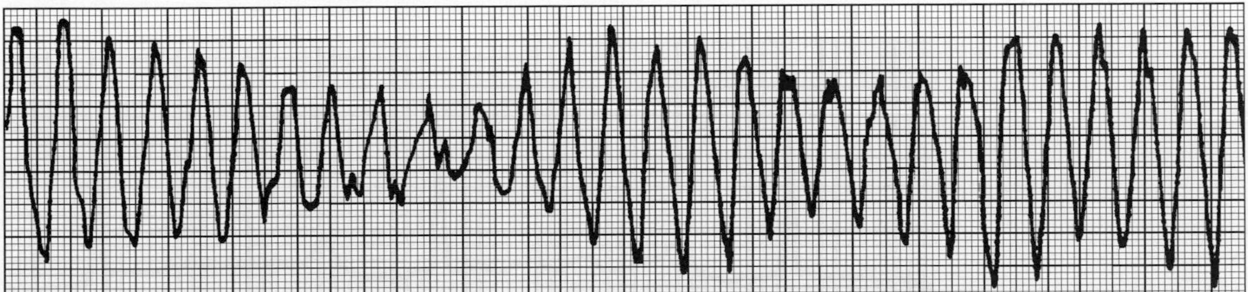

FIGURE 2.1-8. Torsades de pointes.

Note bizarre, twisted point of QRS complexes and varying amplitude.

Etiology of Atrial Fibrillation—

PIRATES

Pulmonary disease
Ischemia
Rheumatic heart disease
Anemia, atrial myxoma
Thyrotoxicosis
Ethanol
Sepsis

Atrial flutter may be confused with atrial fibrillation at high rates. Atrial flutter is distinguished by regular, distinct P waves in a sawtooth pattern.

Rapid atrial fibrillation is often difficult to identify. Adenosine can be used to temporarily slow a rapid supraventricular rhythm.

Signs and Symptoms

- Sensation of **palpitations** or skipped beats.
- **Light-headedness**, fatigue comes from the fact that without the "atrial kick" that the atrial contraction provides, the cardiac output falls.
- May develop chest pain.
- **Thrombus** can develop in dyskinetic atrium and then subsequently embolize to cause transient ischemic attack **(TIA) or stroke.**

Diagnosis

- **ECG:** Absent P waves. Wavy undulating baseline: R-R interval is variable (see Figure 2.1-9).
- **Other findings:**
  - Pulse is irregularly irregular.
  - Echo: May be used to identify presence of clot in the left atrium.

Treatment

- **Rate control:** Slow rate with digoxin, calcium channel blocker (diltiazem), or beta blocker. Often just controlling rate but not changing rhythm can control symptoms. For these patients who stay in A-fib (or flip in and out [paroxysmal A-fib]), anticoagulation is necessary to prevent stroke.
- **Rhythm control:** In some cases the goal is to convert back to sinus rhythm. If patient has been in A-fib < 48 hours and no evidence of ischemia, synchronized cardioversion can be considered (shocking), and amiodarone and beta blockers can help maintain in sinus rhythm after conversion.
- **For unstable patients with any rate or duration of rhythm:** Immediate synchronized cardioversion (shock).

Wolff-Parkinson-White Syndrome (WPW)

WPW is a syndrome in which there is an "accessory pathway" that allows the electrical signal to travel from sinus node to ventricle bypassing the A-V node (this is called a "pre-excitation syndrome"), and then back up the normal His-Purkinje system. This results in an abnormal finding on ECG (delta wave—see below) and a risk for certain arrhythmias. *Anti-arrhythmia meds that block the AV-node (adenosine, beta blockers, calcium channel blockers, and digoxin) are contraindicated—will make it worse!*

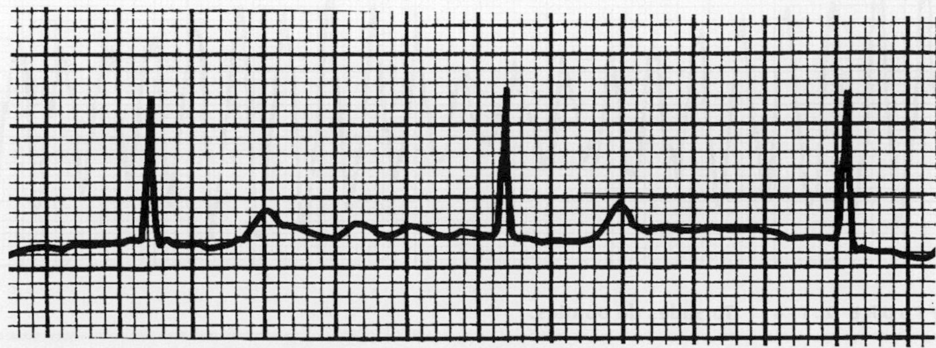

FIGURE 2.1-9. Atrial fibrillation.

Note lack of P wave.

DIAGNOSIS

- **ECG:** Shows a "delta" wave, a slurred upstroke of the QRS complex (see Figure 2.1-10).
- Patients with suspected WPW should have electrophysiologic testing (test that finds the abnormal electrical tract) in the cardiac catheterization lab and radiofrequency ablation of the detected bypass tract.

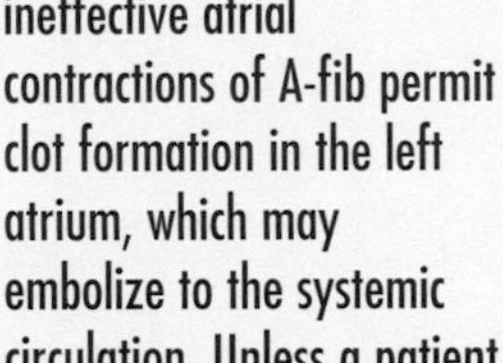

Cardioversion in A-fib: The ineffective atrial contractions of A-fib permit clot formation in the left atrium, which may embolize to the systemic circulation. Unless a patient is unstable, anticoagulate prior to cardioversion.

TREATMENT

- **Unstable patients** with WPW and rapid atrial fibrillation with rapid ventricular response require emergent synchronized cardioversion.
- **Stable patients** with WPW and atrial fibrillation or wide-complex SVT are treated with procainamide, amiodarone, or sotalol.

Heart Block

- **First-degree** (see Figure 2.1-11):
  - Prolonged PR interval (> 0.20 s).
  - No treatment required, not usually a problem!
- **Sccond-degree** (two types—Mobitz I and II):
  - **Mobitz I (Wenckebach),** less dangerous (see Figure 2.1-12).
    - Progressive PR prolongation with progressive shortening of the R-R interval until a beat is dropped.
    - **Only if symptoms,** treat with atropine or temporary pacing.
  - **Mobitz II,** more dangerous (see Figure 2.1-13).
    - Fixed prolonged PR interval followed by a nonconducted beat at a regular interval.
    - Treat with atropine, temporary pacing, and permanent pacemaker.
    - **Dangerous**—always place pacemaker!
    - Important to treat quickly, as this can rapidly degenerate into complete heart block.
- **Third-degree** (complete heart block):
  - Independent atrial and ventricular activity (see Figure 2.1-14) (total asynchrony).
  - **Emergency**—treat symptomatic patients with atropine and temporary pacing, followed by permanent pacemaker.
  - Always needs pacemaker (dangerous rhythm).

Don't give ABCD (adenosine, beta blockers, calcium channel blocker, or digoxin) to someone with WPW. ***Procainamide*** is the classic choice.

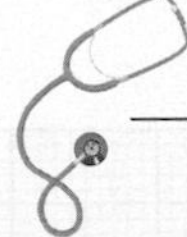

Causes of Mobitz I:
- Inferior wall MI
- Digitalis toxicity
- ↑ vagal tone

Causes of Mobitz II:
- Inferior wall or septal MI
- Conduction system disease

Causes of third-degree heart block:
- Inferior wall MI
- Digitalis toxicity
- Conduction system disease

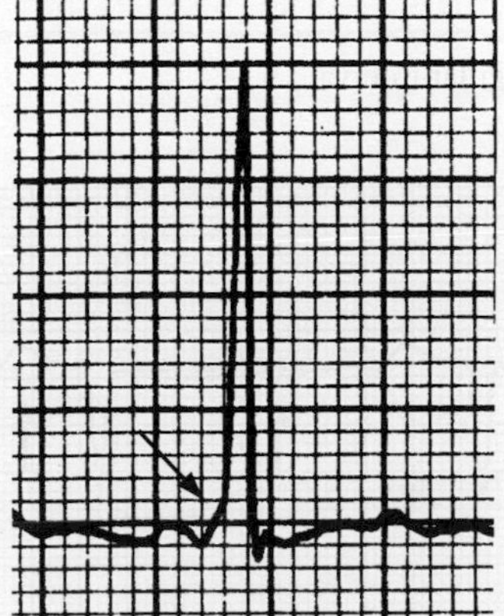

FIGURE 2.1-10. Wolff-Parkinson-White syndrome.

Note slurred upstroke of QRS (arrow) known as the "delta" wave.

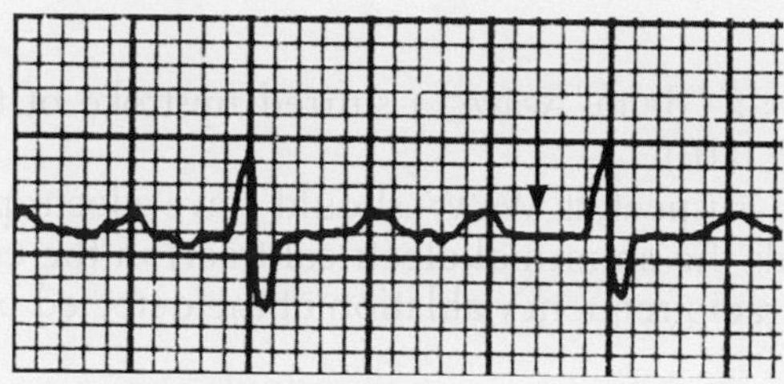

FIGURE 2.1-11. First-degree AV block.

Note pause (arrow) before QRS complex.

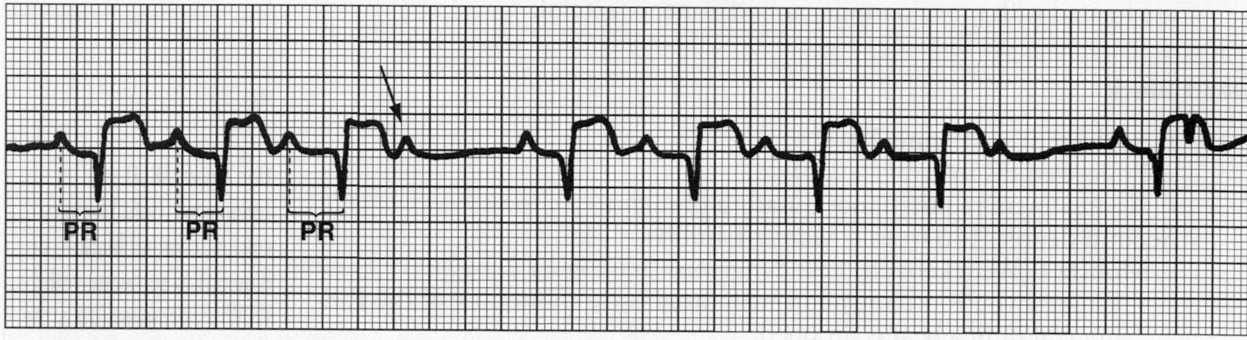

FIGURE 2.1-12. Wenckebach second-degree AV block (Mobitz I).

Note progressive lengthening of PR segment until a QRS complex is dropped. Arrow denotes nonconducted P wave.

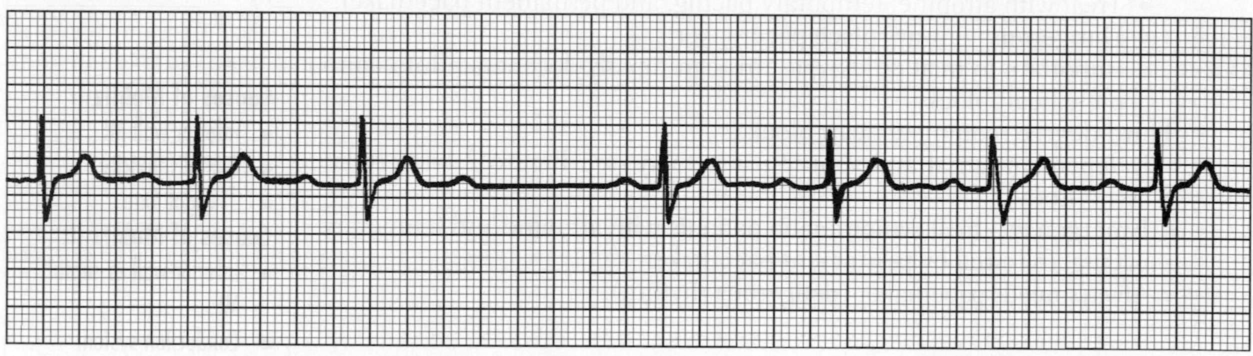

FIGURE 2.1-13. Mobitz II second-degree AV block.

Note constant PR interval followed by a nonconducted P at a regular interval.

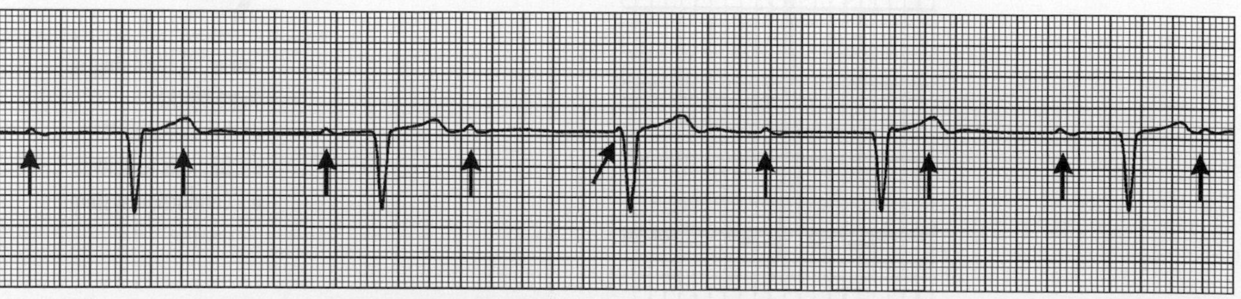

FIGURE 2.1-14. Complete (third-degree) AV block.

Note dissociation between atrial and ventricular rhythms. Arrows denote P waves.

Sinus Bradycardia

- Heart rate < 60.
- Normal P waves and PR intervals.

ETIOLOGY

- Medication (beta blocker, calcium channel blocker, digoxin).
- Inferior wall MI.
- ↑ intracranial pressure.
- Normal variant: Well-trained athletes can have very low resting heart rates.
- Carotid sinus hypersensitivity.
- Hypothyroidism.

SIGNS AND SYMPTOMS

Often asymptomatic; light-headedness and/or syncope can occur.

TREATMENT

- **Asymptomatic patients** do not require immediate treatment: Look for underlying cause.
- **Symptomatic patients:** Atropine +/– pacing.

> ***Causes of Bradycardia— "One INCH"***
>
> If the R-R distance is at least one inch, consider:
> **O**vermedication
> **I**nferior wall MI/ Increased intracranial pressure
> **N**ormal variant
> **C**arotid sinus hypersensitivity
> **H**ypothyroidism

HYPERTENSION

Defined as systolic BP > 140 or diastolic BP > 90 on two separate occasions (see Table 2.1-4).

EPIDEMIOLOGY

Twenty-five to thirty-five percent of adults have hypertension.

ETIOLOGY

- **Primary:** Essential hypertension (primary, idiopathic)—90% is this!
- **Secondary causes:**
  - Renal parenchymal disease (chronic pyelonephritis).
  - Renal artery stenosis.
  - Primary hyperaldosteronism (Cushing's and Conn's syndromes).
  - Pheochromocytoma.
  - Eclampsia and preeclampsia.
  - Coarctation of the aorta (congenital).

TABLE 2.1-4. Definition of Hypertension (JNC-7).

HYPERTENSION	SYSTOLIC BLOOD PRESSURE	DIASTOLIC BLOOD PRESSURE
Normal	< 120	< 80
Prehypertension	120–139	80–89
Stage 1	140–159	90–99
Stage 2	> 160	> 100

If patients do not fit into a discrete category, use the highest (worst) one.

CARDIOLOGY

PATHOPHYSIOLOGY

For primary, it is simply due to normal cardiac output with ↑ peripheral vascular resistance.

RISK FACTORS

- Diabetes
- High-sodium diet
- Obesity
- Tobacco use
- Family history of hypertension
- Black race
- Male gender

> Hypertension due to **pheochromocytoma** is characterized by ectopic production of epinephrine and norepinephrine, causing wide swings in blood pressure.

> What drug do you use for a diabetic patient with hypertension? ACE inhibitor (it will protect the kidneys also).

SIGNS AND SYMPTOMS

- Most patients with hypertension have no symptoms.
- Severe hypertension may present with:
  - Light-headedness.
  - Morning occipital headaches.
  - Epistaxis.
  - Hematuria.
  - Blurred vision.
  - Angina.
  - Congestive heart failure.

EVALUATION

- Blood pressure in both arms, repeated if abnormal.
- Funduscopic examination to look for AV nicking, retinal hemorrhage, papilledema.
- Auscultation for renal artery bruits.
- ECG may show LVH or left ventricular strain.
- Urinalysis to look for active sediment, hematuria.
- Blood urea nitrogen (BUN)/creatinine, serum potassium (evidence of renal insufficiency).

TREATMENT

For repeated elevated blood pressure measurements:

- **Nonpharmaceutical:**
  - Dietary changes: High fruits, vegetables, and low-fat dairy products, low total and saturated fats, low salt.
  - Weight loss, physical exercise.
- **Drug therapy:**
  - Low-dose thiazide diuretics are first choice for stage 1 hypertension.
  - Low-dose ACE inhibitor, calcium channel blockers, or beta blockers are also effective.
  - Two- or three-drug therapy for patients not initially controlled.

COMPLICATIONS

Hypertension ↑ risk of:

- Stroke
- MI
- Atrial fibrillation
- Heart failure

- Peripheral vascular disease
- Renal disease
- Retinopathy

An active urinary sediment contains blood, protein, and red and white cell casts.

A 24-year-old woman with preeclampsia treated with IV drip of magnesium complains of difficulty breathing and has diminished reflexes. **Next step?** Stop magnesium and give IV calcium. (High magnesium levels result in cardiac suppression)

The **mean arterial pressure (MAP)** is: (2dBP + sBP) / 3.

Hypertensive Emergency

Malignant hypertension is characterized by severely elevated blood pressure accompanied by end-organ damage. New-onset neurologic signs, papilledema, chest pain or heart failure, and renal failure should alert the physician to the need for rapid blood pressure reduction.

Diagnosis

Presence of end-organ damage (ECG changes, new-onset renal failure, active urinary sediment, intracranial bleed, etc.).

Use parenteral blood pressure–lowering agents only if end-organ damage is found, due to the risk of rapid reduction in coronary and cerebral perfusion with rapidly lowered blood pressure.

Treatment

ICU monitoring is required. Reduce the mean arterial pressure by no more than 20%. Common intravenous agents include:

- Labetalol.
- Nitroprusside.
- If pheochromocytoma is the cause, use phentolamine.
- For preeclampsia-related hypertension, use magnesium or hydralazine.

Aortic Dissection

- Usually associated with a transverse tear through the intima and internal media of the aortic wall.
- Can → death by extension of the intimal tear to a full-thickness tear with hemorrhage into the extravascular space, dissection into the pericardium with tamponade, or extension into the branch arteries, including coronary arteries, carotids, mesenteric, renal, and iliac arteries.

A patient presenting to the ER with tearing chest pain and has different blood pressures in each arm. **Next step?** Start an IV beta blocker ASAP (with or without nitrates). **Think:** Aortic dissection and order emergency CT angiogram to confirm.

Classification

- **DeBakey classification:**
  - Type I: Ascending plus part of distal aorta (most common).
  - Type II: Ascending aorta only.
  - Type III: Distal aorta only.
- **Stanford classification:**
  - Type A: Ascending aorta or both ascending and descending.
  - Type B: Descending aorta only.

Etiology

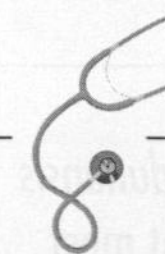

Aortic dissection due to syphilis occurs because the *Treponema* infects the vasa vasorum of the aorta.

- **Hypertension.**
- Connective tissue disease: **Marfan's** (classic test question!) and Ehlers–Danlos syndromes.

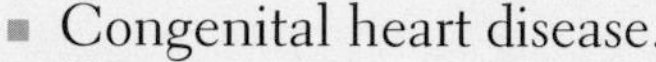

- Congenital heart disease.
- Trauma.
- Pregnancy (third trimester).
- Aortic coarctation: Turner's syndrome, idiopathic.
- Cocaine use (hypertension), syphilis.

> ***Causes of aortic dissection—***
>
> ***PATC³H***
>
> **P**regnancy
> **A**ortic coarctation
> **T**rauma
> **C**ocaine, **C**ongenital, **C**onnective tissue
> **H**ypertension

Signs and Symptoms

- Severe "*tearing*" chest pain, may radiate to back.
- Unequal pulses distally for descending aortic dissection.
- Aortic regurgitation murmur transmitted down right sternal border with ascending aortic dissection.

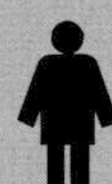

A middle-aged man comes to the ER with severe hypertension and a tearing pain in his back. **What do you do?** Control hypertension with labetolol and do a CT-dissection study to rule out aortic dissection.

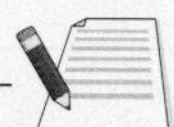

> Always get a chest film when you suspect MI—some of these patients will have aortic dissection, and thrombolysis may kill them. If there is a widened mediastinum, do not give lytics!

Diagnosis

- If aortic dissection is strongly suspected despite negative studies, the gold standard is aortic angiogram.
- **Other findings with other tests:** Helical CT with IV contrast or transesophageal echocardiography can also diagnose; may show dissection with extravasation of blood, intimal flap.
- **CXR:** Can be normal but often shows **widened mediastinum**, apical pleural capping, and loss of the aortic knob.

Treatment

- Blood pressure control is crucial! Use beta blocker + nitroprusside to keep SBP below 120, as long as the patient can maintain organ perfusion.
- Immediate surgical repair for type A dissection (ascending aorta).
- Medical stabilization for type B dissection (descending aorta).

Complications

- MI: Dissection or obstruction of coronary arteries.
- Stroke: Dissection or obstruction of carotids.
- Aortic regurgitation: Dissection through aortic root.
- Cardiac tamponade: Dissection into pericardium which fills with blood and compresses heart.

BACTERIAL ENDOCARDITIS

> *Staphylococcus lugdunensis* is the organism that most often causes aggressive endocarditis requiring surgical intervention.

Localized infection of the endocardium characterized by vegetations involving the valve leaflets or walls. It is best categorized by the infecting organism, which determines the course of the disease. It can also be classified as acute or subacute.

- **Acute bacterial endocarditis** (ABE):
  - Infection of **healthy valves** by high-virulence organisms.
  - Produces metastatic foci (embolizes).

- Usually fatal if not treated within 6 weeks.
- Most common organism is *Staphylococcus aureus.*
- **Subacute bacterial endocarditis (SBE):**
  - Seeding of **previously damaged valves or abnormal** (rheumatic heart disease, congenital valve defects: mitral valve prolapse) by low-virulence organisms.
  - May not *always* result in embolic phenomena.
  - Most common organism is *Streptococcus viridans.*
  - Mitral valve is most often affected.

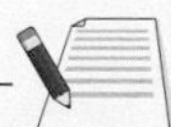

The organism that most often causes endocarditis in IV drug users? ***Staph aureus.***

ETIOLOGY

- **Acute**: *S aureus,* gram-negative organisms.
- **Subacute:** *S viridans,* other oral flora, group A beta-hemolytic strep, enterococci, *Staphylococcus epidermidis.*
- **Special conditions:**
  - **IV drug users:** *S aureus,* streptococci, enterococci, *Candida.*
  - **Prosthetic valves** (10–20% of cases): *S aureus, S viridans,* gram-negative bacilli, fungi.
  - **Nosocomial infections:** Indwelling venous catheters, hemodialysis, CT surgery.

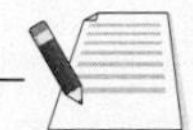

Right-sided acute bacterial endocarditis often affects the tricuspid valve and septic pulmonary emboli are common. ***Think: IV drug users.***

There is a strong association between *Streptococcus bovis* endocarditis and colonic neoplasms.

CARDIOLOGY

SIGNS AND SYMPTOMS

- ABE:
  - Acute onset of fever, chills, rigors.
  - New cardiac murmur.
  - Metastatic infections—meningitis, pneumonia.
- SBE:
  - Gradual onset of fever, sweats, weakness, arthralgia, anorexia, weight loss, and cutaneous lesions.
  - New cardiac murmur.
  - Splenomegaly.
  - Petechiae: Multiple nonblanching red macules on upper chest and mucous membranes.
- **Other findings:**
  - **Osler's nodes:** *Tender* violaceous subcutaneous nodules on fingers and toes (see Figure 2.1-15).
  - **Splinter hemorrhages:** Fine linear hemorrhages in middle of nail bed (see Figure 2.1-16).
  - **Janeway lesions:** Multiple hemorrhagic *nontender* macules or nodules on palms and soles (see Figure 2.1-17).
- **Roth's spots:** Retinal hemorrhages seen on funduscopy.
- Conjunctival hemorrhages.

DIAGNOSIS

Duke's criteria (patient must have 2 major, 1 major + 3 minor, or 5 minor criteria for diagnosis):

- **Major criteria:**
  - Two positive blood cultures taken at least 12 hours apart, or 3+ positive cultures taken at least 1 hour apart with typical organisms.
  - Echocardiography—vegetations are pathognomonic, but their absence does not rule out endocarditis; transesophageal echo is more sensitive.

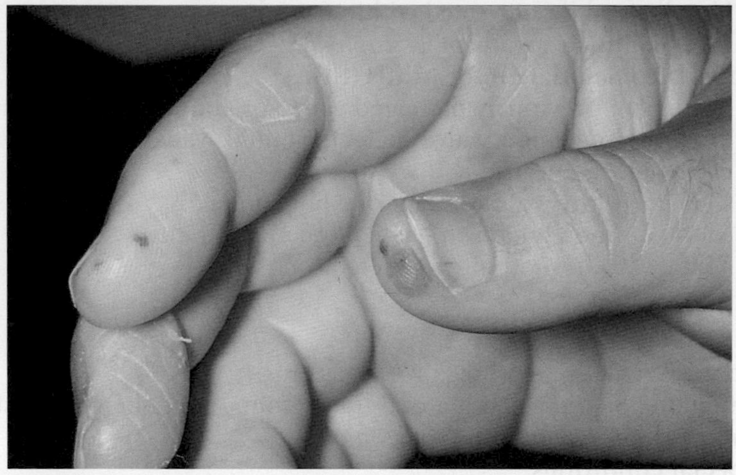

FIGURE 2.1-15. Osler's node.

(Photo contributor: Armed Forces Institute of Pathology, Bethesda, Maryland. Reproduced, with permission, from Knoop KJ, Stack LB, Storrow AB. *Atlas of Emergency Medicine*. 3rd ed. New York: McGraw-Hill, 2010: 375.)

- Minor criteria:
  - Predisposing lesion on valve or IV drug use.
  - Fever > 38°C.
  - Arterial emboli (Janeway lesions).
  - Osler's nodes, Roth's spots.
  - Positive blood cultures not meeting major criteria.
  - Echocardiogram suspicious for endocarditis but not meeting major criteria.

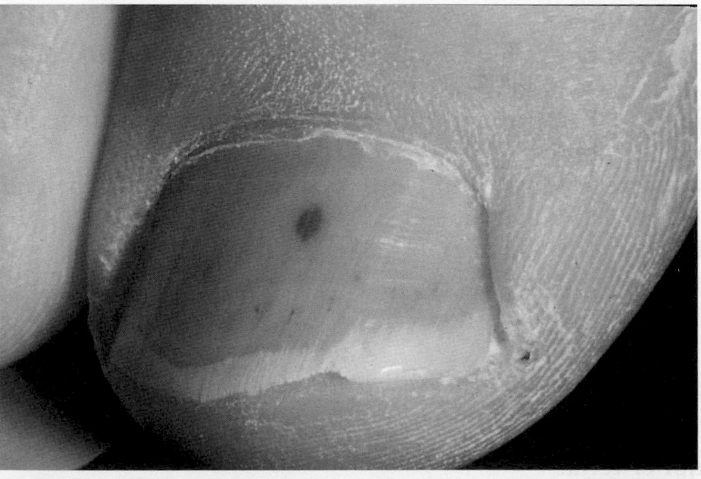

FIGURE 2.1-16. Splinter hemorrhage.

(Photo contributor: Armed Forces Institute of Pathology, Bethesda, Maryland. Reproduced, with permission, from Knoop KJ, Stack LB, Storrow AB. *Atlas of Emergency Medicine*. 3rd ed. New York: McGraw-Hill, 2010: 375.)

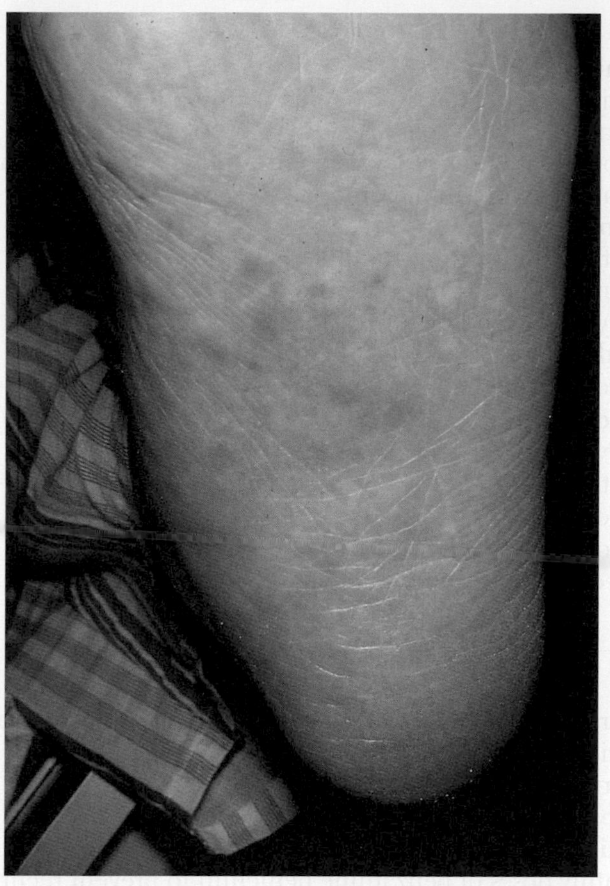

FIGURE 2.1-17. Janeway lesion.

(Photo contributor: Department of Dermatology, Wilford Hall USAF Medical Center and Brooke Army Medical Center, San Antonio, Texas. Reproduced, with permission, from Knoop KJ, Stack LB, Storrow AB. *Atlas of Emergency Medicine.* 3rd ed. New York: McGraw-Hill, 2010: 374.)

TREATMENT

- Streptococci: Penicillin G or ceftriaxone × 4 weeks.
- Staphylococci: Nafcillin or oxacillin × 4 weeks.
- MRSA: Vancomycin × 4 weeks.

RHEUMATIC FEVER

- **Rheumatic fever (RF)** is a systemic immune process that usually occurs secondary to pharyngeal streptococcal infection.
- **Rheumatic heart disease (RHD)** is the occurrence of valvular abnormalities due to immune complex deposition in valve leaflets generated by rheumatic fever.

Most common valve affected by RHD is mitral, followed by aortic, then tricuspid.

ETIOLOGY

Recent streptococcal infection of pharynx.

Diagnosis

- **Laboratory findings:**
  - Positive antistreptolysin-O (ASLO) antibody titers.
  - Elevated ESR.
- Diagnosis of rheumatic fever requires presence of two major criteria or one major and two minor criteria.
  - **Major criteria:**
    - Arthritis (migratory, multiple joints).
    - Carditis (endo-, myo-, peri-).
    - Erythema marginatum rash.
    - Subcutaneous nodules.
    - Sydenham's chorea.
  - **Minor criteria:**
    - Fever.
    - Arthralgias.
    - Elevated ESR.
    - Prolonged PR interval.
    - Recent streptococcal pharyngitis.

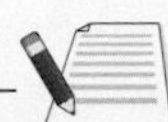

The reason for treating strep throat is to prevent the complication of rheumatic fever, not due to worry of the pharyngitis itself, which would resolve without antibiotics.

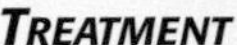

Treatment

- **Acute:**
  - Course of penicillin to eradicate throat carriage of group A streptococci.
  - Aspirin for arthritis.
  - Steroids for carditis.
- **Chronic:**
  - Monthly doses of benzathine penicillin to prevent recurrences.
  - Follow-up with cardiologist in severe cases.

DYSLIPIDEMIA

About half of all cases of coronary artery disease are associated with disorders of lipid metabolism. Formulas for calculating lipid levels:

- LDL = TC – HDL – VLDL
- VLDL = Trig/5
- Total cholesterol (TC):
  - Normal: < 200
  - Borderline: 200–240
  - High: > 240
- Normal HDL: 30–100

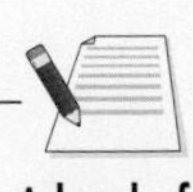

A level of HDL > 60 is cardioprotective.

Major Lipoproteins

- Chylomicrons: Transport cholesterol from the gut in the bloodstream.
- Chylomicron remnants: Left over after lipoprotein lipase liberates free fatty acids from chylomicrons for use in tissues.
- Very low-density lipoprotein (VLDL): Secreted from the liver; carries cholesterol in the bloodstream.
- Intermediate-density lipoprotein (IDL): Metabolized from VLDL.

- LDL: Metabolized from IDL, it carries cholesterol in the bloodstream to tissues.
- HDL: Uptakes free cholesterol secreted by tissues and transports it to the liver.

A high-risk cardiac patient who is on a statin and has a good LDL but a low HDL should be started on fibrate.

Isolated Hypercholesterolemia

- Familial hypercholesterolemia: Elevated LDL (type IIa).
- Familial defective apo B100: Elevated LDL (type IIa).
- Polygenic hypercholesterolemia: Elevated LDL (type IIa).

Isolated Hypertriglyceridemia

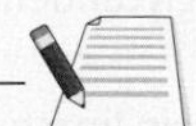

Patients with very high triglyceride levels (> 1,000) are at risk of devoloping pancreatitis.

- Familial hypertriglyceridemia: Elevated VLDL (type IV).
- Familial lipoprotein lipase deficiency: Elevated chylomicrons (type I, V).
- Familial apo CII deficiency: Elevated chylomicrons (type I, V).

Combined Hypertriglyceridemia and Hypercholesterolemia

- Combined hyperlipidemia: Elevated VLDL, LDL (type IIb).
- Dysbetalipoproteinemia: Elevated VLDL, IDL (type III).

Physical Findings

- Xanthelasma: Painless, nonpruritic raised yellow plaques that occur on eyelids near inner canthi.
- Xanthoma: Reddish brown papules on scalp, face, trunk, and flexor surfaces of limbs.

Diagnosis

- Serum lipoprotein analysis is done after a 12-hour fast.
- One-time sample cholesterol levels may not represent true levels in the following circumstances:
  - Weight loss
  - Pregnancy
  - Major surgery
  - Severe illness
- *Note:* In patients who have MI, lipoprotein levels obtained within the first 24 hours will more closely approximate true pre-MI levels than later levels, which may not return to baseline for several weeks.
- For cholesterol levels, see Table 2.1-5.

Treatment of Hypercholesterolemia

Goals of treatment:

- For a patient with 0–1 risk factors (low risk), keep LDL ≤ 160.
- For a patient with 1–2 risk factors (moderate risk), keep LDL ≤ 130.
- For a patient with known atherosclerotic heart disease (high risk), keep LDL ≤ 70.
- For treatment strategies, see Table 2.1-6.

TABLE 2.1-5. Cholesterol Levels Associated with Familial Disease

	Type	Total Cholesterol Level (mg/dL)	LDL Level	VLDL	Chylomicrons
Familial hypercholesterolemia	IIa	275–500	High	Normal	Normal
Familial defective apo B100	IIa	275–500	High	Normal	Normal
Polygenic hypercholesterolemia	IIa	240–350	High	Normal	Normal
Familial hypertriglyceridemia	IV	250–750	Normal/High	High	Normal/High
Familial lipoprotein lipase deficiency	I, (I,V)	> 750	Normal/High	Normal/High	High
Familial apoprotein CII deficiency	I, (I,V)	> 750	Normal/High	Normal/High	High
Familial combined hyperlipidemia	IIb	250–500	High	High	Normal/High
Dysbetalipoproteinemia	III	250–500	Normal	High	Normal/High

TABLE 2.1-6. Treatment of Hypercholesterolemia

Treatment	Mechanism	Results
Diet therapy	Therapeutic Lifestyle Changes (TLC) diet ▪ Total fat 25–30% total calories ▪ Polyunsaturated fat < 10% ▪ Monounsaturated fat < 20% ▪ Carbohydrate 50–60% ▪ Fiber 20–30 g/day ▪ Protein 15% total calories ▪ Saturated fat < 10% ▪ Dietary cholesterol < 300 mg/day	Step 2 diet reduces total cholesterol by 10–12%. Exercise variably raises HDL. If diet therapy and exercise fail by 6 weeks, progress to medications.
Statins	Statins are HMG-CoA reductase inhibitors and act to ↓ LDL and ↑ HDL.	Can lower LDL cholesterol by 35% and raise HDL by ~8%.
Bile acid sequestrants	Cholestyramine and colestipol bind bile acids in the gut.	Reduces LDL cholesterol by 15–20%.
Nicotinic acid	Reduces lipolysis in adipose tissue, inhibits hepatic synthesis of cholesterol.	Can reduce LDL cholesterol by ~20% over 6 months. Side effects include cutaneous flushing, abdominal pain, nausea.
Fibrinates	Best for reducing triglycerides (in VLDL and chylomicrons).	↑ HDL by 5–30%.

COMMON CARDIAC MEDICATIONS

	Medication	Main Clinical Uses	Adverse Effects
Class I: Sodium channel blockers	Lidocaine	Suppresses ventricular dysrhythmias.	Mild: drowsiness, confusion, ataxia. Severe: psychosis, seizures, AV block, respiratory depression.
	Quinidine	Suppresses ventricular dysrhythmias, atrial premature beats, A-fib.	Cinchonism: tinnitus, hearing loss, visual changes, delirium, psychosis. Also causes GI upset, promotes torsades de pointes (prodysrhythmic). Potentiates many other medications.
	Procainamide	Suppresses ventricular dysrhythmias and A-fib, A-flutter, WPW.	Myocardial depression, prolonged QT and QRS, torsades de pointes, V-fib.
Class II: Beta blockers	Propranolol	SVT, thyrotoxicosis, acute MI, hypertension.	All beta blockers can cause bronchoconstriction; use with caution in asthmatics. Hypotension, light-headedness, fatigue, depression, and elevation of triglycerides can occur.
	Metoprolol	SVT, acute MI, hypertension.	
	Esmolol	SVT, thyrotoxicosis.	
	Labetalol	Hypertension.	
Class III: Prolongs action potentials	Amiodarone	VT, VF, A-fib, WPW.	Bradycardia, AV block, peripheral neuropathy, pulmonary fibrosis, corneal deposits, skin discoloration, hepatotoxicity. Due to high iodine content, can cause hypo- or hyperthyroidism.
	Bretylium	Ventricular dysrhythmias.	Transient hypertension, hypotension.
	Sotalol	AV reentry SVT, WPW	Bradycardia, CHF, peripheral edema.

	Medication	Main Clinical Uses	Adverse Effects
Class IV: Calcium channel blockers	Verapamil	Mild to moderate hypertension.	Calcium channel blockers reduce inotropy and are contraindicated in patients with heart failure, 2nd- or 3rd-degree heart block.
	Diltiazem	Mild to moderate hypertension.	
	Amlodipine, nifedipine	Mild to moderate hypertension.	
Other antidysrhythmic agents	Adenosine	Supraventricular tachycardia.	Transient asystole, hypotension, flushing.
	Digoxin	Rate control of atrial tachydysrhythmia, increased inotropy for CHF.	Toxicity can occur in therapeutic range. Vomiting, anorexia, confusion, visual changes, AV block, PVCs, VT, VF. Hyperkalemia is seen with acute poisoning. Hypokalemia lowers threshold for toxicity (remember, many drugs used for CHF can cause hypokalemia). Chronic therapy can cause gynecomastia.
	Magnesium	Torsades de pointes, hypertension due to preeclampsia.	Hypotension, flushing, CNS changes, decreased reflexes, respiratory collapse.
	Epinephrine	Asystole, anaphylaxis, pressor.	May cause ischemia.
Inotropic agents	Dopamine	Increases inotropy, chronotropic, pressor.	Increases peripheral vasoconstriction at doses > 5–10 μg/kg/min.
	Dobutamine	Increases inotropy.	Associated with reflex arterial vasodilatation and tachycardia.
Chronotropic agents	Atropine	Asystole, symptomatic bradycardia.	Anticholinergic.
Venous/coronary dilators	Nitroglycerin	Venous and coronary artery dilator, can be used for malignant hypertension.	Hypotension, headache.
Antihypertensive agents	Nitroprusside	Malignant hypertension.	Can cause hypotension, cyanide toxicity, methemoglobinemia.
	Minoxidil	Severe hypertension.	Can cause hypotension, tachycardia, hair growth.

	Medication	Main Clinical Uses	Adverse Effects
	Hydralazine	Moderate to severe hypertension, particularly in the setting of preeclampsia and eclampsia. Hydralazine is a direct vasodilator.	Can cause tachycardia, angina, lupus-like syndrome with a malar rash that disappears after discontinuing the drug.
	Clonidine	Central-acting agent for hypertension.	Hypotension, rebound hypertension after halting medication.
	Phentolamine	Parenteral alpha blocker used for hypertension due to pheochromocytoma, cocaine.	Hypotension, tachycardia, light-headedness.
	Prazosin	PO alpha blocker used for mild to moderate hypertension.	
	ACE inhibitors	Hypertension (decrease preload and afterload), nephroprotective CHF. Decrease cardiovascular events and mortality in high-risk patients > 55 years old.	All ACE inhibitors are variably associated with cough and angioedema and can cause acute renal failure in patients with bilateral renal artery stenosis. Hyperkalemia.
	Angiotensin receptor blockers	Hypertension. Unclear magnitude of renal protection compared to ACE inhibitors.	Side effects similar to ACE inhibitors but less cough.
Antiplatelet agents	Aspirin	Used to prevent MI in patients with risk factors, can improve mortality from MI by about 25%.	Associated with GI bleed. Some patients can have hypersensitivity reaction to aspirin.
	2b,3a inhibitors	Intravenous adjunct to heparin and thrombolysis in setting of acute MI; best use still being investigated.	Can be associated with excessive bleeding.
Antithrombotic agents	Warfarins	Long-term prevention of clots in deep vein thrombosis (DVT), A-fib, stroke, and others.	Warfarins have an initial procoagulant effect. When anticoagulating as an inpatient, use heparin coverage initially. For outpatients, start at very low doses and raise gradually.
	Heparins	Myocardial infarction, pulmonary embolism, deep venous thrombosis.	Both low-molecular-weight and unfractionated heparins can be associated with excessive bleeding.

	Medication	Main Clinical Uses	Adverse Effects
Thrombolytic agents	Streptokinase	Myocardial infarction, pulmonary embolism, embolic cerebrovascular accident (CVA).	Relatively low cost. Cannot be used more than once within a 6-month period. Associated with hemorrhage at various sites.
	Tissue plasminogen activator	Myocardial infarction, pulmonary embolism, embolic CVA.	High cost. Associated with hemorrhage at various sites.

CARDIOLOGY

HOW TO PRESENT AN ELECTROCARDIOGRAM (ECG)

First, confirm that the ECG belongs to your patient. If possible, compare to a previous tracing. Then, present in a systematic manner:

1. *Rate* (see Figure 2.1-18): The rate is [number of] beats per minute (bpm):
   - The ECG paper is scored so that one big box is 0.20 seconds. These big boxes consist of five little boxes, each of which is 0.04 seconds.
   - A quick way to calculate rate when the rhythm is regular is the mantra: **300, 150, 100, 75, 60, 50** (= 300 / # large boxes), which is measured as the number of large boxes between two QRS complexes. Therefore, a distance of one large box between two adjacent QRS complexes would be a rate of 300, while a distance of five large boxes between two adjacent QRS complexes would be a rate of 60.
   - For irregular rhythms, count the number of complexes that occur in a 6-second interval (30 large boxes) and multiply by 10 to get a rate in bpm.
2. *Rhythm*: The rhythm is [sinus]/[atrial fibrillation]/[atrial flutter] or other:
   - If p waves are present in all leads and upright in lead I and inverted in lead AVR, then the rhythm is sinus. Lack of p waves suggests a disorganized atrial rhythm, a junctional rhythm, or a ventricular rhythm. A ventricular rhythm (V-fib or V-tach) is an unstable one

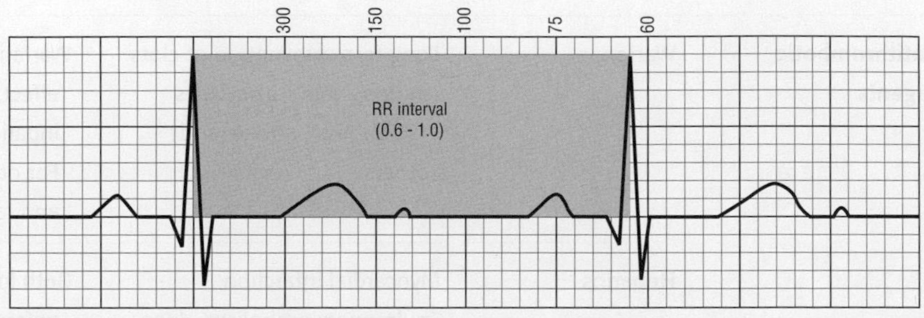

FIGURE 2.1-18. Calculating rate.

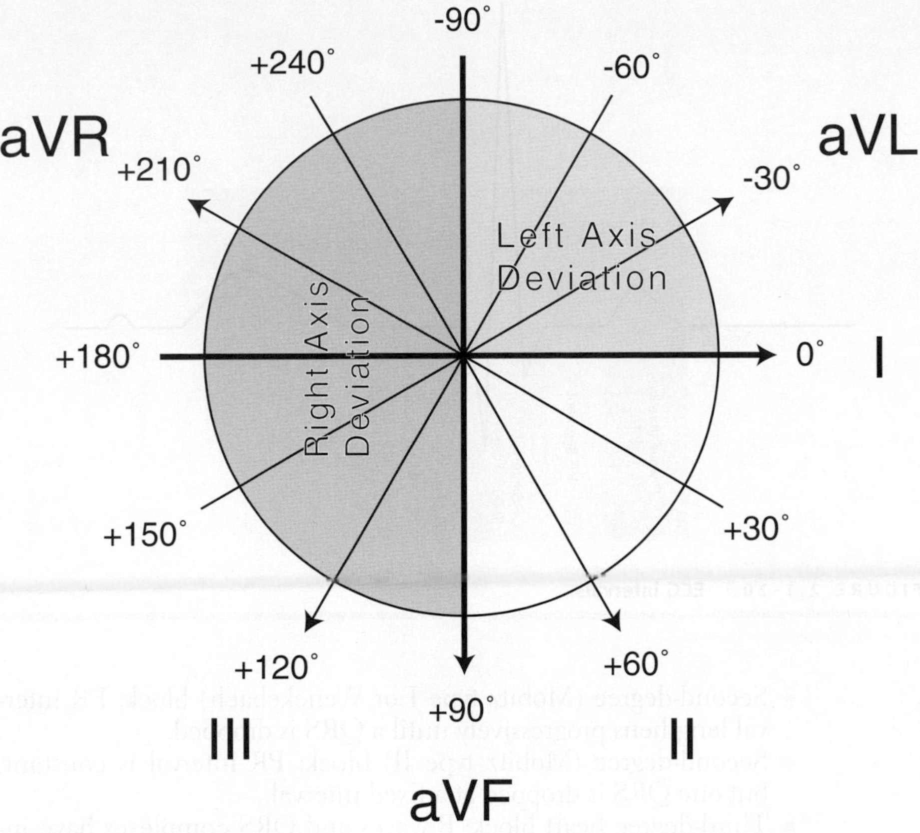

FIGURE 2.1-19. ECG axes.

(could spell imminent death), and you should be getting ready for advanced cardiac life support (ACLS).

- Normal sinus rhythm is usually a regular narrow-complex rhythm with each QRS complex preceded by a p wave.

3. *Axis* (see Figure 2.1-19): The axis is [normal]/[deviated to the right]/[deviated to the left]:
   - If I and aVF are both upright or positive, then the axis is normal.
   - If I is upright and aVF is upside down, then there is left axis deviation (LAD).
   - If I is upside down and aVF is upright, then there is right axis deviation (RAD).
   - If I and aVF are both upside down or negative, then there is extreme RAD.
4. *Intervals* (see Figure 2.1-20): The [PR]/[QRS] intervals are [normal]/[short-ened]/[widened]:
   - Normal PR interval = 0.12 to 0.20 seconds:
   - Short PR is associated with Wolff-Parkinson-White syndrome (WPW).
   - WPW syndrome is characterized by a "delta" wave, or slurred upstroke of QRS complex.
   - Long PR interval is associated with heart block, of which there are three types:
     - First-degree block: PR interval > 0.20 seconds (one big box).

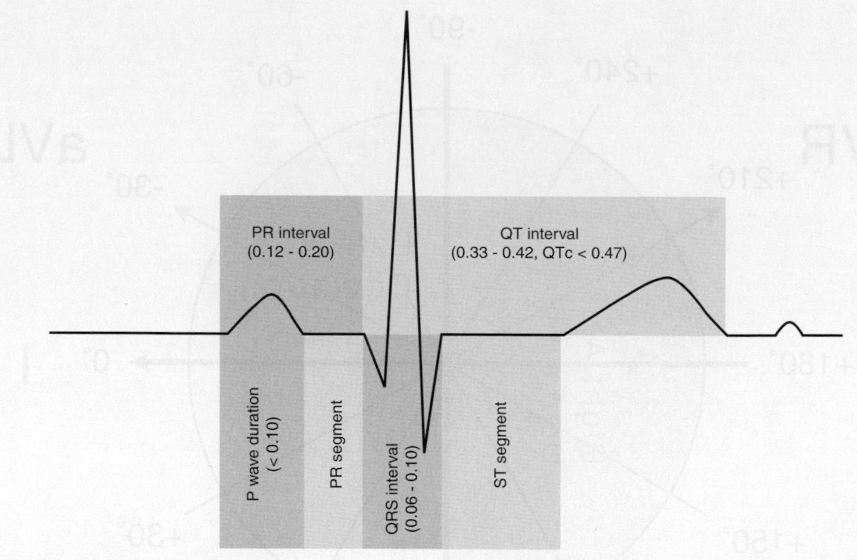

FIGURE 2.1-20. ECG intervals.

- Second-degree (Mobitz type I or Wenckebach) block: PR interval lengthens progressively until a QRS is dropped.
- Second-degree (Mobitz type II) block: PR interval is constant, but one QRS is dropped at a fixed interval.
- Third-degree heart block: P waves and QRS complexes have independent rates, no association is noted between P waves and QRS complexes.

- Normal QRS interval ≤ 0.12 seconds: Prolonged QRS is seen when the beat is initiated in the ventricle rather than the sinoatrial node, when there is a bundle branch block, and when the heart is artificially paced with longer QRS intervals. Prolonged QRS is also noted in tricyclic overdose and Wolff-Parkinson-White syndrome.

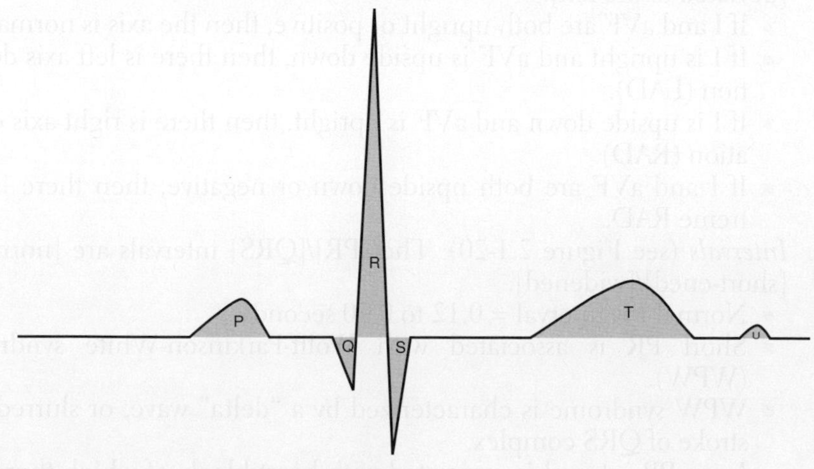

FIGURE 2.1-21. ECG wave morphology.

5. *Wave morphology* (see Figure 2.1-21):
   a. *Ventricular hypertrophy:* There [is/is no] [left/right] [ventricular/atrial] hypertrophy. There are multiple criteria for determining right (RVH) and left ventricular hypertrophy (LVH). A few are listed here:
      - *Clues for LVH:*
        - $R_I > 15$ mm
        - $R_{I, II \text{ or } aVF} > 20$ mm
        - $R_{a\,VL} > 11$ mm
        - R_{V5} or $R_{V6} > 26$ mm
        - $R_I + S_{III} > 25$ mm
        - R + S in V lead > 45 mm
        - $S_{V1} + R_{V5}$ or $R_{V6} > 35$ mm
      - *Clues for RVH:*
        - $R_{V1} > 7$ mm
        - $S_{V1} < 2$ mm
        - R/S ratio in $V_1 > 1$
        - RAD of 110° or more
   b. *Atrial hypertrophy:*
      - Right atrial hypertrophy: Tall or peaked p waves in limb or precordial leads.
      - Left atrial hypertrophy: Broad or notched p waves in limb leads.
   c. *Ischemic changes:* There [are/are no] S-T wave [depressions/elevations] or [flattened/inverted] T waves. Presence of Q wave indicates an old infarct.
   d. *Bundle branch block:* There [is/is no] [left/right] bundle branch block. Clues:
      - Presence of RSR′ wave in leads V_1–V_3 with ST depression and T wave inversion goes with RBBB.
      - Presence of notched R wave in leads I, aVL, and V_4–V_6 goes with LBBB.

HIGH-YIELD FACTS IN

Endocrinology

Type 1 Diabetes Mellitus

- Type 1 diabetes is characterized by absolute insulin deficiency from selective autoimmune destruction of the pancreatic beta cells, which are responsible for producing insulin.
- It accounts for < 10% of all diabetes cases and mainly affects lean children, teenagers, and young adults. Usually diagnosed before age 30.

Etiology

- **Type 1A diabetes:** Autoimmune-mediated diabetes. There are strong genetic associations with linkage to the HLA DQA and DQB genes. Several autoantibodies directly against the beta cells or their products are usually detectable:
  - Anti–islet cell autoantigen (anti-ICA).
  - Anti–glutamic acid decarboxylase (anti-GAD).
  - Anti-insulin antibodies.
  - Antibody to the tyrosine phosphatase IA-2.
- **Type 1B diabetes:** Idiopathic, with no autoimmune markers, occurs more commonly in Asian or African ancestry.

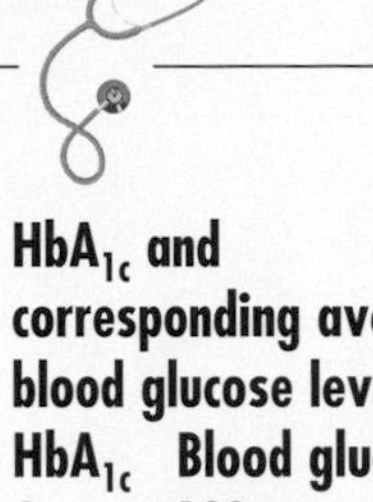

HbA_{1c} and corresponding average blood glucose levels:

HbA_{1c}	Blood glucose
6	120
7	150
8	180
9	210
	(Increments of 30)

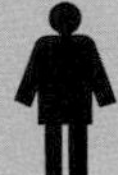

A woman presents with a recurrent vaginal candidiasis that is refractory to treatment. *Think: Diabetes mellitus.* **Next step:** Get a finger stick for blood glucose.

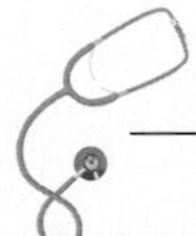

The only treatment for Type 1 DM patients is insulin (both long and short acting), administered by subcutaneous injection. Oral hypoglycemics have no role in management because these patients have no functioning pancreatic beta cells.

Signs and Symptoms

Usually presents with symptomatic hyperglycemia or diabetic ketoacidosis (discussed later).

- Polyuria.
- Polydipsia.
- Weight loss.
- Dehydration.
- Blurred vision.
- Fatigue.
- Foot ulcers.
- Can get restrictive cardiomyopathy without coronary artery disease.

Diagnosis

- Confirmed with a fasting serum glucose of > 126 mg/dL.
- Glycosuria (causes an osmotic diuresis that leads to dehydration).
- HbA_{1c} is a measure of glucose control over the past 3 months. Most complications can be prevented if the HbA_{1c} level is kept below 7%.

Treatment

Treated solely with insulin (see Table 2.2-1 for types); oral agents have no role in its management.

TABLE 2.2-1. Insulin Preparations and Their Pharmacokinetic Properties

Preparation	Onset	Peak (hr)	Duration (hr)
Rapid-acting			
Insulin lispro	10–15 min	1–2	3–5
Insulin aspart	10–15 min	1–2	3–5
Short-acting			
Regular	30–60 min	2–4	4–8
Intermediate-acting			
Neutral Protamine Hagedorn (NPH)	1–3 hrs	4–10	10–18
Lente	2–4 hrs	4–12	10–20
Long-acting			
Insulin detemir	2–3 hrs	No peak	Up to 24 hrs
Insulin glargine	2–3 hrs	No peak	24 hrs

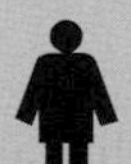

A 60-year-old diabetic who was recently started on insulin came back with complaints of high finger sticks in the early morning with recurrent nightmares. *Think: Somogyi effect.* **What will you do?** Change to longer acting insulin at night to avoid 3 AM hypoglycemia.

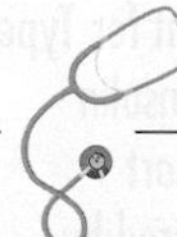

Measure finger-stick glucose levels 5×/day:

- Morning fasting
- Breakfast postprandial
- Lunch postprandial
- Dinner postprandial
- Before bed

Postprandial is 2 hours after the meal.

Initiating Therapy

- Patients are usually hospitalized at the time of initial diagnosis (because often present with DKA which is dangerous) and are treated with regular insulin.
- The average total daily dose of regular insulin is used as the initial dose of outpatient insulin therapy (be conservative so as not to induce hypoglycemic episodes).
- Divide the total daily dose to give two-thirds before breakfast and one-third before dinner if using NPH or 70/30 preparations.
- Initially, the patient should monitor finger-stick glucose levels five times a day and keep a record of the levels:
  - Choose the regimen that is easiest for the patient to follow while maintaining good blood glucose control.
  - **Type I DM patients must always take insulin to avoid ketosis, even if fasting** (may decrease dose).

DAWN PHENOMENON

An exaggeration of the normal tendency of the plasma glucose to rise in the early morning hours before breakfast, probably secondary to an increase in growth hormone (GH) secretion.

SOMOGYI EFFECT

- Characterized by nighttime hypoglycemia followed by a dramatic increase in fasting glucose levels and increased plasma ketones.
- If Somogyi phenomenon is suspected, patients should check their blood glucose around 3 AM Hypoglycemia at this time confirms diagnosis.
- **The morning hyperglycemia is a rebound effect.**
- Replacement of intermediate-acting insulin with long-acting insulin at bedtime can prevent this effect (want to try to avoid peaking of insulin effect in the middle of the night).

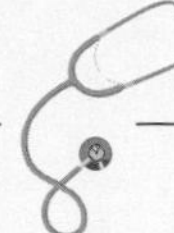

If a patient has hypoglycemic finger sticks in AM, decrease the bedtime NPH, even if the bedtime finger sticks are high.

Type 2 Diabetes Mellitus

- Type 2 diabetes is characterized by variable degrees of **insulin deficiency and insulin resistance.**
- It accounts for > 90% of diabetes cases in the United States. Usually diagnosed after age 30, but increasingly seen in adolescents and children due to rising incidence of obesity and sedentary lifestyle.
- Concordance rate for type 2 DM in monozygotic twins is > 90% (< 50% in type 1).
- Commonly associated with obesity, and often presents after period of weight gain.

A patient presents with persistent morning hyperglycemia, despite steadily increasing his nighttime NPH insulin dose. He also complains of frequent nightmares. His wife brings him in because she witnessed him having a seizure in the middle of the night. *Think: Somogyi effect.* **Next step:** Check 3 AM blood glucose.

ETIOLOGY

- Hyperglycemia is caused by:
  - Impaired secretion of insulin.
  - Decreased cellular responsiveness to insulin.
  - Impaired inhibition of hepatic gluconeogenesis.
- The syndrome of insulin resistance (**metabolic syndrome**—see below) associated with hyperglycemia leading to obesity, hypertension, hyperlipidemia, and coronary artery disease.
- Glucose toxicity: Hyperglycemia itself can induce impaired glucose tolerance and increased hepatic glucoseogenesis.

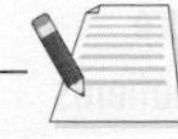

It is important for diabetics to have their feet frequently inspected to look for small cuts that may develop into ulcers. Due to neuropathy, diabetics can often have significant foot pathology and not feel anything.

SIGNS AND SYMPTOMS

- Patients may be asymptomatic.
- Presenting complaint is often a complication of their diabetes, such as a soft tissue infection. Can also present with signs of hyperglycemia.

- Increased susceptibility to fungal infections (cell-mediated immunity is impaired by acute hyperglycemia).
- Patients with type 2 DM will suffer from DKA only in rare instances (called ketosis-prone or atypical type 2 diabetes).
- The nonketotic hyperglycemic-hyperosmolar coma (NKHC) is more common in type 2 DM, but still rare.

Diabetics have increased susceptibility to infections due to decreased efficacy of granulocytes despite normal number:

- *Pseudomonas*
- Mucormycoses
- Actinomycoses
- Aspergillosis (eosinophilic pneumonia with asthma; treat with steroids)
- Renal abscesses (with urinary tract infections)

DIAGNOSIS

Requires any one of the following:

- Random glucose > 200 mg/dL in the presence of symptoms.
- Asymptomatic patients require a fasting glucose of > 126 mg/dL on two separate occasions.
- If patients have fasting glucose levels of > 100 mg/dL and < 126 mg/dL, an oral glucose tolerance test is indicated.
- Positive oral glucose tolerance test is a plasma glucose > 200 mg/dL at 2 hours after ingesting 75 g of glucose in solution.

TREATMENT

- Initial management should consist of **education**, diet, and exercise to achieve weight control.
- Patient education increases compliance with diet, exercise, and medication therapy. Discussions should involve when to seek medical attention, side effects of medications, proper foot care, ophthalmology visits, and symptoms of hyper- and hypoglycemia.
- If glycemic control cannot be obtained with diet and exercise, start oral hypoglycemic.
- Combination of low-dose insulin secretogogues (Glyburide) plus low-dose insulin sensitizers (metformin) may improve HbA_{1c} with few side effects but DPP-4 inhibitors are also being increasingly used in the initial therapeutic regimen.
- Patients not controlled with oral hypoglycemics alone may require insulin.
- Glucose-lowering drugs: See Table 2.2-2.

Metabolic Syndrome

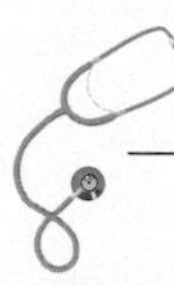

Metformin and thiazolidinediones are contraindicated in patients with advanced heart failure.

A constellation of findings that lead to increased risk of cardiovascular disease such as myocardial infarction, stroke, and death. With the growing epidemic of obesity, the prevalence of metabolic syndrome is rapidly increasing even among adolescents and children. The definition of metabolic syndrome in adults includes at least three of the following:

1. Fasting plasma glucose ≥ 100 mg/dL (6.1 mmol/L).
2. Abdominal obesity: waist girth > 102 cm (> 40 in) for men and > 88 cm (> 35 in) for women.
3. Serum TG > 150 mg/dL (1.7 mmol/L).
4. HDL-C < 40 mg/dL (1 mmol/L) for men; < 50 mg/dL (1.3 mmol/L) for women.
5. Blood pressure ≥ 130/85 mm Hg or on medications.

TABLE 2.2-2. Glucose-Lowering Drugs

Sulfonylureas: glimepiride, glyburide, glipizide	■ HgA_{1C} change: Moderately effective, lower blood glucose by 20% and A_{1C} by 1–2%. ■ Mechanism: Stimulates insulin secretion from the pancreas. ■ Benefits: Extensive experience; low cost; daily dosing. ■ Risks/Concerns: Hypoglycemia especially with renal disease; weight gain; may impede ischemic preconditioning.
Meglitinides: repaglinide (Prandin), nateglinide (Starlix)	■ HgA_{1C} change: Reduce A_{1C} by 1–2%. ■ Mechanism: Increase insulin production by the pancreas. ■ Benefits: Less hypoglycemia, targets postprandial glucose, mimics physiological insulin secretion. ■ Risks/Concerns: Short-acting glucose lowering drugs, should be taken before each meal; slightly less effective compared to sulfonylureas.
Biguanides: metformin	■ HgA_{1C} change: Reduce A_{1C} by 1–2%. ■ Mechanism: Decreases liver's glucose production and slightly increases muscle glucose uptake. ■ Benefits: No weight gain; no hypoglycemia when used alone (it may even lead to initial weight loss). ■ Risks/Concerns: Major side effects are GI symptoms; most serious side effect is lactic acidosis (50% mortality). ■ Contraindications: Within 24–48 hours of injection of radiographic contrast material; renal disease with GFR < 60 mL/min or creatinine > 1.5 (increased risk of lactic acidosis); liver disease; CHF; excessive alcohol intake. ■ *Note: Unless contraindicated, it is the first choice for an oral hypoglycemic agent.*
Thiazolidinediones: troglitazone, rosiglitazone, pioglitazone	■ HgA_{1C} change: Reduce A_{1C} by 0.5–1.4%. ■ Mechanism: Decreases insulin resistance at the muscle and liver. ■ Benefits: No hypoglycemia; may improve HDL cholesterol and triglycerides. ■ Risks/Concerns: Slow onset of action (take 4–6 weeks to see an effect on blood glucose); weight gain (subcutaneous insulin-sensitive fat); fluid retention; major side effects is hepatotoxicity, which requires liver monitoring; expensive. ■ Contraindications: Class III and IV heart failure and liver disease. Recently, there has been a concern for increased cardiovascular disease that lead to FDA warning.
Alpha-glucosidase inhibitors: acarbose, miglitol	■ HgA_{1C} change: Reduce A_{1C} by 0.5–1.0%. ■ Mechanism: Slows the digestion of carbohydrates. ■ Benefits: No weight gain; no hypoglycemia when used alone. ■ Risks/Concerns: Major side effects are GI symptoms (transient diarrhea, nausea, and abdominal pain); caution use with IBD, intestinal obstructions; expensive.
DPP-4 Inhibitors: sitagliptin (Januvia)	■ HgA_{1C} change: Reduce A_{1C} by 0.5–1.0%. ■ Mechanism: Increases insulin production and decreases the liver's production of glucose. ■ Benefits: No weight gain; less hypoglycemia. ■ Risks/Concerns: Low side effect profile–URI symptoms, nausea, and diarrhea; require dose adjustment in renal insufficiency; expensive.

(continues)

TABLE 2.2-2. Glucose-Lowering Drugs *(continued)*

GLP-1 analog: exenatide (Byetta)	▪ HgA_{1C} change: Reduce A_{1C} about 0.8%. ▪ Mechanism: Enhances insulin secretion, decreases liver's glucose output, and may suppress appetite. ▪ Benefits: Weight loss; less hypoglycemia. ▪ Risks/Concerns: Nausea and vomiting; hypoglycemia risk increased when combined with sulfonylurea; hypertriglyceridemia.
Pramlintide (Symlin):	▪ Synthetic analog of the human hormone amylin that is cosecreted normally with insulin. ▪ New class of agents, was approved as adjunctive therapy in patients with type 1 or 2 diabetes mellitus. ▪ It is used in patients who fail to achieve good glycemic control, despite intensive insulin therapy, with or without metformin and/or sulfonylureas. ▪ Its use is associated with weight loss.

Acute Complications of Diabetes Mellitus

DKA is a complication mostly associated with type 1 DM, while nonketotic hyperglycemic hyperosmolar syndrome (HHS) is associated with type 2 DM. However, there is some overlap between type 1 and type 2.

The major acute complications of diabetes are the hyperglycemic and hypoglycemic emergencies. Hyperglycemic emergencies include diabetic ketoacidosis (DKA) and hyperglycemic hyperosmolar syndrome (HHS).

Diabetic Ketoacidosis

Metabolic acidosis due to ketoacid accumulation secondary to severely depressed insulin levels.

Etiology

- Severe insulin deficiency causes the body to switch from metabolizing carbohydrates to metabolizing and oxidizing lipids.
- Usually precipitated by lapse in insulin treatment, acute infection, major trauma, or stress.

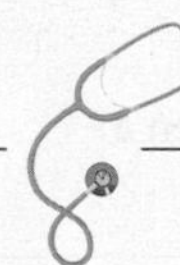

DKA is the most life-threatening acute complication of diabetes, and is often the presenting syndrome of type 1 DM, but can also occur in type 2 DM, especially in people of color.

Pathophysiology

- Insulin deficiency causes hyperglycemia, which induces an osmotic diuresis **(severe dehydration).**
- Profound dehydration, sodium loss, and potassium loss occurs.
- The body believes there is no glucose because the cells aren't getting any, which triggers the oxidation of free fatty acids from adipose tissue. The liver converts these free fatty acids into an alternative energy source: **ketones** (acetoacetic acid and beta-hydroxybutyric acid), which causes the metabolic ketoacidosis.
- There is respiratory compensation for this metabolic acidosis (fast breathing [ie, Kussmaul], blowing off CO_2).
- **Other findings:**
  - Acetone is produced from spontaneous decarboxylation of acetoacetic acid. The acetone is disposed of by respiration and its odor is present on the patient's breath (fruity odor).
  - *Pseudohyponatremia* (not real hyponatremia) is due to a normal response to the osmotic shifts of severe hyperglycemia. The sodium reading in the lab value does not accurately represent what the true sodium is. The "corrected" sodium concentration is obtained by adding 1.6 mEq of sodium for each 100 mg/dL of glucose above normal.

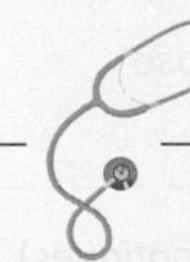

When calculating the anion gap in DKA, use the actual Na, not the corrected Na.

Signs and Symptoms

- **Polyuria** and **polydypsia**, nausea, vomiting and vague abdominal pain.
- Lethargy and fatigue are later components.
- May progress to coma.
- Signs of dehydration are present, and patients may be hypotensive and tachycardic.
- Kussmaul respirations (rapid deep breaths) may be present.
- Acetone (fruity) odor may be present on the patient's breath.

Diagnosis

- Anion gap metabolic acidosis (ketones are unmeasured ions) serum pH < 7.30.
- Hyperglycemia.
- Hyperketonemia.
- Usually, the diagnosis can be presumed at the bedside if patient's urine is strongly positive for ketones and the finger-stick glucose is high.
- Glucose is usually between 400 and 800 mg/dL.
- Initially, potassium is high due to acidosis, but drops with treatment (insulin drives K^+ into cells).

Treatment

- Goals of treatment are to remove ketones and correct the acidosis.
  - You must follow the anion gap as a measure; correction of acidosis is a critical endpoint (correction of high glucose does not mean DKA is over!). Stopping insulin and fluids when glucose is normal but acidosis is still present is a critical mistake!).
  - Can give bicarbonate in fluid to help when severe acidosis, but controversial.
- Aggressive fluid resuscitation to correct volume deficit.
- Correct hyperglycemia with insulin drip. Insulin is required in DKA even after blood glucose returns to normal range. Continue to give insulin and glucose-containing IV fluids.
- Correct underlying causes (eg, infection).
- Bicarbonate may be used to correct severe acidosis (rarely necessary).
- This is a critical patient—usually requires admission to intensive care unit (ICU).

Prognosis

- Mortality rate is approximately 10%.
- Hypotension or coma present at admission are negative prognostic indicators.
- Major causes of death are circulatory failure, hypokalemia, and infection.

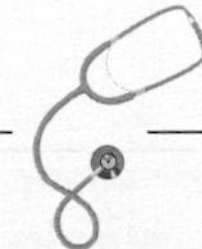

DKA is a life-threatening condition and must be recognized early and treated correctly.

Hyperglycemic Hyperosmolar Syndrome

- Hyperglycemic hyperosmolar syndrome (HHS) is defined by a plasma osmolarity > 320 mOsm/L and a plasma glucose level > 600 mg/dL but a **normal bicarbonate level, normal PH,** and no significant evidence of ketosis.
- Occurs in patients with **type 2 DM.** The diagnosis is considered in any elderly patient with altered mental status and dehydration, particularly with known diabetes.

PATHOPHYSIOLOGY

- Patients usually have a period of symptomatic hyperglycemia before the syndrome develops.
- When fluid intake becomes insufficient, **extreme dehydration** ensues because of the hyperglycemia-induced osmotic diuresis.

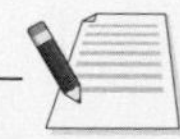

HHS most commonly occurs in patients unable to affect their own environment (eg, nursing home residents) or in elderly residents with impaired thirst mechanism and lack of access to water.

ETIOLOGY

- Medication noncompliance.
- Severe infection or sepsis.
- Dehydration.
- Diuretics.
- Glucocorticoids.

SIGNS AND SYMPTOMS

- Altered mental status.
- Signs of profound dehydration.
- Seizures and transient neurologic deficits may occur.

DIAGNOSIS

- Serum glucose levels are usually > 1,000 mg/dL (much higher than in DKA).
- Serum osmolarity is usually around 385 mOsm/kg.
- Blood urea nitrogen (BUN)/creatinine levels are markedly increased from prerenal azotemia.

In hyperglycemic hyperosmolar syndrome, the preservation of vascular volume is critical. Normal saline is the initial fluid of choice and it should be initiated even before insulin.

TREATMENT

Goal of treatment is to expand the intravascular volume to stabilize vital signs and improve circulation and urine output:

- **Aggressive hydration**! Infuse 2–3 L of normal saline over 1–2 hours.
- Once vital signs have stabilized, change fluid to D_5 ½ NS and monitor vital signs, urine output, serum electrolytes, and BUN/creatinine carefully.
- Electrolytes should be monitored, especially potassium because the concentration may fall as urine output is restored and renal function improves. Begin potassium replacement with the initial infusion of D_5 ½ NS, and keep serum potassium at 4 mEq/L or more.
- Insulin should be administered only after plasma expansion has been initiated. If insulin is given before plasma expansion, it drives glucose into the cells, exacerbating volume depletion.
- Monitor patient for signs and symptoms of cerebral edema, which may occur if the osmolarity is corrected too quickly.
- If insulin is deemed necessary in the initial resuscitation, 5% glucose should be added to the infusion to prevent hypoglycemia when the serum glucose reaches 250 mg/dL.

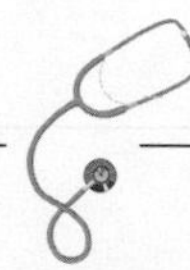

Hypoglycemia is the most common cause of altered mental status in hospitalized patients.

HYPOGLYCEMIA

Abnormally low serum glucose level that causes sympathetic stimulation followed by altered mental status.

Etiology

- **Drug-induced** (most common cause): Insulin, sulfonylureas.
- **Alcohol.**
- Insulinomas.
- Adrenal insufficiency.
- Insulin receptor antibodies.
- Severe liver or renal disease.
- Endotoxic shock.
- Hypopituitarism with deficiency of both GH and cortisol.

Pathophysiology

- Glucose transport across the blood-brain barrier is regulated by adrenergic nervous system activity (resulting in ↑ GH and cortisol secretion and ↓ insulin secretion).
- Glucagon is secreted by the pancreatic alpha cells. It increases plasma glucose levels and stimulates gluconeogenesis in the liver.
- The adrenergic outflow causes the typical sympathetic stimulatory symptoms of hypoglycemia and the lack of glucose to the brain results in altered mental status.

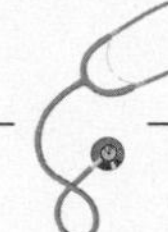

Hypoglycemia due to oral hypoglycemic agents lasts about 24 hours. Patients with sulfonylurea (and/or long-acting insulin analogues) overdose should be admitted to the hospital for 24 hours for monitoring and continuous glucose administration.

Signs and Symptoms

- History of insulin or sulfonylurea treatment.
- Adrenergic symptoms: Diaphoresis, anxiety, tremor, feeling faint, palpitations, and hunger.
- Central nervous system (CNS) manifestations: Confusion, inappropriate behavior (sometimes mistaken for alcohol intoxication), visual problems, stupor, and coma.

For alcoholics and people with malnutrition, always give thiamine prior to glucose to prevent Wernicke's encephalopathy.

Diagnosis

- Abnormally low serum glucose is < 50 mg/dL.
- Distinguish medication-induced vs. endogenous cause: Send C-peptide level to distinguish between endogenous (high C-peptide) and exogenous (low C-peptide) insulin because synthetic insulin has no C-peptide.

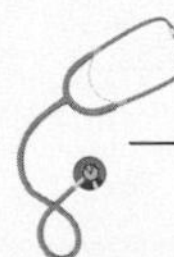

Whipple's triad of hypoglycemia:

1. Plasma glucose < 60 mg/dL
2. Symptoms of hypoglycemia
3. Improvement of the symptoms with administration of glucose

Treatment

- Once hypoglycemia is confirmed or if serum glucose level is not immediately available, obtain IV access and administer IV fluids with glucose.
- Only if patient's mental status is okay should you try giving food (PO); otherwise, they may aspirate.
- Whenever dextrose is administered for hypoglycemia, and alcoholism or nutritional deficiency is suspected, administer **thiamine** prior to glucose to prevent **Wernicke's encephalopathy.**
- Continue checking glucose levels, as they can drop again quickly (rebound hypoglycemia), or if from a medication, it may have a long half-life and still be on board.
- If hypoglycemia is refractory to glucose administration, consider adrenal insufficiency and give steroids.

Chronic Complications of Diabetes Mellitus

DIABETIC RETINOPATHY

ETIOLOGY

The highly vascular retina is commonly involved in long standing diabetes. Diabetes is responsible for most cases of legal blindness in adults in the United States.

PROGRESSION

1. **Background diabetic retinopathy:** Early changes, include hard exudates, microaneurysms, and minor hemorrhages on funduscopic examination.
2. **Preproliferative retinopathy:** Presence of "cotton-wool spots," which are indicative of retinal infarcts.
3. **Neovascularization/proliferative retinopathy:** Abnormal vessels form on the retina can cause damage. They are abnormal in both appearance and structure and are prone to hemorrhage (retinal and vitreous hemorrhage).

DIAGNOSIS

Regular and careful screening by opthalmologist is necessary to detect the early changes of diabetic retinopathy.

TREATMENT

- Control blood glucose level.
- Blood pressure reduction is beneficial.
- Controlling plasma lipids may also slow the progression of eye disease.
- Ophthalmologist can do laser ablation of abnormal vessels.

DIABETIC NEPHROPATHY

ETIOLOGY

Diabetes is the most common cause of renal failure in the United States. Diabetic nephropathy begins with a period of glomerular hyperfiltration and intraglomerular hypertension. Subsequently, glomerular injury develops with the eventual loss of filtration capacity, leading to azotemia.

PROGRESSION

Progresses from a small amount of a small protein (microalbumin) to large amounts of a large protein.

1. Microalbuminuria (30–300 mg/d).
2. Macroalbuminuria (> 300 mg/d).
3. Frank nephrotic syndrome (> 3.5 g/d).

DIAGNOSIS

Annual measurement of microalbumin-to-creatinine ratios on spot urine samples, and serum creatinine concentrations to screen for diabetic kidney disease.

TREATMENT

- Aggressive blood pressure control, particularly with ACE inhibitor or angiotensin II receptor blockers.
- Control glucose level.

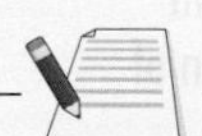

ACE inhibitors reduce albuminuria and slow the progression of renal disease in diabetic patients with and without hypertension.

Diabetic Foot

Etiology

Diabetic patients frequently have peripheral vascular disease and peripheral neuropathy. These place the diabetic foot at extreme risk for ulceration, infection, and, ultimately, possible amputation.

Signs and Symptoms

- Cold feet.
- Claudication, leg discomfort on ambulation (relieved with rest).
- Numbness, burning, or tingling sensation of the hands and feet, in a glove and stocking distribution.

Diagnosis

- Frequent, careful examination of the feet.
- Detect sensory deficits in the foot (Monofilament test).

Treatment

- Glucose control is critical.
- Use comfortable, protective, and well-fitting shoes and plain cotton socks.
- Ongoing foot care by a podiatrist is important.
- Aggressive treatment of the diabetic foot ulcer or infection with broad-spectrum antibiotics, often for longer periods of time. Debridement if necessary.

Counterregulatory Hormones

Counterregulatory hormones are hormones that counteract insulin action. Therefore, they can cause insulin resistance and diabetes if there is too much of them, or they can rise in response to hypoglycemia (too much insulin). High-yield facts and potential questions include:

- **Glucagon:**
  - The most important and fastest to act. It acts on the liver to increase gluconeogenesis and glycogenolysis.
  - Glucagon (1 mg IM) is used to resuscitate hypoglycemic coma if you cannot get IV access. (Never give anything by mouth, including glucose gel.)
  - Will not work in a patient who is alcoholic with liver failure. Alcohol will suppress gluconeogenesis, and glycogen stores are impaired in severe liver disease.
  - Loss of the glucagon response to hypoglycemia occurs after a long period of diabetes, especially type 1, leading to hypoglycemia unawareness.
  - Too much glucagon (glucagonoma) will present with new-onset diabetes, weight loss and characteristic rash (necrolytic migratory erythema).
- **Catecholamine:**
  - Too much insulin leads to hypoglycemia; catecholamines rise, giving the signs and symptoms of hypoglycemia such as tachycardia, sweating, and anxiety.
  - Pheochromocytoma patients (too much catecholamine) have an ↑ risk of hyperglycemia and diabetes.

- **Cortisol:**
  - Too much cortisol, as in Cushing's syndrome or in treatment of various diseases such as asthma, leads to hyperglycemia and diabetes.
  - Too little cortisol, as in Addison's disease, leads to hypoglycemia.
- **Growth hormone:**
  - A high level of GH in the early morning leads to hyperglycemia (dawn phenomenon).
  - A high level of GH in acromegaly is associated with hyperglycemia and diabetes in nearly half of cases.
  - In addition to measuring IGF_1, screen for acromegaly by conducting an oral glucose tolerance test to see if the GH will be suppressed in response to insulin release by the glucose given. If there is no suppression, the test is positive for acromegaly.
  - Neonatal hypoglycemia is a cardinal sign of GH deficiency.
- **Placental secretion hormones,** including GH, corticotropin-releasing hormone, progesterone, and human placental lactogen, could lead to gestational diabetes in susceptible individuals, which is why diabetes screening during pregnancy is conducted when these hormone levels are at their peak—around the 24th week of gestation.

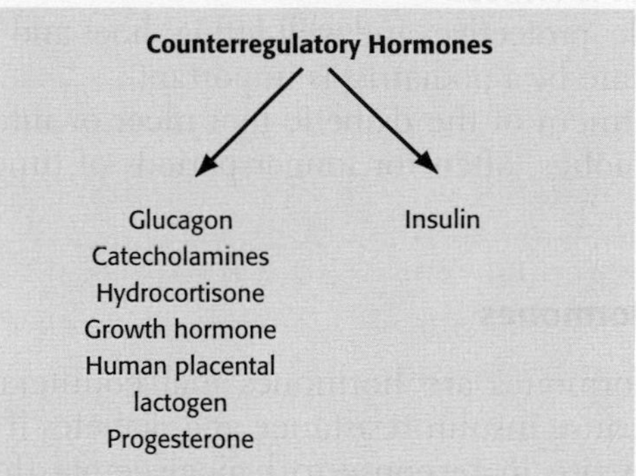

DISORDERS OF THE PITUITARY GLAND

ENDOCRINOLOGY

Pituitary adenomas are part of multiple endocrine neoplasia (MEN) type I (pituitary, pancreas, parathyroid).

Pituitary Tumors

- Anterior pituitary (adenohypophysis): Derivative of Rathke's pouch.
- Posterior pituitary (neurohypophysis): Composed of hypothalamic neuronal axon terminals, storage and release site for hormones produced by these neurons.
- For specific hormones, see Table 2.2-3.

Pathology

- Constitute ~ 10% of intracranial tumors.
- Most are benign, slow growing.
- Anterior pituitary: Craniopharyngiomas, adenomas.
- Posterior pituitary: No primary tumors.
- Metastases and meningiomas are occasionally seen.
- Pathology/manifestations arises from:
  - Excess hormone production.
  - Compression of suprasellar structures.
  - Destruction of normal pituitary parenchyma.
  - Compression of pituitary stalk → ↑ prolactin due to loss of inhibition by dopamine.

TABLE 2.2-3. Pituitary Hormones and Their Functions

Anterior Lobe	Main Stimulatory Actions	Hypothalamic Stimulus
Adrenocorticotropic hormone (ACTH, corticotropin)	▪ Growth and secretion of adrenal cortex to make cortisol and sex hormones	▪ CRH
Growth hormone (GH, somatotropin)	▪ Secretion of somatomedin C (insulin-like growth factor) ▪ Body growth	▪ GRH
Thyroid-stimulating hormone (TSH, thyrotropin)	▪ Growth of thyroid gland ▪ Production of T_3 and T_4	▪ TRH
Follicle-stimulating hormone (FSH)	▪ Spermatogenesis in the male ▪ Ovarian follicle growth in the female	▪ GnRH
Luteinizing hormone (LH)	▪ Testosterone secretion in the male ▪ Ovulation in the female	▪ GnRH
Prolactin	▪ Milk production ▪ Maternal behavior	▪ PRH (stimulates) ▪ Dopamine (inhibits)
Melanocyte-stimulating hormone (MSH)	▪ Skin pigmentation	
Posterior Lobe		**Releasing Stimulus**
Antidiuretic hormone (ADH; vasopressin, AVP)	▪ Retains sodium and water, producing concentrated urine	▪ Osmoreceptors
Oxytocin	▪ Milk letdown ▪ Contractions of labor	▪ Touch receptors in uterus, genitalia, and breast

Pituitary Adenomas

- **Prolactinoma** is the most common pituitary tumor. It can present with galactorrhea or amenorrhea. Women usually present earlier than men. Prolactin levels correlate with tumor size. Treat with dopamine agonists (bromocriptine).
- **Nonfunctioning tumors** are the second most common pituitary tumors. Symptoms include visual changes or slightly high prolactin levels due to mass effect, which disrupts the inhibitor signal that dopamine has on prolactin-producing cells. Treat with surgery.
- Less common pituitary adenomas include **somatotrophs** (GH; see Acromegaly), **corticotrophs** (ACTH), and **thyrotrophs** (TSH).
- **Pituitary microadenomas** (< 10 mm) are found in ~15% of asymptomatic women by MRI; in the absence of progression (assessed by follow-up MRI), they are clinically insignificant.

Craniopharyngiomas

- Arise from embryologic remnants of Rathke's pouch.
- Most common tumors of suprasellar region in children.
- Solid or cystic; usually calcified.

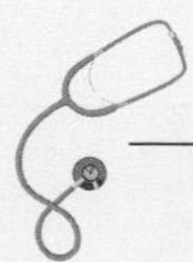

Patients rarely complain of "tunnel vision" (bitemporal hemianopsia) or a deficit when the defect is confined to the temporal visual fields. They more typically just report increased clumsiness or bumping into things.

Neurologic Symptoms

- Headache.
- Compression of optic chiasm:
  - Superior bitemporal quadrantanopsia: Early visual defect, since compression begins on inferior surface of chiasm.
  - Bitemporal hemianopsia ("tunnel vision"): Classic finding, occurs when tumor has reached significant size.
- Signs of increased intracranial pressure (ICP) are rare, as tumors are usually diagnosed before they reach the requisite dimensions.

Diagnosis of Pituitary Adenomas/Craniopharyngiomas

- **Magnetic resonance imaging (MRI):** More sensitive than CT, can detect microadenomas; use with gadolinium contrast.
- **Computed tomography (CT):** More sensitive than x-ray.
- **X-ray:** May show enlargement of sella; craniopharyngiomas may show calcifications in suprasellar regions.
- **Hormone studies:** Detect excesses or deficiencies, give information about type of tumor; useful when tumor cannot be detected radiographically.
- If a patient presents with manifestations of a specific disease (such as acromegaly, Cushing's, etc.), always start with hormonal workup prior to diagnostic imaging. That is because of the high prevalence of incidentalomas in the general population.

Treatment of Pituitary Adenomas/Craniopharyngiomas

- Dopamine agonists for prolactinomas (dopamine inhibits prolactin).
- Surgery: Indicated whenever there are neurologic symptoms.
- Radiotherapy: Can reduce size of tumor without surgery, sometimes used as surgical adjunct.
- Hormone replacement for hypopituitarism.

Acromegaly

- Type of pituitary adenoma also, but diagnosis and treatment are somewhat specific.
- Disorder marked by progressive enlargement (megaly) of peripheral (acral) body parts resulting from excess GH production.

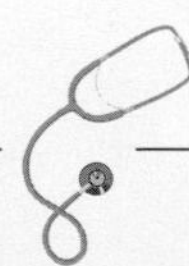

Acromegaly: The changes in a patient's appearance occur over many years and may not be apparent to the patient or his family. Old photos may suggest the diagnosis.

Etiology

- Pituitary somatotroph (cells that make GH, or somatotropin) adenoma is by far the most common cause.
- Ectopic GH secretion; hypothalamic tumors secreting growth hormone–releasing hormone (GHRH) are rare.

Signs and Symptoms

- Progressive enlargement of peripheral body parts, particularly head, hands, and feet.
- Progressive and irreversible organomegaly, especially cardiomegaly.

- Often, patients present with decompensated heart failure prior to diagnosis.
- Impaired glucose tolerance due to the anti-insulin actions of GH.
- Hyperphosphatemia due to GH's influence on tubular resorption of phosphate.
- Gigantism in children due to excess linear growth prior to epiphyseal closure.

DIAGNOSIS

- Lack of GH suppression by glucose load.
- **Serum insulin-like growth factor I (IGF-I) levels** is the best single test for diagnosis of acromegaly. It is made by the liver under stimulation by GH, elevated in acromegalics and does not fluctuate as does GH itself.
- **GH levels** are highly variable so testing will yield inaccurate results. Always check IGF-I if acromegally is suspected.

TREATMENT

- Surgery (transsphenoidal or transfrontal adenectomy, depending on the size and location of the tumor).
- Radiation therapy (takes 6–10 years to work).
- Dopamine agonist such as bromocriptine (preferred because of lower cost) or somatostatin analog such as octreotide.
- GH receptor blocker such as pegvisomant (Somavert).

Hypopituitarism

- **Tumors** causing dysfunction either by invasion, replacement, or compression. It can affect normal pituitary parenchyma, pituitary stalk, and hypothalamic parenchyma.
- **Surgical destruction** of pituitary or hypothalamus: Either therapeutic or as a result of an unrelated neurosurgical procedure.
- **Sheehan's syndrome:** Pituitary gland enlarges during pregnancy due to hyperplasia of lactotrophs without commensurate increase in blood supply; if hypotension occurs during childbirth, pituitary infarction can result.
- **Systemic** (rare): Hemochromatosis, sarcoid, lymphocytic hypophysitis (more common in women in late pregnancy and postpartum).
- **Infectious** (rare): Tuberculosis (TB), neurosyphilis.

A 29-year-old woman presents with inability to lactate after childbirth. Delivery was complicated by blood loss and hypotension. *Think: Sheehan's syndrome.* **Next step:** Check prolactin level and MRI with contrast of head.

SIGNS AND SYMPTOMS

- **ACTH deficiency**: See Adrenal Insufficiency section.
- **GH deficiency:** Growth retardation in children.
- **Prolactin:**
  - Deficiency: Failure to lactate after childbirth.
  - Excess: Amenorrhea and galactorrhea in women, ↓ libido and gynecomastia in men.

Drugs that inhibit dopamine activity also cause hyperprolactinemia: tricyclic antidepressants, prochlorperazine, haloperidol, methyldopa, metoclopramide, cimetidine.

- **TSH deficiency:** See Hypothyroidism section.
- **Luteinizing hormone (LH)** and **follicle-stimulating hormone (FSH) deficiency:** Amenorrhea and genital atrophy in women, ↓ libido in men.
- In slow-growing tumors, GH, FSH, and LH levels are affected early; ACTH and prolactin levels decline only with advanced disease.
- **Antidiuretic hormone (ADH) deficiency:** known as diabetes insipidus (discussed in separate section below).

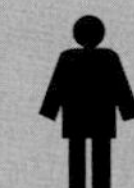

A 36-year-old woman complains of amenorrhea for 1 year, increasingly bad headaches, clumsiness, and sporadic nipple discharge; beta-hCG levels are normal. *Think: Prolactinoma.* **Next step:** Check serum prolactin level, MRI brain.

Drugs that inhibit dopamine activity also cause hyperprolactinemia: tricyclic antidepressants, prochlorperazine, haloperidol, methyldopa, metoclopramide, cimetidine.

DIAGNOSIS

The following circumstances must be considered when interpreting pituitary hormone levels:

- ACTH levels must be taken with serum cortisol levels; if cortisol is high, ACTH is probably low due to feedback inhibition. Insulin-induced hypoglycemia stimulates ACTH secretion and is an effective test of the entire hypothalamic-pituitary-adrenal axis. Test is administered similarly to GH provocation described below.
- Prolactin levels are normally elevated in the third trimester and in breast-feeding mothers.
- GH levels are pulsatile and decline to minimal levels by age 30. Evaluation requires stimulation testing: Insulin or levodopa stimulate a burst in serum GH, serum levels are drawn at 30, 60, and 90 minutes post stimulus and compared to normal values.
- Thyroid-stimulating hormone (TSH) must be taken with serum triiodothyronine (T_3) and thyroxine (T_4); if they are normal or high, TSH is probably low due to feedback inhibition.
- In women, LH and FSH levels vary with the menstrual cycle, so the timing of the levels is important; postmenopausal women have high LH and FSH levels normally.
- ADH levels normally vary according to plasma osmolality; testing is discussed in Diabetes Insipidus section.
- Evaluation of target organ function is usually required: Tests include imaging studies, hormone levels, and response to exogenous pituitary hormones.

TREATMENT

- Address underlying cause: Tumor, infection, systemic disease.
- **Hormone replacement:**
  - Cortisol for ACTH deficiency.
  - Prolactin:
    - No treatment for deficiency.
    - Bromocriptine (dopamine agonist; dopamine suppresses prolactin production).
    - Surgery, or radiation for large tumors not responding to dopamine agonists.

- GH for GH deficiency in children.
- Thyroxine for TSH deficiency.
- FSH and LH deficiency can be treated with estrogen/progesterone replacements in women (fertility is usually not restored unless GNRH is given in a pulsatile fashion, via pump) and testosterone replacements in men.
- DDAVP for ADH deficiency.

ANTIDIURETIC HORMONE (ADH) DISORDERS

Diabetes Insipidus (DI)

- Central DI: Inadequate pituitary release of ADH.
- Nephrogenic DI: Lack of renal response to ADH.

Etiology

- **Central DI:**
  - Idiopathic: Accounts for 50% of cases.
  - Posterior pituitary or hypothalamic damage (tumor, trauma, neurosurgery).
  - Systemic: Sarcoidosis, neurosyphilis, encephalitis.
- **Nephrogenic DI:**
  - Familial.
  - Chronic renal disease.
  - Sickle cell anemia (renal papillary necrosis).
  - Hypokalemia.
  - Hypercalcemia.
  - Drugs: Lithium, demeclocycline, methoxyflurane.

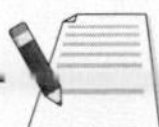

Psychogenic polydipsia: Psychiatric disorder of compulsive water drinking most common in young to middle-aged women. Presents with polyuria and dilute urine, distinguished from DI by *low* plasma osmolality.

Signs and Symptoms

- Polyuria (3–15 L/day).
- Thirst.
- Dilute urine (specific gravity < 1.005).

Diagnosis

- High plasma osmolality (280–310 mOsm/L) due to incomplete compensation for the inability to resorb free water.
- Water deprivation followed by exogenous ADH:
  - Central DI: Low urine Osm → high urine Osm
  - Nephrogenic DI: Low urine Osm → low urine Osm
  - Normal: High urine Osm → high urine Osm
- Infusion of hypertonic saline normally results in a sharp ↓ in urine output; patients with DI do not respond.

Treatment

- **Desmopressin (DDAVP)**: Analog of ADH, useful in **central DI.**
- **Thiazide diuretics**: Paradoxically ↓ urine output in patients with DI by increasing sodium and water resorption in the proximal tubule leading to ↓ water delivery to the ADH responsive sites in the collecting ducts. They are the only therapy useful in **nephrogenic DI.**

ENDOCRINOLOGY

- **Chlorpropamide**: Oral hypoglycemic with side effect of potentiating secretion and action of endogenous ADH. Partial function must exist for this therapy to be of use.

Syndrome of Inappropriate Antidiuretic Hormone Secretion (SIADH)

Excess production of ADH.

ETIOLOGY

- Idiopathic overproduction via the hypothalamic–posterior pituitary axis: Often associated with disorders of the central nervous system (encephalitis, stroke, head trauma) and pulmonary disease (TB, pneumonia).
- Ectopic production by malignant tumors, particularly small cell lung cancer and pancreatic carcinoma.
- Pharmacologic stimulation of the hypothalamic-pituitary axis: Carbamazepine, chlorpropamide, clofibrate, vincristine.

SIGNS AND SYMPTOMS

Attributable to hyponatremia—see chapter on fluid and electrolytes.

DIAGNOSIS

- Hyponatremia.
- Low serum osmolality.
- High urinary sodium.
- Osmolality of urine > serum.
- Normal adrenal and thyroid functions.

TREATMENT

- Fluid restriction.
- Hypertonic saline in severe hyponatremia.
- Demeclocycline: Due to causing nephrogenic DI, reserved for cases not responding to fluid restriction.
- Newer agents are direct vasopressin (V2) receptor antagonists: **the vaptans.**
  - IV conivaptan approved for use in volume overloaded hyponatremic states.
  - New oral agent **tolvaptan** recently received FDA approval for treatment of hyponatremia.

THYROID DISORDERS

Hyperthyroidism

Causes of large tongue (macroglossia):

- Acromegaly
- Myxedema
- Amyloidosis

Increased synthesis and secretion of free thyroid hormones resulting in hypermetabolism.

EPIDEMIOLOGY

- Ten times more common in women than in men.
- Annual incidence is 1 in 1000 women.

Etiology

- Graves' disease (most common cause, 80% of cases in the United States).
- Toxic multinodular goiter.
- Toxic adenoma (Plummer's disease).
- Iatrogenic (lithium therapy), inadvertent toxic ingestion, or factitious (thyrotoxicosis factitia).
- Transient hyperthyroidism (subacute thyroiditis).
- Ectopic thyroid hormone secretion (struma ovarii).

Pathophysiology

High levels of free thyroid hormones increase levels of cellular metabolism and cause multiple effects, resulting in a general state of hypermetabolism.

Signs and Symptoms

- Heat intolerance, sweating.
- Palpitations (hyperthyroidism is a common cause of atrial fibrillation).
- Weight loss.
- Tremor.
- Nervousness and anxiety.
- Weakness and fatigue.
- Diarrhea/hyperdefecation.

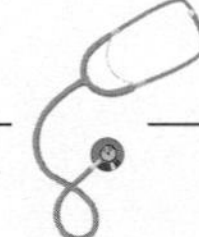

Serum TSH is the most sensitive test for thyroid dysfunction.

Diagnosis

Measure TSH, free T_4, and free T_3 (if the T_4 level is normal) (see Table 2.2-4).

TABLE 2.2-4. Laboratory Evaluation of Thyroid

Thyroid State	T_4	FT_4	T_3	FT_3	TSH	TRH
Hypothyroidism						
1°	↓	↓	↓	↓	↑	↑
2°	↓	↓	↓	↓	↓	N
3°	↓	↓	↓	↓	↓/N	↓
Peripheral unresponsiveness	↑/N	↑/N	↑/N	↑	↓/N	↑/N
Hyperthyroidism						
Pituitary tumor (secretes TSH)	↑	↑	↑	↑	↑	↓
Graves' disease	↑	↑	↑	↑	↓	↓
T_3 thyrotoxicosis	N	N	↑	↑	↓	↓
T_4 thyrotoxicosis	↑	↑	N	N	↓	↓
Toxic nodular goiter	↑	↑	↑	↑	↓	↓

ENDOCRINOLOGY

TREATMENT

Depends on underlying disorder (see below for specifics).

Thyroid Storm

- Exaggerated manifestation of hyperthyroidism with fever, CNS, CV, and GI dysfunction.
- Mortality is high (20–50%) even with the correct treatment.

ETIOLOGY

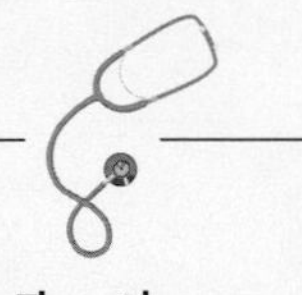

Thyroid storm and myxedema coma are life-threatening medical emergencies.

- Infection.
- Trauma and major surgical procedures.
- DKA.
- MI, cerebrovascular accident (CVA), pulmonary embolism (PE).
- Withdrawal of antihyperthyroid medications, iodine administration, thyroid hormone ingestion.
- Idiopathic.

SIGNS AND SYMPTOMS

Overactivated sympathetic nervous system causes most of the signs and symptoms of this syndrome:

- Fever > 101°F.
- Tachycardia (out of proportion to fever).
- High-output congestive heart failure (CHF) and volume depletion.
- Exhaustion.
- GI manifestations: Diarrhea, abdominal pain.
- Continuum of CNS alterations (from agitation to confusion when moderate, to stupor or coma with or without seizures when most severe).
- Jaundice is a late and ominous manifestation.

DIAGNOSIS

- This is a clinical diagnosis, and since most patients present in need of emergent stabilization, treatment is initiated empirically.
- Patients may have inadequately treated hyperthyroidism.
- May also occur in the setting of unintentional or intentional toxic ingestion of synthetic thyroid hormone in the hypothyroid patient.

TREATMENT

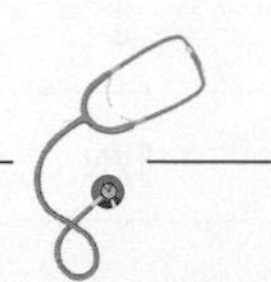

Never send any thyroid storm patient for a procedure involving iodine contrast before giving **propylthiouracil.**

- **Treat the manifestations.**
- **Primary stabilization:**
  - **Airway protection.**
  - Oxygenation.
  - Assess circulation (pulse/BP) and continuous cardiac monitoring.
  - IV hydration.
  - Beta-blocker therapy (eg, propranolol) to block adrenergic effects and block peripheral conversion of T_4 to T_3.
  - Treat fever with acetaminophen and cooling blanket (not aspirin, which displaces T_4 from thyroid binding protein).
- **Addressing the thyroid hormone itself:**
  - **Propylthiouracil** (PTU) or **methimazole** to block synthesis of new thyroid hormone.

- **Iodine** to decrease release of preformed thyroid hormone. Do not give iodine until the PTU has taken effect (1.5 hours) because more thyroid hormone will otherwise be produced using the iodine given.
- **Corticosteroids** also given to prevent peripheral conversion of T_4 to T_3 and to treat "relative" adrenal failure occurring due to high metabolic rate.
- Treat any possible precipitating factors that may be present (eg, MI, infection, etc.).

Graves' Disease

Autoimmune disease causing hyperthyroidism due to antibody which stimulates TSH receptor.

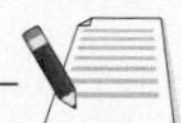

Graves' disease is the most common cause of hyperthyroidism.

PATHOPHYSIOLOGY

- Antibody is produced that interacts with the receptor for TSH resulting in continuous excess secretion.
- Cause of the exophthalmos (infiltrative opthalmopathy) in Graves' is unknown, but is thought to be due to immunoglobulins that interact with self-antigens in the extraocular muscles and on orbital fibroblasts.

Graves' (and Hashimoto's thyroiditis) are sometimes associated with other autoimmune diseases (type I diabetes mellitus, vitiligo, myasthenia, pernicious anemia, collagen diseases).

SIGNS AND SYMPTOMS

- Diffusely enlarged thyroid.
- Exophthalmos.
- Pretibial myxedema.
- Tachycardia, palpitations.
- In elderly patients the presentation is less classic. Apathy can be present without the common hyperactivity signs (apathetic hyperthyroidism). Cardiovascular features may be prominent and hyperthyroidism may not be suspected initially.

DIAGNOSIS

- High radioactive iodine uptake on a radionuclide scan. (If uptake is present but low, then diagnosis is thyroiditis or factitious hyperthyroidism.)
- Elevated free thyroid hormones (T_3, T_4).
- Undetectable TSH levels.
- High TSH receptor antibodies to confirm diagnosis and assess severity.

TREATMENT

- **Long-term antithyroid therapy:**
  - Usually accomplished with **propylthiouracil (PTU).**
  - Methimazole is as effective as PTU when administered at one-tenth of the PTU dosage.
  - PTU has the advantage of inhibiting the peripheral conversion of T_4 to T_3, thus there is usually a more rapid symptomatic improvement. However, euthyroid state is achieved more quickly with methimazole.
  - *Complications:* Leukopenia (check CBC before initiating therapy). Stop medication if absolute PMN drops below 1500 cells/μL. If patient develops fever or sore throat, he or she should be instructed to seek medical care.
  - **Methimazole is contraindicated in pregnancy—use PTU.**

ENDOCRINOLOGY

- **Radioactive iodine ablation therapy:**
  - Can produce the same effects as surgery without the surgical complications.
  - Commonly results in hypothyroidism over time.
  - **Complications:** Radiation thyroiditis commonly appears within 7–10 days after therapy and is associated with accelerated release of thyroid hormone into the blood. Rarely, this results in thyrotoxic crisis.
- **Beta blockers:**
  - Propranolol is the most commonly used. Atenolol could also be used in once a day dosage.
  - Should be used only as adjunctive therapy because it does not treat the underlying problem.
- **Subtotal thyroidectomy:**
  - Still used for younger patients or when ablation therapy is unsuccessful.
  - Delayed complications include hypoparathyroidism (can be life threatening) and hypothyroidism.

Hypothyroidism

- TSH levels greater than twice the upper limit of normal in primary hypothyroidism.
- Can be (1) clinically evident hypothyroidism with classic physical findings or (2) subclinical hypothyroidism detectable only upon laboratory analysis.

Epidemiology

- Clinically evident hypothyroidism occurs in 2% of women and in 0.2% of men.
- The incidence increases with age, usually between 40 and 60.

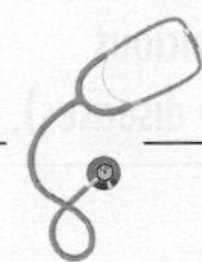

Hashimoto's thyroiditis (chronic lymphocytic thyroiditis) is the most common cause of hypothyroidism in North America.

Etiology

- **Primary hypothyroidism** (thyroid gland dysfunction):
  - Hashimoto's thyroiditis.
  - Previous treatment for hyperthyroidism.
  - Painless thyroiditis.
  - Radiation therapy to the neck (for other malignancy).
  - Iodine deficiency or excess.
  - Medications (lithium is the most common).
  - Prolonged treatment with iodine-containing substances.
- **Secondary hypothyroidism** (pituitary dysfunction):
  - Postpartum necrosis (Sheehan's syndrome).
  - Space-occupying pituitary neoplasm.
  - Infiltrating disease (TB) causing TSH deficiency.
- **Tertiary hypothyroidism** (deficiency in TRH secretion; hypothalamic dysfunction):
  - Granuloma.
  - Neoplasm.
  - Hypothalamic radiation.

Muscle weakness and cramps occur in both hyper- and hypothyroidism. In hyperthyroidism, CPK will be normal. In hypothyroidism, it will be elevated.

Signs and Symptoms

- Fatigue, lethargy, weakness.
- Constipation, weight gain (usually > 15 pounds).

ENDOCRINOLOGY

- Muscle weakness, cramps, arthralgias.
- Cold intolerance.
- Slow speech with hoarse voice (from myxedematous changes in vocal cords).
- Slow thinking with poor memory.
- Skin: Dry, coarse, thick, and cool; nonpitting edema of the skin and eyelids.
- Hair: Brittle and coarse; loss of outer one-third of eyebrows.
- Thyroid gland: May or may not be palpable (depending on the etiology of the hypothyroidism).
- Heart: Distant heart sounds may be present if pericardial effusion is present. Bradycardia may occur.
- Neurologic: **Delayed relaxation phase of deep tendon reflexes** (very specific). Cerebellar ataxia can be present. Peripheral neuropathies with paresthesias; carpal tunnel syndrome.
- Musculoskeletal: Muscular stiffness and weakness.

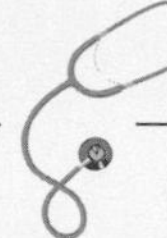

Consider evaluating thyroid function tests in any patient with hypercholesterolemia.

DIAGNOSIS

- See Table 2.2-4 for results of thyroid tests.
- Also, **in Hashimoto's thyroiditis:** May show **increased antithyroglobulin and antimicrosomal antibody titers.**
- The TRH stimulation test is useful in distinguishing secondary from tertiary hypothyroidism.

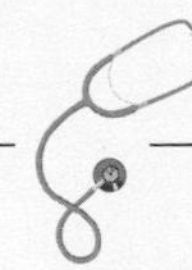

Thyroid peroxidase autoantibodies (TPO Ab) are indicative of autoimmune thyroid disease and have predictive value for progression to overt hypothyroidism or development of drug-induced thyroid dysfunction.

TREATMENT

- Start therapy with low-dose levothyroxine and increase dose every 6–8 weeks, depending on the patient's response (*start low, go slow*).
- Elderly patients and patients with coronary artery disease should be started on a low dose of levothyroxine because high doses may precipitate angina pectoris.
- **Monitoring therapy:**
  - In 1° hypothyroidism, it is adequate to measure the TSH level, which should fall well within the normal range.
  - In 2° hypothyroidism, measure the T_4 level, which should fall well within the normal range.

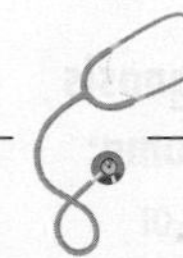

Hypothermia **is often missed by tympanic thermometers. Use a rectal probe if hypothermia is suspected.**

Subclinical Hypothyroidism

Elevated TSH level with normal thyroid hormone levels in the absence of overt clinical symptoms.

CLINICAL COURSE

This is not usually a precursor to 1° hypothyroidism. There are usually two distinct patterns:

- Patients who will eventually develop 1° hypothyroidism: Patients with both elevated TSH and detectable antithyroid antibodies often progress to clinically evident hypothyroidism.
- Euthyroidism with reset thyrostat: Permanent state without definitive progression to 1° hypothyroidism. Probably due to subtle damage to the thyroid gland from another cause.

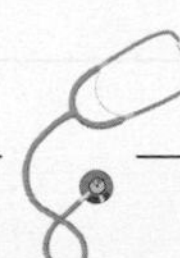

Infection is a common precipitant of myxedema coma; pan-culture and empiric antibiotic therapy with broad-spectrum antibiotics is recommended for all affected patients.

TREATMENT

Thyroid replacement therapy is necessary only in the following circumstances:

- All patients with TSH > 10.
- Patients with TSH > 5 and goiter or antithyroid antibody.

Myxedema Coma

Life-threatening complication of hypothyroidism with profound lethargy or coma usually accompanied by hypothermia. Mortality is 20–50% even if treated early.

ETIOLOGY (PRECIPITATING FACTORS)

- Sepsis.
- Prolonged exposure to cold weather.
- CNS depressants (sedatives, narcotics).
- Trauma or surgery.

SIGNS AND SYMPTOMS

- Profound lethargy or coma is obvious.
- Hypothermia: Rectal T < 35°C (95°F).
- Bradycardia or circulatory collapse.
- Hypoventilation with respiratory acidosis.
- Delayed relaxation phase of deep tendon reflexes, areflexia if severe (this is important clue).

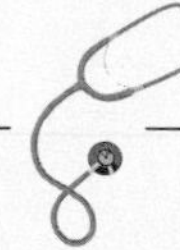

Differential diagnosis of myxedema coma:
Severe depression or primary psychosis
Drug overdose or toxic exposure
CVA
Liver failure
Hypoglycemia
CO_2 narcosis
CNS infection

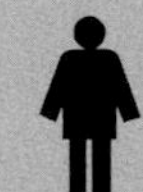

A 75-year-old female presents with progressive obtundation and nonarousal. Core temperature is 35°C; cold, doughy skin; delayed deep tendon reflex relaxation phase. Urine analysis with many leukocytes and gram-negative rods. *Think: Myxedema coma.*

DIAGNOSIS

Lab tests for the patient presenting with signs and symptoms of myxedema coma (in descending order):

- TSH, T_3, T_4, free thyroxine (FT_4).
- Cortisol level.
- Complete blood count (CBC) with differential.
- Serum electrolytes.
- Blood urea nitrogen (BUN) and creatinine.
- Blood glucose.
- Blood and urine cultures.
- Urine toxicology screen.
- Serum transaminases and lactic dehydrogenase (LDH), creatine phosphokinase (CPK).
- Arterial blood gas (ABG) to rule out hypoxemia and CO_2 retention.
- Carboxyhemoglobin.
- Chest radiograph.
- Brain CT.

ENDOCRINOLOGY

TREATMENT

- Airway management with mechanical ventilation if necessary (ABCs, etc).
- Pharmacologic therapy:
  - Intravenous levothyroxine.
  - Glucocorticoids (until coexisting adrenal insufficiency is excluded).
- Prevent further heat loss.
- Monitor patient in intensive care unit.
- IV hydration (D_5 ½ NS).
- Rule out and treat any precipitating causes (antibiotics for suspected infection).

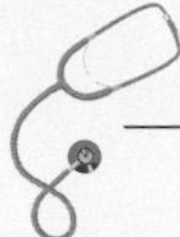

Corticosteroids are given empirically in myxedema coma before T_4 is given due to concern that associated Addison's disease exists. Giving only T_4 could precipitate an addisonian crisis.

Thyroiditis

- Inflammation of the thyroid.
- Can be divided into three common types (Hashimoto's, subacute, and silent) and two rarer forms (suppurative and Riedel's).

A patient who comes in with fever, anxiety, and a painful neck should be worked up for thyroiditis (pain!). Thyroid function tests will show decreased TSH with increased T_4 but decreased uptake on iodine scan. **Next step?** *Prescribe an NSAID or steroid.*

ETIOLOGY

- **Hashimoto's thyroiditis:** Autoimmune disorder that involves CD4 lymphocyte-mediated destruction of the thyroid. The lymphocytes are specific for thyroid antigens. Cause for activation of these cells is unknown.
- **Subacute thyroiditis:** Possibly a postviral condition because it usually follows a viral upper respiratory infection (URI). Not considered an autoimmune reaction.
- **Silent thyroiditis:** Usually occurs **postpartum** and is thought to be autoimmune mediated.
- **Suppurative thyroiditis:** Usually a bacterial infection, but fungi and parasites have also been implicated in some cases. Commonly seen in HIV-positive patients with *Pneumocystis jiroveci* pneumonia (PCP).
- **Riedel's thyroiditis:** Fibrous infiltration of the thyroid of unknown etiology; also called fibrous thyroiditis.

Workup of someone with recent onset of hyperthyroid symptoms (anxiety, heat intolerance) and a painful neck shows: decreased TSH and increased free T_4 and decreased uptake on iodine scan. *Next step: NSAID/ steroid (this is thyroiditis).*

SIGNS AND SYMPTOMS

- **Hashimoto's:** There may be signs of hyper- or hypothyroidism depending on the stage. Usually, there is diffuse, firm enlargement of the gland, but it may be of normal size if the disease has progressed.
- **Subacute:** Tender, enlarged gland, severe neck pain, often mistaken for pharyngitis. Fever and signs of hyperthyroidism are initially present. Hypothyroidism may develop. Very high erythrocyte sedimentation rate (ESR).
- **Silent:** Similar to subacute except there is no tenderness of the gland (painless thyroiditis).
- **Suppurative:** Fever with severe neck pain. Focal tenderness of involved portion of the gland.
- **Riedel's:** Slowly enlarging rock-hard mass in the anterior neck. Tight, stiff neck. Must differentiate from thyroid cancer. Hypothyroidism may occur if advanced. Fibrosis may involve mediastinum.

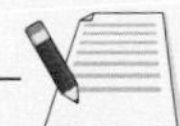

The thyroid in Hashimoto's is nontender, which distinguishes it from other forms of thyroiditis.

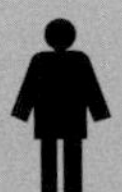

A 35-year-old female with a history of hyperthyroidism and a recent flu presents with neck pain and an elevated ESR. *Think: Subacute thyroiditis.* **Next step:** Check thyroid function tests.

Diagnosis

- **History:**
  - Presentation following viral URI is suggestive of subacute thyroiditis.
  - Presentation after penetrating injury to the neck is suggestive of suppurative processes.
  - Postpartum presentation is suggestive of silent thyroiditis.
- **Laboratory examination:**
  - TSH and FT_4 may be normal or indicative of hypo- or hyperthyroidism.
  - White blood count (WBC) with differential should be obtained to look for leukocytosis and left shift (subacute and suppurative).
  - Antimicrosomal antibodies are present in > 90% with Hashimoto's and 50–80% with silent thyroiditis.
  - Serum thyroglobulin levels are elevated in subacute and silent thyroiditis (test is very nonspecific).
- **Imaging studies:** Radioactive iodine uptake (RAIU) can be useful to distinguish Graves' disease (increased RAIU) from subacute thyroiditis (decreased RAIU), in a hypothyroid patient.

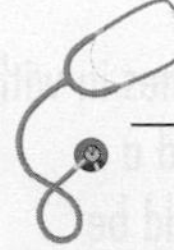

Differential diagnosis of thyroiditis:
The hyperthyroid stage of Hashimoto's, subacute, or silent thyroiditis, may mimic Graves' disease.
Riedel's must be differentiated from thyroid cancer.
Subacute thyroiditis can be mistaken for oropharyngeal, tracheal infections, or for suppurative thyroiditis.

Treatment

- Treat hypothyroidism, if present, with levothyroxine for 6–8 weeks. Reevaluate the TSH level, particularly in postpartum thyroiditis that might be manifested as depression.
- Control symptoms of hyperthyroidism, if present, with propranolol.
  - Pain management in patients with subacute thyroiditis should be accomplished with nonsteroidal anti-inflamatory drugs (NSAIDs). If ineffective, begin a tapering course of steroids.
- IV antibiotics and abscess drainage, if present, should be performed in suppurative thyroiditis.
  - **Do not** give PTU or methimazole in thyroiditis—the mechanism is release of preformed hormone from inflamed gland, *not* overproduction of hormone by the gland.

Prognosis

- **Hashimoto's:** Most patients do not completely recover their total thyroid function.
- **Subacute:** Hypothyroidism persists in 10%.
- **Silent:** Hypothyroidism persists in 6%.
- **Suppurative:** Full recovery is common.
- **Riedel's thyroiditis:** Hypothyroidism occurs when the entire gland undergoes fibrosis.

Evaluation of a Thyroid Nodule

Epidemiology

- Common (1% of men and 5% of women).
- Incidence ↑ after age 45.
- History of neck irradiation (increased CA risk).
- Family history of pheochromocytoma, thyroid CA, or hyperparathyroidism (MEN II) increases suspicious for cancer.

Signs and Symptoms

- Dysphagia, hoarseness (indicative of malignant infiltration).
- Physical exam: Likelihood of malignancy increases with nodule > 2 cm, regional lymphadenopathy, fixation to tissues, age < 40, male sex, family history of thyroid cancer, history of head and neck irradiation.

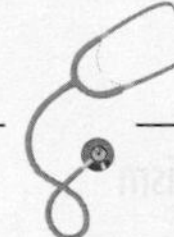

If thyroidectomy is planned, obtain a thyroglobulin level after surgery. A return to normal following thyroidectomy suggests the absence of metastatic thyroid tissue.

Diagnosis (see Figure 2.2-1)

- Fine-needle aspiration is the best initial study. Accuracy can be > 90%.
- Thyroid ultrasound is performed to evaluate the size and number of thyroid nodules. It also evaluates whether the nodules are cystic or solid.
- Thyroid scan with technetium 99m–labeled iodine (RAIU) classifies nodules as hyperfunctioning (hot nodules, less likely to be malignant) or hypofunctioning (cold nodules, more likely to be malignant).

Thyroid Cancer

Epidemiology

- Incidence ~ 9/100,000.
- 2:1 female predominance.
- Increases with age and plateaus after age 50.
- Worse prognosis if < 20 years old or > 65 years old.

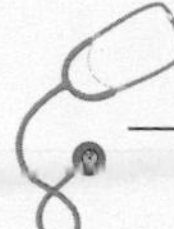

Measurement of serum thyroglobulin is useful for following thyroid cancers in response to treatment, but a serum thyroglobulin level is not useful in distinguishing benign from malignant nodules.

Risk Factors

- History of childhood head or neck irradiation.
- Large nodule (> 4 cm).
- Enlarging neck mass.
- Family history.

Classification

Two types—follicular (epithelial) and parafollicular:

- **Epithelial** (three histologic types):
  - Papillary: Most common, has best prognosis.
  - Follicular: Early metastasis.
  - Anaplastic: Rare, worst prognosis.

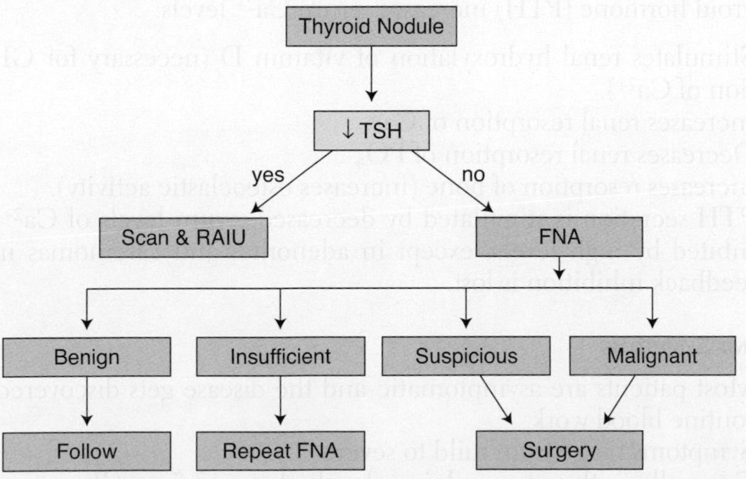

FIGURE 2.2-1. Initial approach to the thyroid nodule.

Causes of hypercalcemia:
Hyperparathyroidism
Bone metastases
Sarcoidosis
Hyperthyroidism
Thiazide diuretics
Immobilization
Paget's disease (only if patient is immobilized)

A patient who is post thyroid surgery has symptoms of muscle aches, weakness, and perioral parasthesias. *Think: Hypocalcemia from hypoparathyroid* (either damaged by clamping off thyroid vessels or accidentally excised).

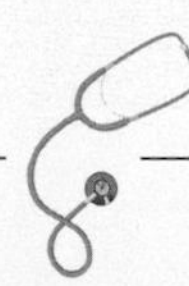

Before you send a patient with 1° hyperparathyroidism to surgery, make sure you are not dealing with familial benign hypocalciuric hypercalcemia (FBHH). Urine calcium is usually < 50 mg/24 hr. It is autosomal dominant with 100% penetrance and is benign. No treatment, only reassurance, of patient and family members. Family history of kidney stones may be a tip-off.

- **Parafollicular** (also called medullary thyroid cancer):
  - Calcitonin is increased from parafollicular C-cells.
  - Seen in MEN IIa and IIb.

TREATMENT

- Thyroidectomy.
- Radioiodine ablation of residual cancer and micrometastasis.
- Oral T_4 suppressive therapy after surgery, to suppress TSH that is thought to promote thyroid growth.
- Careful monitoring of TSH and thyroglobulin levels (a rise indicates recurrence of the cancer).

PARATHYROID DISORDERS

Hyperparathyroidism

- **Primary:** Hypersecretion of parathyroid hormone (PTH) by the parathyroid glands (*the rest of the section refers to 1° only*).
- **Secondary:** Glandular hyperplasia and elevated PTH in an appropriate response to hypocalcemia (due to renal failure, GI disturbances, etc.).
- **Tertiary:** Continued elevation of PTH after the disturbance causing 2° hyperparathyroidism has been corrected.

EPIDEMIOLOGY

- Most common in middle-aged and elderly women.
- Common: Present in 0.1% of the population.

ETIOLOGY

- Parathyroid adenoma: 85%, 1 gland involved.
- Parathyroid hyperplasia: 14%, all four glands involved.
- Parathyroid carcinoma: 1%, 1 gland involved.
- Associated with MEN I and IIa (10% of cases).
- Neck irradiation increases risk.

PATHOPHYSIOLOGY

Parathyroid hormone (PTH) increases serum Ca^{2+} levels:

- Stimulates renal hydroxylation of vitamin D (necessary for GI absorption of Ca^{2+}).
- Increases renal resorption of Ca^{2+}.
- Decreases renal resorption of PO_4^-.
- Increases resorption of bone (increases osteoclastic activity).
- PTH secretion is stimulated by decreased serum levels of Ca^{2+} and inhibited by high levels, except in adenomas and carcinomas in which feedback inhibition is lost.

SIGNS AND SYMPTOMS

- Most patients are asymptomatic and the disease gets discovered during routine blood work.
- Symptoms range from mild to severe.
- Generally, with **serum calcium** levels above 13.5 mg/dL, patients experience fatigue, polyuria, weakness, nausea, vomiting, abdominal pain,

and changes in mental status from confusion to lethargy to obtundation and coma.

- Milder elevations in calcium can result in mild neurocognitive impairment.

DIAGNOSIS

- Elevated serum Ca^{2+}, low serum PO_4^-.
- High serum PTH.

TREATMENT

- Older asymptomatic patients with serum $Ca^{2+} < 12$ should just be followed for progression.
- **Surgery:**
  - Adenomas should be excised.
  - In hyperplasia, all four glands are removed and a small portion is reinserted in an easily accessible place such as the forearm, so that it can function, but if hyperplasia recurs, subsequent surgical intervention is simplified.
- **Emergency measures:**
  - Hydration with normal saline (salt leads to increased urinary calcium excretion), followed by furosemide diuresis.
  - Bisphosphonates to block bone resorption (IV pamidronate).
  - Calcitonin acts rapidly but loses its efficacy after several days.

Hypoparathyroidism

Condition characterized by PTH deficiency.

ETIOLOGY

- Idiopathic.
- DiGeorge syndrome: Congenital aplasia or hypoplasia of thymus caused by missing gene on chromosome 22. Findings include hypoparathyroidism (parathyroid hypoplasia, heart defects, and deficiency of T cells and cell-mediated immunity (CMI).
- Postsurgical (ie, thyroidectomy).
- Infiltrative carcinoma.
- Irradiation.
- Hypomagnesemia (magnesium is necessary for parathyroid gland to secrete PTH).

EPIDEMIOLOGY

Equal incidence in men and women.

> A 30-year-old woman presents with perioral paresthesias and a long QT interval on electrocardiogram (ECG). She recently had surgery for a thyroid goiter. *Think: Hypoparathyroidism* (due to neck surgery with probable accidental resection of the parathyroids). **Next step:** Check serum calcium, PTH, and vitamin D levels.

Vitamin D acts on the intestines to increase absorption of calcium and phosphate. It is formed in the skin via sunlight as a previtamin and is converted to an inactive intermediate (25-OH vitamin D) in the liver before being converted to its active form 1,25-$(OH)_2$ vitamin D (calcitriol) in the kidney.

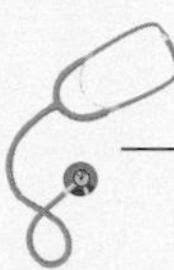

Pseudohypoparathyroidism presents the same as hypoparathyroidism, except that the pathophysiology in pseudohypoparathyroidism is tissue resistance to PTH, so that PTH is high (distinguishing feature). Pseudohypoparathyroidism is associated with Albright's hereditary osteodystrophy (round facies, short stature, short fourth metacarpal bone, and subcutaneous calcification).

Addisonian or adrenal crisis is an acute complication of adrenal insufficiency characterized by shock, dehydration, confusion, vomiting, hyponatremia, hyperkalemia, and hypoglycemia. It is precipitated by sepsis, hemorrhage, trauma, and other stressors.

SIGNS AND SYMPTOMS

Signs and symptoms of hypocalcemia (see also chapter on nephrology and acid-base disorders):

- Seizures.
- Perioral paresthesia.
- Fasciculations, tetany, and muscle weakness.
- CNS irritability, confusion and seizure.
- Chvostek's and Trousseau's signs.
- Bronchospasm.
- Anxiety, psychosis.

DIAGNOSIS

- Low serum calcium.
- High serum phosphorus.
- Normal or low PTH.
- Normal 25-OH vitamin D.
- Low 1,25-$(OH)_2$ vitamin D.
- QT prolongation on ECG.

TREATMENT

- Treat severe, life-threatening hypocalcemia with intravenous calcium.
- Maintenance therapy with calcitriol and oral calcium supplementation.

ADRENAL DISORDERS

Adrenal Insufficiency

- Primary insufficiency (Addison's disease) is due to a problem with the adrenal gland itself, in which it does not produce hormones.
- In secondary insufficiency, the adrenal gland is intact, but the pituitary does not produce ACTH, so that there is no stimulus for the adrenal gland to secrete its hormones.
- Tertiary insufficiency is due to hypothalamic failure.

EPIDEMIOLOGY

More common in women (2:1), in its autoimmune form.

ETIOLOGY

- **Primary insufficiency (Addison's disease):**
  - Autoimmune (80%).
  - Tuberculosis (15%).
  - Neoplastic disease.
  - Sarcoidosis.
  - Amyloidosis.
  - Blastomycosis.
  - Hemochromatosis.
  - AIDS.
  - Adrenal hemorrhage due to trauma, anticoagulants, or coagulopathies.
  - Waterhouse-Friederichsen syndrome (fulminant septicemia).
  - Adrenalectomy.
- **Secondary insufficiency:**
  - Suppression of hypothalamic-pituitary-adrenal axis by exogenous steroids (most common).

- Sheehan's syndrome (postpartum pituitary necrosis).
- Pituitary infarct/tumor.
- Autoimmune destruction of pituitary.

ANATOMY

- The adrenal cortex consists of three zones (GFR):
  - Outer—**zona glomerulosa:** Produces aldosterone (mineralocorticoids).
  - Middle—**zona fasciculata:** Produces cortisol (glucocorticoids).
  - Inner—**zona reticularis:** Produces androgens and estrogens (sex hormones).
- The adrenal medulla produces catecholamines.

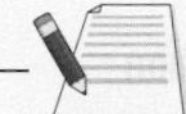

Primary adrenal insufficiency results in increased levels of ACTH. Melanocyte-stimulating hormone (MSH) and ACTH are cleaved from the same propeptide, so elevated ACTH results in increased skin pigmentation.

PATHOPHYSIOLOGY

- **Aldosterone:**
  - Produced when angiotensin II (stimulated by renin secretion from the kidney), acts on the zona glomerulosa to convert corticosterone to aldosterone.
  - Principal function is to increase renal sodium reabsorption in the distal tubule and collecting ducts, causing secretion of potassium and hydrogen ions.
  - Deficiency results in hyperkalemia and hyponatremia.
- **Cortisol:**
  - Stimulates gluconeogenesis by increasing protein and fat catabolism and decreasing utilization of glucose and tissue sensitivity to insulin.
  - Promotes anti-inflammatory state via inhibition of arachidonic acid, inhibition of interleukin-2 production, and inhibiting release of histamine from mast cells.
  - Has widespread effects on carbohydrate and protein metabolism.
  - Acts to counteract the effects of insulin and maintain blood glucose levels.
  - Governs body water distribution.
  - Enhances the pressor effects of catecholamine on heart muscle and blood vessels.
  - Inhibits inflammatory and allergic reactions.
  - Deficiency results in impairment of body's ability to handle stress.

SIGNS AND SYMPTOMS

- Hyperpigmentation of mucosa, areolae, hand creases, knees, elbows, and knuckles (1° only).
- Salt craving (1° only).
- Orthostatic hypotension.
- Weakness.
- Anorexia.
- Weight loss.
- Abdominal pain.

> An 18-year-old man with hemophilia A who was recently mugged (receiving multiple blows to the back and abdomen) is now complaining of dizziness, abdominal pain, dark patches on his elbows and knees, and uncontrollable cravings for pizza and French fries. *Think: 1° adrenal insufficiency.* **Next step:** ACTH stimulation test.

ENDOCRINOLOGY

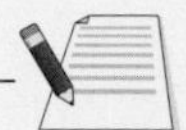

Secondary adrenal insufficiency can be distinguished from Addison's disease by:

- Absence of hyperpigmentation
- Normal aldosterone secretion
- Other signs of hypopituitarism such as hypothyroidism and hypogonadism suggest presence of pituitary lesion or tumor

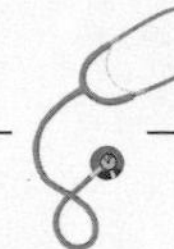

The most common source of glucocorticoid excess is exogenous corticosteroid therapy.

Diagnosis

- ACTH (Cortrosyn) test:
  - Give test dose of ACTH and measure serum cortisol levels at 0, 30, and 60 minutes. A peak level < 18–20 μg/dL suggests adrenal insufficiency.
  - Measuring the plasma ACTH after test will tell you whether it is primary adrenal insufficiency (high ACTH) or secondary adrenal insufficiency (low or normal ACTH).
- Hyperkalemia, hyponatremia, extracellular fluid (ECF) volume contraction and metabolic acidosis due to aldosterone deficiency (1° only).
- Hypoglycemia (more common in 2° adrenal failure due to GH deficiency as well).
- Anemia.
- Elevated BUN and creatinine.
- Elevated ACTH, low serum cortisol.

Treatment

- Glucocorticoid replacement for all patients.
- Instruct patients to increase their glucocorticoid dose in times of stress and infection.
- Patients with Addison's disease should also receive mineralocorticoid replacement therapy.

Adrenal Excess: Cushing's Syndrome

- **Cushing's syndrome:** Symptoms caused by excess cortisol production.
- **Cushing's disease:** Cushing's syndrome caused by excess ACTH secretion by pituitary.

Addison's Disease	Cushing's Disease
Cortisol deficiency	Cortisol excess
Patient is thin	Patient is obese
Hyponatremia	Hypernatremia
Hyperkalemia	Hypokalemia
Metabolic acidosis	Metabolic alkalosis
Hypotension	Hypertension
Hypoglycemia	Hyperglycemia (or diabetes)
Lymphocytosis	Lymphopenia
Eosinophilia	No eosinophilia

Epidemiology

More common in females.

ETIOLOGY

- Exogenous corticosteroid therapy.
- Pituitary tumors (Cushing's disease).
- Adrenal adenomas.
- Ectopic ACTH production (such as small cell lung carcinoma, pheochromocytoma, medullary thyroid carcinoma, and carcinoids).

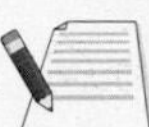

Small cell lung carcinoma is frequently associated with ectopic ACTH production.

SIGNS AND SYMPTOMS

- Hypertension.
- Facial plethora.
- Hair loss.
- Central obesity (apple-shaped habitus, moon facies, thin extremities).
- Hump on back of neck (Buffalo's hump).
- Fragile, easily bruised skin.
- Abdominal purplish striae.
- Proximal muscle weakness.
- Hirsutism.
- Emotional lability.
- Osteoporosis.

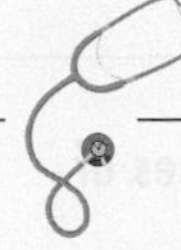

Patients with ectopic ACTH production often do not have all the mentioned symptoms; they usually have only hypertension and muscle weakness due to hypokalemia.

DIAGNOSIS

Twenty-four-hour urinary free cortisol is a reliable test for screening and should be done twice and be three times higher than the upper limit of normal for confirmation.

- **Overnight dexamethasone suppression test:**
  - Dexamethasone 1 mg is given at midnight, plasma cortisol measured at 8 AM.
  - If < 2 μg/100 mL, excludes Cushing's as a diagnosis.
- **High-dose dexamethasone suppression test:**
  - Give 8 mg dexamethasone at midnight, then measure serum cortisol and at 8 AM.
  - If ACTH is undetectable or decreased and there is no cortisol suppression, likely adrenal etiology.
  - If ACTH is normal or increased and there is no cortisol suppression, likely ectopic ACTH etiology.
  - If ACTH is high with partial cortisol suppression, likely pituitary etiology (Cushing's syndrome) where the pituitary is only relatively resistant to negative feedback.
- **Other findings:**
  - Increased 24-hour urinary free cortisol (> 100 μg/24 hr).
  - Hypokalemia, hypochloremia, metabolic alkalosis.
  - Hyperglycemia, hypercholesterolemia.
  - CT of adrenals to look for mass.
  - MRI of pituitary to look for mass.
  - Malignancy workup if ectopic ACTH production is suspected.
  - In equivocal cases, petrosal venous sampling will be needed to demonstrate pituitary ACTH hypersecretion.

Screening tests for Cushing's syndrome in clinically suspect patients include the 24-hour urine free cortisol test and the overnight dexamethasone-suppression test.

Cushing's disease can be distinguished from Cushing's syndrome by the presence of hyperpigmentation (only in Cushing's disease).

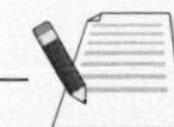

The most sensitive screening test for primary aldosteronism is the plasma aldosterone-plasma renin activity ratio.

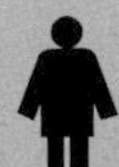

A 42-year-old woman on long-term steroids for asthma has excess adipose tissue in her neck and upper trunk, a wide "moon face," and very fine hair. *Think: Cushing's syndrome* (due to exogenous steroids).

ENDOCRINOLOGY

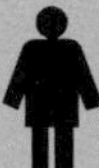

A 44-year-old woman has hypertension, muscle cramps, and excessive thirst. *Think: Hyperaldosteronism.*

Secondary causes of hypertension:
Renovascular hypertension
Primary aldosteronism
Pheochromocytoma
Cushing's syndrome
Renal disease
Acromegaly

TREATMENT

- **Pituitary adenomas** (see Figure 2.2-2):
  - Transsphenoidal surgery.
  - Pituitary irradiation for children and cases refractory to surgery.
- **Adrenal adenoma:** Unilateral resection, followed by 3–12 months of glucocorticoid replacement (normal adrenal needs time to come out of suppression).
- **Bilateral adrenal hyperplasia:** Bilateral resection with lifelong replacement of glucocorticoids and mineralocorticoids.
- **Ectopic ACTH production:**
  - Treat underlying disease.
  - Remove source of neoplasm if possible.

Hyperaldosteronism

- Isolated excess production of aldosterone.
- Also called Conn's syndrome.

EPIDEMIOLOGY

- One to two percent of all patients with hypertension.
- Most frequent in ages 30–60.
- Adrenal tumor more common in women.

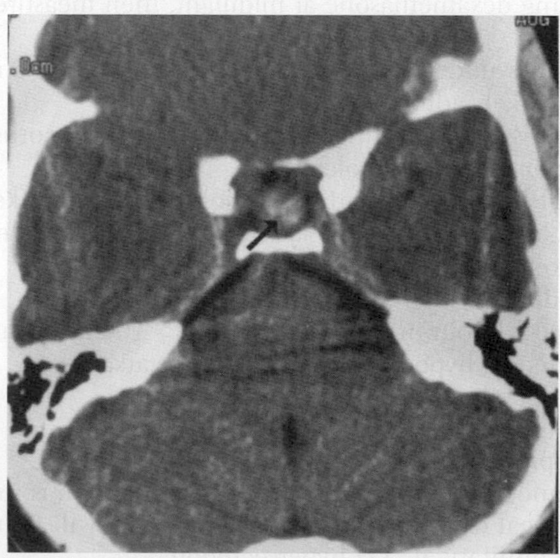

FIGURE 2.2-2. Pituitary adenoma (arrow).

(Reproduced, with permission, from Lee SH, Rao K, Zimmerman RA. *Cranial MRI and CT*, 4th ed. New York: McGraw-Hill, 1999: 653.)

A young man is evaluated with persistent hypertension. He was diagnosed at a routine examination. His blood pressure has remained high despite diet, weight loss, and compliance with therapy, which includes four BP medications. *Think: Secondary hypertension.*

ETIOLOGY

- Unilateral aldosterone producing adenoma (most common cause).
- Bilateral hyperplasia of zona glomerulosa (idiopathic).

SIGNS AND SYMPTOMS

- Usually asymptomatic.
- Hypertension.
- May see signs of hypokalemia (muscle cramps, palpitations).

DIAGNOSIS

- Measure plasma aldosterone to plasma renin activity ratio; a ratio > 20 suggests hyperaldosteronism.
- Other findings:
  - Hypokalemia, hypernatremia, and metabolic alkalosis.
  - High serum aldosterone, low renin levels.
  - Twenty-four-hour urine high in potassium and aldosterone.
  - Evidence of adrenal mass on abdominal CT.
  - Aldosterone escape: After initial edema and weight gain, patients usually diurese and shed the edema.

TREATMENT

- Adrenalectomy for tumor.
- Medical management for hyperplasia:
  - Spironolactone (potassium sparing) or ACE inhibitors to control blood pressure.
  - Low-sodium diet.
  - Maintenance of ideal body weight, regular exercise, smoking cessation.

Pheochromocytoma–

Rule of 10s

10% are extra-adrenal
10% are bilateral
10% are malignant
10% are familial
10% are pediatric
10% calcify
10% recur after resection

Multiple endocrine neoplasia type I: (3Ps)

Pituitary tumors
Pancreatic islet tumors
Hyperparathyroidism due to Parathyroid hyperplasia

Pheochromocytoma

Tumor of the adrenal medulla resulting in catecholamine excess.

EPIDEMIOLOGY

Equal incidence in men and women. Tumors in women are three times as likely to be malignant.

ETIOLOGY

- MEN types IIa and IIb.
  - MEN IIa: Pheochromocytoma, parathyroid hyperplasia, and medullary thyroid cancer.
  - MEN IIb: Pheochromocytoma, medullary thyroid CA, and mucosal neuromas.

5H's

Headache
Hypertension
Hot (diaphoretic)
Heart (palpitations)
Hyperhidrosis

- Neurofibromatosis.
- Von Hippel–Lindau disease: Pheochromocytoma, retinal angiomas, CNS hemangioblastomas, renal cell carcinoma, pancreatic pseudocysts, ependymal cystadenoma.

SIGNS AND SYMPTOMS

- Patients experience "paroxysmal attacks" of high blood pressure.
- Physical exam usually normal outside of an attack.
- Symptoms of catecholamine (sympathetic) excess will predominate during an attack.
- Tremor.
- Anxiety.
- Weight loss.

A 38-year-old woman on labetalol presents with poorly controlled hypertension, frequent headaches, and palpitations. *Think: Pheochomocytoma.* **Next step:** Stop labetalol and check urine catecholamines and serum metanephrines.

The classic triad of symptoms for pheochromocytoma consists of hypertension with the triad of headaches, palpitations, and diaphoresis.

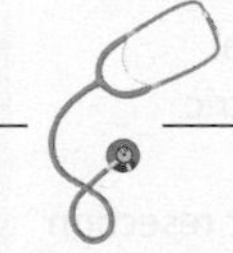

Patients with pheochromocytoma may carry an incorrect diagnosis of anxiety disorder.

DIAGNOSIS

- Elevated 24-hour urine catecholamines and metanephrines.
- Fractionated plasma free metanephrines.
- CT or MRI to look for adrenal mass, if negative with clinical impression and biochemical tests being positive, obtain MIBG scan. MIBG is a compound that resembles metanephrine and is taken up by phochromocytoma tissue.

TREATMENT

- Surgical resection.
- Alpha-adrenergic blockade (may also add beta blocker).

BONE DISORDERS

Osteomalacia

- Disease of impaired bone mineralization.
- Termed *rickets* in the pediatric population.

Urinary excretion of metanephrine, normetanephrine, and catecholamines may be used to confirm the presence of excess catecholamine production.

ETIOLOGY

- Decreased Ca^{2+} absorption.
- Dietary calcium deficiency: Rare, avoidance of dairy products.
- GI disorders: Malabsorption syndromes, gastrectomy, dumping syndrome.
- Vitamin D deficiency.
- Hepatobiliary and pancreatic disease: Loss of bile acids or pancreatic lipase reduce absorption of fat-soluble vitamins.
- Extremely low-fat diets.

- Renal osteodystrophy: Decreased renal hydroxylation of vitamin D.
- Decreased serum PO_4^-.
- Renal tubular acidosis, Fanconi's syndrome, hypophosphatasia.

SIGNS AND SYMPTOMS

- Bone pain.
- Weakness.
- Difficulty walking: Broad-based waddling gait with short strides.
- Thoracic kyphosis.

DIAGNOSIS

- **Radiographs:**
  - Show diffuse, nonspecific osteopenia.
  - Vertebrae may be biconcave from compression by intervertebral disks.
  - Pseudofractures (radiolucent lines perpendicular to bone cortex).
- **Labs:**
  - Ca^{2+} and PO_4^- low to normal.
  - High alkaline phosphatase.
  - PTH may be elevated in response to low Ca^{2+}.

TREATMENT

- Address underlying disorder.
- Calcium, vitamin D supplements.

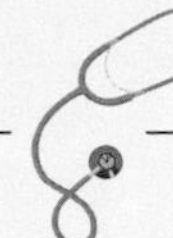

Prior to surgery for tumor resection, patient must be properly alpha blocked with phenoxybenzamine or other alpha blockers to prevent intraoperative hypertensive crisis. Also, prior to starting beta-blocker therapy, alpha blockers must be on board to prevent unopposed alpha receptor stimulation.

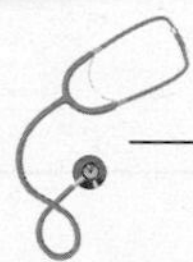

Abnormalities of vitamin D synthesis and metabolism are common in osteomalacia.

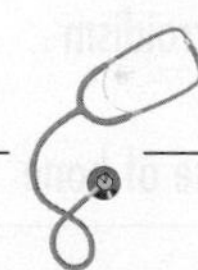

Oncogenic osteomalacia can be cured with removal of the tumor.

Osteoporosis

Systemic disorder resulting in a reduction of bone mass that leads to increased risk of fracture.

EPIDEMIOLOGY

Risk factors for osteoporosis include:

- Female and elderly.
- Postmenopause.
- Family history of osteoporosis.
- Cigarette smoking.
- Thin body habitus.
- Sedentary lifestyle.

PATHOPHYSIOLOGY

- Reduction in bone mass occurs due to an imbalance between bone acquisition and bone reabsorption.
- There is no change in the ratio of mineral to organic bone.
- Histology: Decreased cortical thickness and decreased number and size of cancellous bone trabeculae (especially horizontal).
- **Clinical findings:**
- Osteoporosis is asymptomatic until fracture occurs.
- Vertebral body fractures:
  - Pain in the lumbar region.
  - Acute in onset.
  - Radiating to the flank.

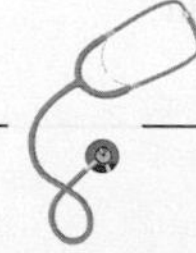

Bone Mineral Density Scoring

T score > −1 = normal bone mass

T score −2.5 to −1 = osteopenia

T score ≤ −2.5 = osteoporosis

ENDOCRINOLOGY

- Usually occur after sudden bending or lifting.
- Radiation of the pain down one leg is common.
- Spinal cord compression is rare.

- Hip fractures:
  - Most serious complication.
  - Most resulting from a fall from a standing position.
  - Incidence of fracture increases with age in both men and women.
- **Laboratory findings:**
  - Serum calcium and phosphorus usually *normal*.
  - Alkaline phosphatase is increased after fractures but is usually normal if fractures aren't present.
  - Bone-specific alkaline phosphatase assays are useful for monitoring response to therapy.
  - Twenty percent of postmenopausal women have hypercalciuria.

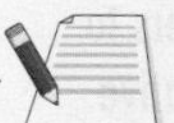

Bone mineral densitometry is the only reliable method for measuring bone mass; osteoporosis is present when the T score is < – 2.5.

Diagnosis

- Since bone loss is a universal process of aging, 2° osteoporosis should be diagnosed definitively and other causes should be ruled out.
- Biconcavity of vertebral bodies with pathologic fractures is highly suggestive of osteoporosis.
- Bone densitometry establishes the diagnosis.
- Measure bone mineral density using dual x-ray absorptiometry (DEXA) scan (not a bone scan).
- **Indications for measurement of bone mass:**
  - Women age ≥ 65 years.
  - Postmenopausal women age < 65 years who have at lease one risk factor for osteoporosis other than menopause.
  - Postmenopausal women who present with fractures.
  - Women who are considering therapy for osteoporosis and for whom bone mineral densitometry tests results would influence this decision.
  - Women who have been receiving hormone replacement therapy for a prolonged period.
  - Radiographic findings suggestive of osteoporosis or vertebral deformity.
  - Corticosteroid therapy for > 3 months.
  - Primary hyperparathyroidism.
  - Treatment for osteoporosis (to monitor therapeutic response).

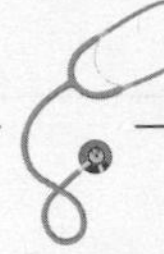

Differential in osteoporosis:
- Malignancy: Multiple myeloma, lymphoma, leukemia, and metastatic carcinoma
- Hyperparathyroidism
- Osteomalacia
- Paget's disease of bone

Treatment of osteoporosis is determined by bone mass and risk factors for osteoporosis.

Prevention and Therapy

- Prevention of low bone mass by adequate dietary calcium and weight-bearing exercise. These measures increase peak bone mass earlier in life and prevent accelerated bone loss later in life.
- Estrogen replacement therapy prevents rapid bone loss and subsequently decreases rate of fractures.
- Calcitonin decreases bone reabsorption.
- Bisphosphonates (alendronate) increase density of spinal bone and decreases incidence of fractures when used in conjunction with vitamin D and calcium supplementation.

Bisphosphonates and teriparatide are the agents that decrease nonvertebral fractures in osteoporosis.

Paget's Disease of Bone

Chronic disease of adult bone in which localized areas of bone become hyperactive and the normal bone matrix is replaced by softened and enlarged bone.

ETIOLOGY

Cause is unknown, but it is suspected that a viral infection plays a role.

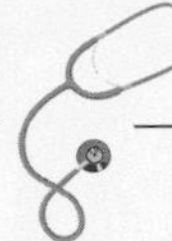

When alkaline phosphatase is elevated, send gamma-glutamyl transpeptidase (GGT) to determine if hepatic or bone (elevated in liver but not bone).

EPIDEMIOLOGY

- Rare for age > 40 years.
- 3:2 male predominance.

PATHOPHYSIOLOGY

- Hyperactive bone turnover.
- Increased bone formation.
- Pelvis, femur, skull, tibiae, and vertebrae all affected.
- Enlarged multinucleated osteoclasts.

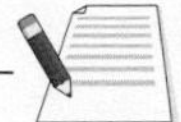

Paget's disease is associated with elevated serum alkaline phosphatase levels and typical radiographic abnormalities; most patients are asymptomatic.

CLINICAL FINDINGS

- Most patients are asymptomatic; diagnosis is made at autopsy.
- Incidental radiographic findings: Area of hyperlucency surrounded by a hyperdense border.
- Elevated alkaline phosphatase.
- Symptomatic patients:
  - Increasing hat size due to skull involvement.
  - Swelling or lengthening of a long bone, causing gait disturbance.
  - Dull aching pain, usually in the back; may radiate to the buttocks or lower extremities.
  - Rarely hearing loss due to involvement of the ossicles or auditory canal impinging on CN VIII.
- Complications:
  - Pathologic fractures.
  - Rarely "high-output" cardiac failure due to high vascularity of lesions.
  - Urinary stones due to high calcium excretion.
  - Sarcoma occurs in 1% of patients; poor prognosis.

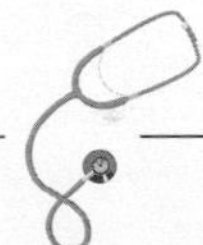

The primary indication for treatment in Paget's disease is the presence of symptoms and lytic involvement of vertebrae, skull, weight-bearing bones, or areas adjacent to major joints.

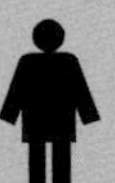

A patient is found to have an elevated alkaline phosphatase during a routine blood test. No other abnormalities were found. Further workup revealed the enzyme to be heat labile. *Think: Paget's disease.*

TREATMENT

- Most patients require no treatment.
- Indications for therapy are excessive pain, neural compression, profound alteration in posture or gait, high-output heart failure, hypercalcemia, and excessive calciuria, with or without renal calculi.
- Indomethacin is usually satisfactory for pain relief.
- Osteotomy is useful in selected cases of anatomic deformity or impingement.
- Bisphosphonates decrease bone reabsorption and are usually well tolerated.
- Calcitonin may be instituted in cases with cardiac failure or neurologic deficits. Calcitonin also has an analgesic effect.

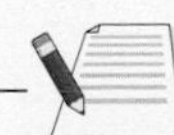

The therapy of choice for uncomplicated Paget's disease is an oral bisphosphonate.

HIGH-YIELD FACTS IN

Gastroenterology

ABDOMINAL PAIN

- **Visceral pain:**
  - Dull, and poorly localized pain.
  - Midline location due to bilateral innervation of organs.
  - Associated with stretching, inflammation, or ischemia, involving bowel walls or organ capsules.
- **Parietal pain:**
  - Sharp, well-localized pain; peritonitis associated with rebound tenderness and involuntary guarding.
  - Pain location correlates with associated dermatomes.
  - Occurs commonly with inflammation, air, frank pus, blood, or bile in or adjacent to the peritoneum.
- **Referred pain:**
  - Pain stimuli generated at an afflicted location are perceived as originating from a site in which there is no current pathology.
  - These sites are usually related by a common embryological origin.
  - The pain can sometimes be perceived in both locations.

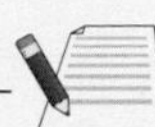

Visceral pain is Vague. Example: Early appendicitis; initially dull, periumbilical pain.

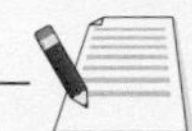

Parietal pain is Pinpoint. Example: Late appendicitis; local inflammation of the peritoneum → tenderness in the right lower quadrant.

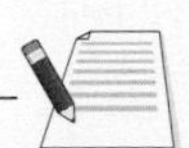

Example of referred pain: Ureteral obstruction can produce pain in the ipsilateral testicle.

Causes of Abdominal Pain

There are no hard-and-fast rules for localizing different types of abdominal pain. The following are classic examples for the exam:

- **Epigastric, upper abdominal pain:**
  - Gastroduodenal: Gastritis, peptic ulcer/perforation.
  - Pancreatic: Acute/chronic pancreatitis.
  - Aorta: Ruptured abdominal aortic aneurysm, dissecting abdominal aortic aneurysm.
  - Cardiac: Angina, myocardial infarction, pericarditis.
- **Right upper quadrant (RUQ):**
  - Hepatobiliary: Cholelithiasis, cholecystitis, cholangitis, hepatitis, abscess.
  - Peptic ulcer.
- **Left upper quadrant (LUQ):**
  - Spleen: Trauma, infarction, abscess, rupture (mononucleosis).
  - Gastric ulcer.
- **Right lower quadrant (RLQ):**
  - Appendicitis
  - Small bowel obstruction
  - Crohn's disease
  - Mesenteric lymphadenitis
  - Meckel's diverticulum
- **Left lower quadrant (LLQ):**
  - Diverticulitis
  - Inflammatory bowel disease
- **Flank pain:**
  - Nephrolithiasis
  - Pyelonephritis
  - Testicular torsion
  - Prostatitis
  - Epididymitis
- **Adnexal (lower abdominal pain):**
  - Ectopic pregnancy
  - Tubo-ovarian abscess

- Pelvic inflammatory disease
- Ovarian torsion
- Salpingitis
- Cystitis

- **Anywhere:**
  - Strangulated hernia
  - Large bowel obstruction
  - Sigmoid volvulus
  - Mesenteric ischemia

Note: All premenopausal women with abdominal pain must have a pregnancy test, even if they say they are not sexually active.

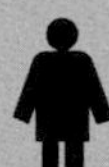

A 45-year-old obese woman complains of fever, RUQ pain, and nausea that is worse when she eats fatty foods. *Think: Cholecystitis.* **Next step:** Check RUQ ultrasound and LFTs.

A 26-year-old woman complains of severe left lower quadrant pain, vaginal bleeding, and light-headedness. Last menstrual period was 6 weeks ago. *Think: Ectopic pregnancy.* **Next step:** Pelvic exam and abdominal ultrasound. Consider OB/GYN and surgical consultation.

Other Causes of Abdominal Pain

- **Abdominal wall:** Hernia, rectus sheath hematoma.
- **Metabolic:** Diabetic ketoacidosis, acute intermittent porphyria, hypercalcemia.
- **Infectious:** Herpes zoster, mononucleosis, HIV.
- **Drugs/toxins:** Heavy metal poisoning, black widow spider envenomation.
- **Other:** Sickle cell anemia, foreign body.

Abdominal Pain in the Elderly

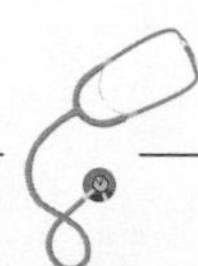

In elderly patients with abdominal pain, always consider vascular causes, including:

- AAA
- Mesenteric ischemia
- Myocardial infarction

Elderly patients who present with abdominal pain must be treated with particular caution. Common problems include:

- Difficulty communicating.
- Comorbid disease.
- Inability to tolerate intravascular volume loss.
- Unusual presentation of common disease.
- May not mount a white blood cell count or a fever.
- Complaint often incommensurate with severity of disease.

Note: Up to 2% of elderly patients with a myocardial infarction (MI) will present with abdominal pain.

VASCULAR PROBLEMS OF THE ABDOMEN

Abdominal Aortic Aneurysm (AAA)

- Dilation of the abdominal aorta usually involves the infrarenal arteries.
- AAAs are the most common site of atherosclerotic aneurysms.
- Men are more frequently affected.
- Acute expansion or leak of an AAA causes pain and may precede rupture, a life-threatening emergency.

RISK FACTORS

- Familial.
- Smoking.
- Atherosclerosis.
- Trauma/infection.
- Aneurysms > 5 cm associated with 20–40% 5-year risk of rupture.

SIGNS AND SYMPTOMS

- Abdominal or back pain.
- Pulsatile mass in abdomen.
- Hypotension (or symptoms of).
- History of vascular disease or atherosclerosis.

DIAGNOSIS

- **Screening:** U.S. Preventive Services Task Force recommends one-time screening with ultrasound (US) in men > 65–75 years of age who ever smoked. Screening of first-degree relatives usually begins at 50 years of age.
- **Ultrasonography, magnetic resonance imaging (MRI) or computed tomography (CT) scan with IV contrast:** Can demonstrate size of aneurysm and location of leak or rupture. May replace angiogram as gold standard.
- **Angiogram:** Usually done when treatment is planned to visualize renal and peripheral arteries. Can underestimate size of aneurysm with mural thrombus. Gold standard.

TREATMENT

- **Medical management:** Control hypertension, smoking cessation, treat coronary artery disease (CAD) and carotid artery disease and serial noninvasive assessment.
- **Surgical management:** Usually when diameter is > 5.0–5.5 cm, rapidly progressive (> 0.5cm/yr), symptomatic, or traumatic/infectious.
- **Dissection/rupture:** Requires emergent surgical repair/consult. All patients should have good IV access along with type and crossmatch of blood for transfusions if necessary.

A 63-year-old man complains of pain in his "kidney" for 3 days. He is a smoker and has a history of MI × 2. He has no back tenderness but you feel a large pulsatile mass in his abdomen. *Think: Abdominal aortic aneurysm.* **Next step:** CT with IV contrast, blood pressure control, consider vascular surgery consult depending on results of CT.

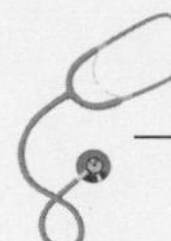

Acute Mesenteric Ischemia vs. Chronic Mesenteric Ischemia

Acute mesenteric ischemia: Sudden onset of abdominal pain due to acute occlusion of mesenteric vessel by emboli or thrombosis; emergency.

Chronic mesenteric ischemia: Episodic, postprandial pain, due to slow narrowing of vessels due to atherosclerosis; weight loss associated; not emergency.

Mesenteric Ischemia

Interruption of intestinal blood flow resulting in abdominal pain and potentially catastrophic intestinal pathology depending on the severity of vascular compromise.

- Ischemia of celiac trunk affects stomach, duodenum and liver.
- Ischemia of superior mesenteric artery (SMA) affects jejunum, ileum, and right colon.
- Inferior mesenteric artery (IMA) affects left colon and rectum.

Causes

- **Atherosclerosis** causing obstruction of SMA, IMA, or celiac artery (chronic).
- Atrial fibrillation causing **embolus** (acute presentation).
- **Hypertension,** diabetes.
- Low-flow state (hypotension, poor cardiac output).
- **Hypercoagulability** (acute thrombus).

Signs and Symptoms

- Severe abdominal **pain out of proportion to exam,** nausea, vomiting and may have rectal bleed.
- History of **gnawing abdominal pain after eating.**
- Labs may show ↑ lactate, metabolic acidosis.

Diagnosis

- Gold standard is **angiography.**
- Spiral CT scan with contrast and magnetic resonance angiography (MRA) of the abdomen also can diagnose.

Treatment

- Maintain tissue perfusion with fluids.
- Surgery revascularization (bypass).

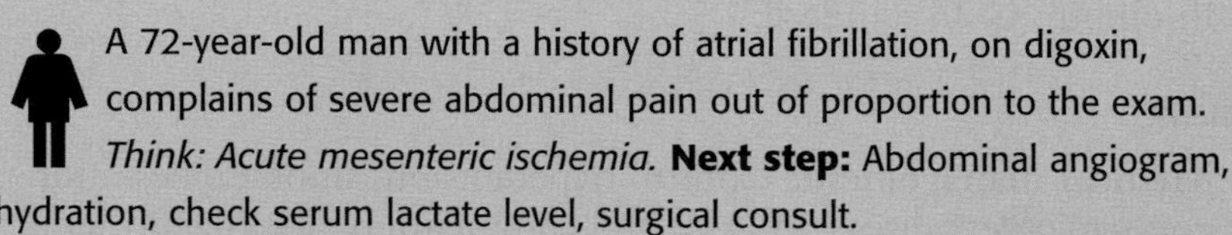

A 72-year-old man with a history of atrial fibrillation, on digoxin, complains of severe abdominal pain out of proportion to the exam. *Think: Acute mesenteric ischemia.* **Next step:** Abdominal angiogram, hydration, check serum lactate level, surgical consult.

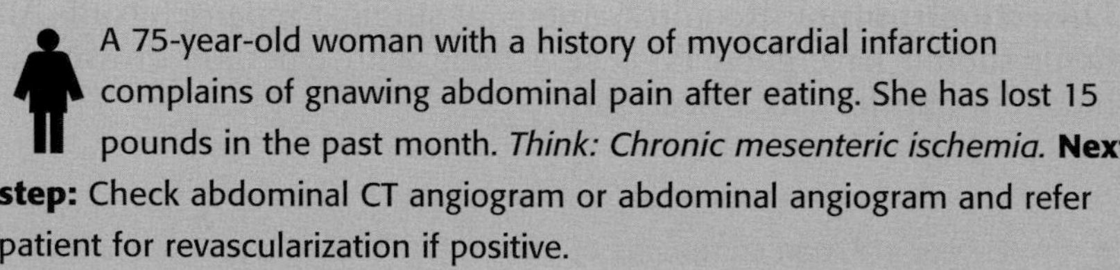

A 75-year-old woman with a history of myocardial infarction complains of gnawing abdominal pain after eating. She has lost 15 pounds in the past month. *Think: Chronic mesenteric ischemia.* **Next step:** Check abdominal CT angiogram or abdominal angiogram and refer patient for revascularization if positive.

Dysphagia

- May be distinguished as mechanical, functional or oropharyngeal.
- Intermittent dysphagia is usually caused by a ring, a web, or a functional cause (motility disorder).
- **Mechanical:** Progressive, associated with weight loss, solid more than liquid. Causes include lyomyoma, squamous cell carcinoma, adenocarcinoma, Barrett's esophagus.
- **Functional:** Intermittent with both solids and liquids. Common causes include achalasia, diffuse esophageal spasms, and scleroderma.
- **Oropharyngeal:** Choking, coughing, or regurgitations result of faulty transfer of bolus from oropharynx to esophagus. Usually structural or neuromuscular causes.

Esophagitis

Inflammation of the esophagus causing pain and discomfort.

Etiology

- Infectious:
  - **Viral:** herpes simplex virus (HSV), varicella-zoster virus (VZV), cytomegalovirus (CMV).
  - **Bacterial:** *Lactobacillus, Streptococcus, Cryptosporidium, Pneumocystis jiroveci* pneumonia (PCP), *Mycobacterium tuberculosis, Candida.*
- Other causes: Radiation, corrosives.

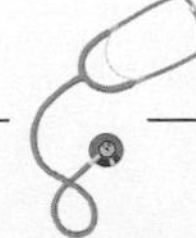

A patient with HIV and odynophagia (pain on swallowing) has esophagitis most likely due to:

- Candida
- CMV
- Herpes

Signs and Symptoms

- Odynophagia.
- Dysphagia.
- Esophageal bleeding.
- Nausea/vomiting.
- Chest pain.
- May be asymptomatic.

Diagnosis

- Either barium esophogram or upper endoscopy.
- Remember some classic findings: HSV, VZV have vesicles; CMV has intranuclear inclusions. Candida will have white plaques.

Treatment

Treat the cause: Gancyclovir for CMV; acyclovir for HSV/VZV; fluconazole for candida.

Esophageal Rupture or Perforation

Iatrogenic or pathologic trauma to the esophagus, which may result in leakage of air and esophageal contents into the mediastinum. Carries a 50% mortality.

Etiology/Types

- **Iatrogenic:** This often occurs in an already diseased esophagus. Comprises 50–75% of cases of esophageal rupture: endoscopy, dilation, Blakemore tubes, intubation of the esophagus, nasogastric tube placement.
- **Boerhaave's syndrome:** A *full-thickness* tear. Generally occurs in the relatively weak left posterolateral wall of distal esophagus. **Due to** forceful vomiting, cough, trauma.
- **Mallory-Weiss syndrome:** A *partial-thickness* tear. Usually occurs in the right posterolateral wall of the distal esophagus and results in bleeding that generally resolves spontaneously. **Due to** forceful vomiting/retching.
- **Foreign body ingestion:** Objects usually lodge near anatomic narrowings—distal to the upper esophageal sphincter, near the aortic arch or at lower esophageal sphincter.

An alcoholic man presents after severe retching, complaining of retrosternal and upper abdominal pain. *Think: Boerhaave's syndrome.* **Next step:** Immediate chest x-ray looking for subcutaneous and/or mediastinal air. Immediate cardiothoracic surgical evaluation if positive.

Signs and Symptoms

- Severe, constant pain in chest, abdomen, and back.
- Dysphagia.
- Dyspnea.
- **Subcutaneous emphysema.**
- Mediastinal emphysema heard as a "crunching sound" with heartbeat (Hammon's crunch).

Diagnosis

- **Chest x-ray:** Left-sided pleural effusion, mediastinal or subcutaneous emphysema.
- **Esophagogram with water-soluble contrast:** Shows extravasation of contrast.
- **Other studies:** Endoscopy, CT, and pleurocentesis (check fluid for low pH and high salivary amylase).

Treatment

Surgical repair of full-thickness tears. Partial-thickness tears may resolve spontaneously.

A 56-year-old man complains of food feeling "stuck" on its way down and vomiting food he ate days ago. His breath is terrible. *Think: Zenker's diverticulum.* **Next step:** Check barium swallow looking for outpouching of esophagus.

Zenker's Diverticulum

Pharyngeal or esophageal pouch due to a defect in the muscular wall of the posterior hypopharynx.

Signs and Symptoms

- Halitosis.
- Regurgitation of food days after eating it ("spit-ups").
- Frequent aspiration.
- Esophageal obstruction.

Diagnosis

Barium swallow or endoscopy.

Treatment

Surgical removal or cricopharyngeal myotomy.

Esophageal Spasm and Achalasia

- **Achalasia:** A neurogenic disorder of esophageal motility with absence of normal peristalsis and impaired relaxation of lower esophageal sphincter (food doesn't get pushed down normally). Thought to arise from scarring in Auerbach's plexus (nerve damage).
- **Diffuse esophageal spasm (DES):** Motility disorder with frequent non-peristaltic contractions. Believed to come from hypoactive inhibitory neurons within Auerbach's plexus. See Table 2.3-1.

Diagnosis

- **Barium swallow** (see Figures 2.3-1 and 2.3-2).
- **Manometry** (measures esophageal pressures): Achalasia will show normal to ↑ pressure at LES with no relaxation upon swallowing; DES will show high-amplitude contractions, possibly including proximal esophagus.

TABLE 2.3-1. Comparison of Achalasia and Diffuse Esophageal Spasm

	Achalasia	Diffuse Esophageal Spasm
Signs and symptoms	Weight loss, cough, diffuse chest pain.	Dysphagia, diffuse chest pain.
Pattern of contraction	Failure of LES to relax on swallowing. ▪ Classic: Simultaneous small wave. ▪ Vigorous: Simultaneous large wave.	Swallow-induced large wave.
Relieved by	Nitroglycerin.	Nitroglycerin.
Barium swallow	"Bird's beak" narrowing of terminal esophagus.	Corkscrew appearance.
Treatment	Nitroglycerin, local botulinum toxin, balloon dilatation, sphincter myotomy.	Nitroglycerin, anticholinergics.

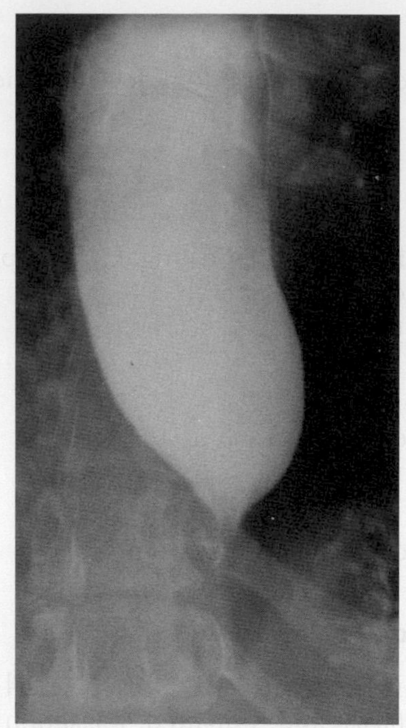

FIGURE 2.3-1. Achalasia.

Barium esophagogram in a patient with achalasia demonstrates a dilated esophagus with a sharply tapered "bird's beak" narrowing. (Reproduced, with permission, from Waters PF, DeMeester TR. Foregut motor disorders and their surgical management. *Med Clin North Am* 65: 1244, 1981.)

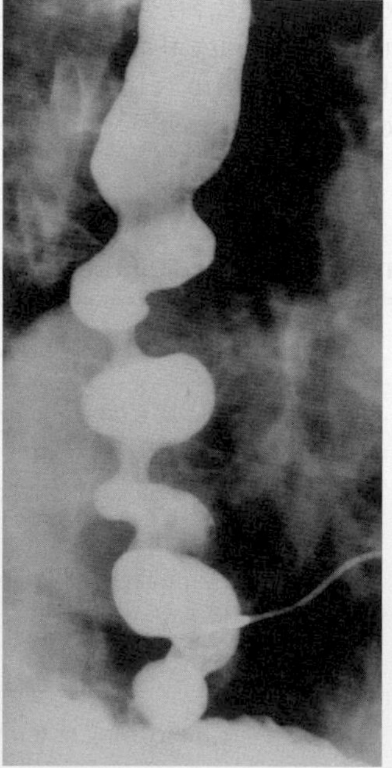

FIGURE 2.3-2. Diffuse esophageal spasm.

Barium esophagogram in a patient with diffuse esophageal spasm demonstrates the characteristic "corkscrew" pattern. (Reproduced, with permission, from Schwartz SI, Fischer JE, Spencer FC, Shires GT, Daly JM. *Schwartz's Principles of Surgery*, 7th ed. New York: McGraw-Hill, 1998: 1129.)

GI Webs and Rings

The following conditions are anatomical obstructions, usually presenting with dysphagia to solids:

- **Plummer-Vinson syndrome:** Hypopharyngeal webs (thin mucosal structures protruding into lumen) associated with iron deficiency anemia.
- **Schatzki's ring:** A narrow lower esophageal ringlike outgrowth associated with dysphagia (see Figure 2.3-3).

Dysphagia to solids *and* liquids often indicates a motility problem (ie, achalasia and esophageal spasm). Dysphagia to *only* solids indicates mechanical obstruction (ie, tumor or Schatzki's ring).

Gastroesophageal Reflux Disease (GERD)

Reflux of acidic gastric contents into the esophagus.

Causes of GERD

- Relaxed or incompetent lower esophageal sphincter (LES).
- Hiatal hernia.
- Delayed gastric emptying.
- ↓ esophageal motility.

Causes of Delayed Gastric Emptying

- Diabetes mellitus.
- Gastroparesis.

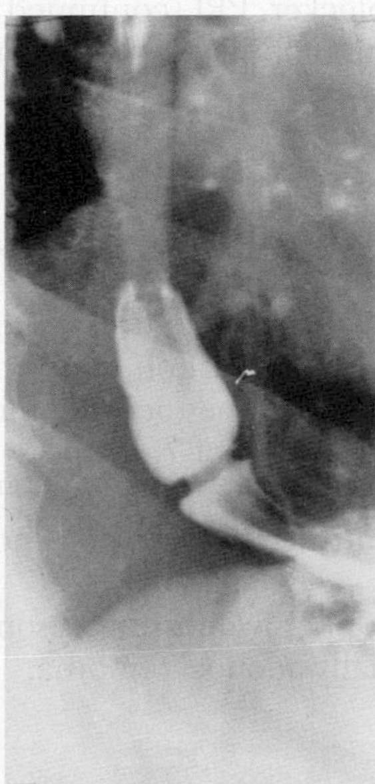

FIGURE 2.3-3. Schatzki's ring.

Barium esophagogram in a patient with Schatzki's ring demonstrates a distal esophageal ring at the gastroesophageal junction. (Reproduced, with permission, from Schwartz SI, Fischer JE, Spencer FC, Shires GT, Daly JM. *Schwartz's Principles of Surgery*, 7th ed. New York: McGraw-Hill, 1998: 1168.)

- Gastric outlet obstruction.
- Anticholinergic use.
- Fatty foods.

Causes of Lowered LES Tone

- Foods (coffee, chocolate).
- Alcohol.
- Cigarettes.
- Drugs (nitrates, calcium channel blockers).
- Hormones (estrogen, progesterone).

Signs and Symptoms

- Substernal burning pain.
- Dysphagia (secondary to stricture formation).
- Hypersalivation, with *sour* taste in mouth (water brash).
- Cough (particularly nocturnal), hoarseness.
- Wheezing.

> Differential of chronic cough:
> - Asthma
> - GERD
> - Postnasal drip

Diagnosis

Often, a trial of proton pump inhibitor (PPI) will be given to relieve symptoms without further workup. However, if "alarm signals" are present (long duration, weight loss, advanced age, nausea, refractory symptoms, guaiac positive), an endoscopy to rule out cancer is *required*.

Treatment

- **Lifestyle modification:** Elevate head of bed, discontinue foods that ↓ LES tone, avoid food < 3 hours before bed.
- **Pharmacologic:** H_2 blocker, PPI (continued indefinitely if severe).
- **Surgical:** Surgical correction such as Nissen fundoplication if all else fails.

Complications of GERD

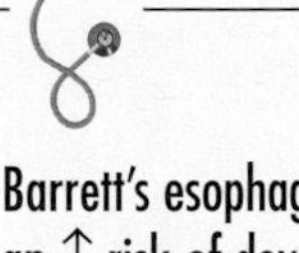

> Barrett's esophagus carries an ↑ risk of development of esophageal adenocarcinoma; numbers vary but about 0.5% chance per year.

- **Esophagitis:** Esophageal damage, bleeding, and friability due to prolonged exposure to gastric contents.
- **Peptic stricture:** Occurs in about 10% of patients with GERD.
- **Barrett's esophagus:** Transformation of normal squamous epithelium to columnar epithelium, sometimes accompanied by an ulcer or stricture. This carries a significant risk of cancerous transformation. High-grade Barrett's requires resection. Other grades of Barrett's require surveillance endoscopy regularly for **life;** Barrett's does **not** regress, even if GERD is successfully treated.
- **Esophageal cancer:** Upper two-thirds of esophagus is usually squamous; lower one-third is usually adenocarcinoma.

DISORDERS OF THE STOMACH

Peptic Ulcer Disease (PUD)

PUD consists of duodenal ulcers (DU) and gastric ulcers (GU).

Common Causes

- *Helicobacter pylori.*
- Nonsteroidal anti-inflammatory drugs (NSAIDs).
- Miscellaneous causes including Zollinger-Ellison syndrome and idiopathic hypersecretion.

Clinical Features

- Burning, gnawing, epigastric pain that occurs with an empty stomach. Pain is relieved within 30 minutes by food. Nighttime awakening with pain (when stomach empties); nausea/vomiting.
- When bleeding, melana or hematochezia is present.
- Associated with blood type O.

Epidemiology

- Two times more common in men.
- Incidence ↑ with age.
- Smoking ↑ risk.

> A patient with known PUD presents with sudden onset of severe epigastric pain. Physical exam reveals guarding and rebound tenderness. *Think: Perforation.* **Next step:** Order a supine and upright abdominal x-ray, looking for free air under the diaphragm.

Physiology Key Concepts

- **Gastrin is made by G cells** in the antrum of stomach and in the duodenum.
- Gastrin release is stimulated by gastrin-releasing peptide.
- Gastrin release is **inhibited by somatostatin.**
- **Gastrin stimulates parietal cells to secrete HCl into the gastric lumen.**
- Parietal cells are stimulated by gastrin, acetyl choline (from vagus nerve) and **histamine.**
- When stimulated, **parietal cells secrete acid into the lumen via a proton pump** that exchanges potassium for protons.
- **Gastrin also stimulates secretion of bicarbonate into the gastric venous circulation** (alkaline tide) and **into the protective gastric mucous gel.**
- Gastric bicarbonate secretion into the mucous gel **is inhibited by nonsteroidal anti-inflammatory drugs (NSAIDs), acetazolamide, alpha blockers, and alcohol.**
- Gel thickness is ↑ **by prostaglandin E** (PGE) and reduced by steroids and NSAIDs.
- **Zollinger-Ellison syndrome (ZE):**
  - A gastrin-secreting tumor in or near the pancreas. ZE can be part of multiple endocrine neoplasia type I (MEN I). Diarrhea is common.

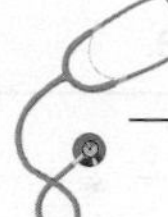

Causes of Peptic Ulcer Disease

NSAIDs and steroids inhibit production of PGE, which helps produce the gastric mucosal barrier.

H pylori produces urease, which breaks down the gastric mucosal barrier.

Gastric ulcers can even occur with achlorhydria.

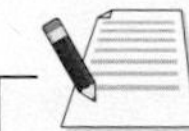

Smoking is a risk factor for gastric ulcer.

- ZE has a triad of PUD, gastric acid hypersecretion, and an elevated gastrin level.

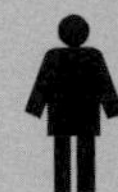

A 52-year-old woman presents due to 3 months of early satiety, weight loss, and vomiting. *Think: Gastric outlet obstruction.*

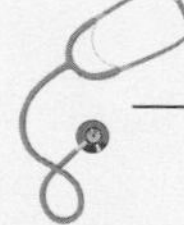

Over 90% of patients with ZE have peptic ulcer disease.

DIAGNOSIS

- **Duodenal ulcer (DU):** Diagnose via endoscopy; however, most symptomatic cases of DU are easily diagnosed clinically. If patient responds to DU therapy, there is no need to do the biopsy.
- ***H pylori*:** Endoscopy with biopsy—allows culture and sensitivity for *H pylori* (organism is notoriously hard to culture—multiple specimens required during biopsy).
  - Serology: Anti–*H pylori* IgG indicates current or prior infection.
  - Urease breath test: $C^{13/14}$ labeled urea is ingested. If gastric urease is present, the carbon isotope can be detected as CO_2 isotopes in the breath.
- **ZE:** Secretin stimulation test—secretin, a gastrin inhibitor, is delivered parenterally (usually with Ca^{2+}), and its effect on gastrin secretion is measured. In ZE syndrome, there is a paradoxical astronomic rise in serum gastrin.
  - Gastrin level (must be taken when off antacid meds): If elevated, test for hyperacidity with gastric pH monitor.

H pylori may colonize 90% of the population—infection does not necessitate disease.

TREATMENT

Mainly depends on the cause:

- **Discontinue** NSAIDs, steroids, and smoking.
- **Triple therapy for *H pylori*** (eg, PPI, amoxicillin, and clarithromycin).
- **Antacid agents:** H_2 blockers and PPIs.
- **If bleeding, endoscopy** is done and sucralfate (enhances mucosal barrier) or misoprostol (prostaglandin analog) is used.
- **Surgery is indicated when ulcer is refractory** to 12 weeks of medical treatment or if hemorrhage, obstruction, or perforation is present.

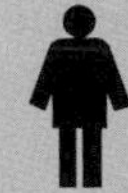

A 33-year-old female smoker presents with burning epigastric pain that is improved after eating a meal. *Think: Duodenal ulcer.* **Next step:** Trial of PPI. If not resolved in 4–6 weeks, then esophagogastroduodenoscopy (EGD).

COMPLICATIONS

- **Bleeding:** 20% incidence.
- **Perforation:** 7% incidence.
  - Posterior perforation of a duodenal ulcer will cause pain that radiates to the back and can cause pancreatitis. A chest or abdominal film will not show free air because the posterior duodenum is retroperitoneal.
  - Anterior perforation will show free air under the diaphragm in 70% of cases (see Figure 2.3-4).

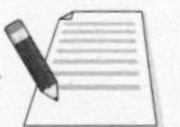

Gastric ulcer pain is typically exacerbated by food. Duodenal ulcer pain is typically relieved by food.

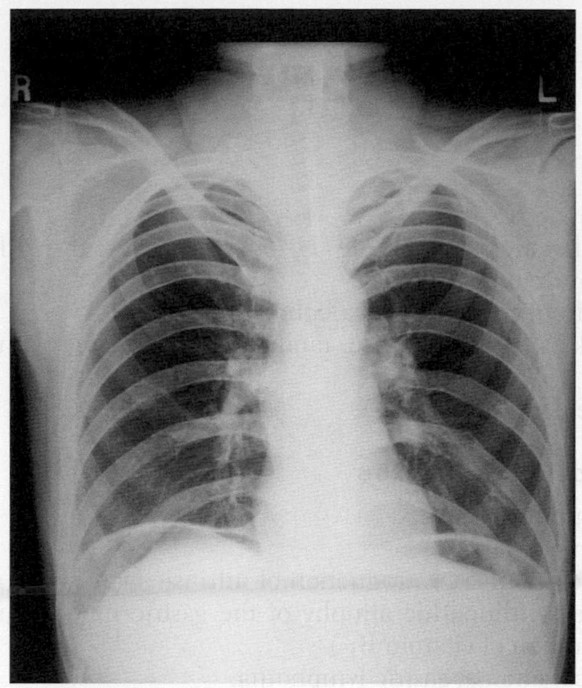

FIGURE 2.3-4. Free air.

Upright chest film in a patient with perforated duodenal ulcer demonstrates free air underneath both right and left hemidiaphragms. (Reproduced, with permission, from Schwartz SI, Fischer JE, Spencer FC, Shires GT, Daly JM. *Schwartz's Principles of Surgery*, 7th ed. New York: McGraw-Hill, 1998: 1195.)

- **Gastric outlet obstruction**, due to scarring and edema (can also be a complication of neoplasm).

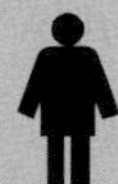

A 45-year-old Japanese male smoker presents with epigastric pain, exacerbated by eating, and weight loss. *Think: Gastric ulcer.* **Next step:** Must get EGD, as patient has weight loss.

Gastritis

Acute or chronic inflammation of the stomach lining.

Etiology

- **↑ acid:** Smoking, alcohol, stress.
- **↓ mucosal barrier:** NSAIDs, steroids, *H pylori*.
- **Direct irritant:** Pancreatic and biliary reflux, infection.
- **Autoimmune.**

Signs and Symptoms

- Burning or gnawing pain usually **worsened with food** and relieved by antacids.
- Vomiting may relieve the pain after eating.

Cimetidine is a p450 inhibitor and, therefore, prolongs the action of drugs cleared in the liver by this system.

Diagnosis

Endoscopy.

Treatment

Similar to PUD:

- Discontinue NSAIDs.
- Triple therapy to eradicate *H pylori* if present (PPI, amoxicillin, clarithromycin).
- Abstain from cigarettes and alcohol.
- H_2 blockers (eg, cimetidine, ranitidine), sucralfate, or misoprostol and PPI.
- Over-the-counter antacids.

Etiologies of gastritis—

GNASHING

Gastric reflux (bile or pancreatic secretions)
Nicotine
Alcohol
Stress
***H**elicobacter pylori* and other infections
Ischemia
NSAIDs
Glucocorticoids (long-term use)

Complications of Chronic Gastritis

- Gastric atrophy.
- Gastric metaplasia.
- Pernicious anemia (↓ production of intrinsic factor from gastric parietal cells due to **idiopathic** atrophy of the gastric mucosa and subsequent malabsorption of vitamin B_{12}).
- Gastric carcinoma, gastric lymphoma.

DISORDERS OF THE PANCREAS

Normal Secretions from the Pancreas

- **Exocrine:** Bicarbonate, amylase, lipase, tyrosine, and other digestive enzymes.
- **Endocrine:** Insulin, glucagon, somatostatin.

Acute Pancreatitis

- Inflammation of the pancreas due to parenchymal autodigestion by proteolytic enzymes.
- Two varieties: Interstitial and necrotizing.
- In severe cases, it can be associated with a *systemic inflammatory response syndrome* (SIRS), which can progress to multiorgan system failure and acute respiratory distress syndrome (ARDS).

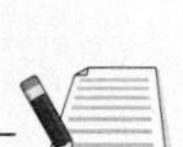

Hypercalcemia can cause pancreatitis, and pancreatitis can cause *hypocalcemia.*

Etiologies

- Gallstones.
- Alcohol.
- Hypertriglyceridemia.
- Complication of endoscopic retrograde cholangiopancreatography (ERCP).
- Drugs: Thiazides, furosemide, estrogen, antiretrovirals.
- Other rare problems: Neoplasm, hypercalcemia, idiopathic.

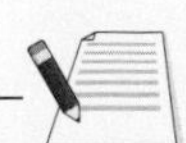

Most common causes of pancreatitis: Gallstones and alcohol.

Signs and Symptoms

- Severe, constant midepigastric or LUQ pain, *radiates to the back.*
- Pain sometimes improved when patient sits up and leans forward.

- Nausea, vomiting.
- Low-grade fever.
- Abdomen is usually tender with guarding, but no rebound.
- **The Grey-Turner sign** (flank discoloration) and Cullen sign (periumbilical discoloration) suggests **retroperitoneal hemorrhage.**

DIAGNOSIS

- Diagnostic markers in blood:
  - **Amylase:** Normally secreted by pancreas to break down carbohydrates. Elevation in pancreatitis, but not specific—can be found in small bowel inflammation, among other settings (in salivary glands, ovaries, testes, muscle).
  - **Lipase:** Normally secreted by the pancreas to break down triglycerides. Elevation in pancreatitis is fairly specific, though also found in gastric and intestinal mucosa. Level two times the upper limit of normal is 90% specific and 80–90% sensitive.
- Diagnostic imaging:
  - **Contrast-enhanced dynamic CT (CECT):** May show degree of pancreatic necrosis.
  - **Abdominal film:** May see calcification of pancreas, which is indicative of chronic pancreatitis, the "sentinel loop" of a localized small bowel ileus, and colon cutoff sign.
  - **Ultrasound:** May identify gallstones as the cause.
  - **ERCP:** Should be avoided in acute cases, but may be useful in endoscopic when associated with jaundice and cholangitis.

Ranson's criteria on admission—

GA LAW

Glucose
Age
LDH
AST
WBC

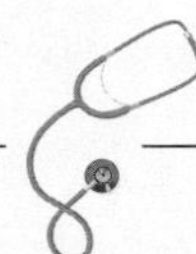

Elevated lipase is more specific than amylase for diagnosing pancreatitis.

A 50-year-old male alcoholic presents with midepigastric pain radiating to the back. He is leaning forward on his stretcher and vomiting. *Think: Pancreatitis.* **Next step:** Establish IV access and start large-volume resuscitation with crystalloid.

TREATMENT

- **IV hydration.**
- **Bowel rest.**
- NG tube for severe nausea, vomiting, or associated ileus.
- Analgesics and antiemetics as needed.
- **Antibiotics** (eg, imipenem) if infection is suspected, or necrosis identified on CT abdomen.

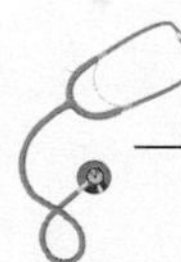

A "sentinel loop" on x-ray is distention and/or air-fluid levels near a site of abdominal distention. In pancreatitis, it is secondary to pancreatitis-associated ileus.

SEQUELAE

- **< 48 hours:** Usually isolated left pleural effusion containing high-amylase peripancreatic fluid.
- **1–4 weeks: Pseudocyst** (diagnosed by CT); if it persists, it can rupture or create a fistula, so surgical drainage is required. Ascites may result from pancreatic duct disruption or leaking pseudocyst.
- **4–6 weeks: Abscess;** requires surgical drainage.

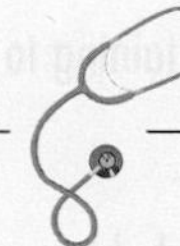

Gastric varices (without esopohageal varices) indicates splenic vein thrombosis, which is a complication of pancreatitis.

PROGNOSIS

Ranson's criteria (see Table 2.3-2).

TABLE 2.3-2. Ranson's Criteria (Predicts Risk of Mortality in Pancreatitis)

On Admission	After 48 Hours
Glucose (serum) > 200	Drop in hematocrit > 10%
Age > 55	↑ in BUN > 5
LDH > 700	Calcium < 8
AST > 250	PO_2 < 60 mm Hg
WBC > 16,000	Base deficit > 4
	Fluid deficit > 6 L

Number of Risk Factors	Mortality
< 3	1%
3 or 4	16%
5 or 6	40%
> 6	Approaches 100%

Chronic Pancreatitis

Recurrent episodes of acute pancreatitis, usually from alcohol abuse (70–80%), which → inflammation, scarring, and duct obstruction.

Other Causes

- Hereditary pancreatitis.
- Protein energy malnutrition may cause chronic pancreatitis.

Signs and Symptoms

- Pain similar to acute pancreatitis.
- Malabsorption.
- Steatorrhea.
- Elevated blood sugars.
- Polyuria.
- Associated with chronic liver disease.

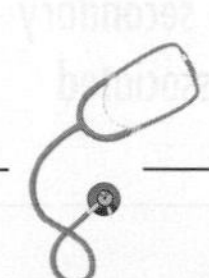

Chole = of or pertaining to bile
Cyst = bladder
Cholecyst = gallbladder
Lith(o) = stones, calculus
Cholang = bile duct
Choledocholithiasis = stones in the bile duct

Diagnosis

Pancreatic calcifications on x-ray or CT abdomen, diabetes, steatorrhea.

Workup

Abdominal x-ray (may show calcifications), trypsin level (low indicates poorly functioning pancreas). If these are inconclusive, do CT and/or ERCP (looking for abnormal duct anatomy). Finally, if all is still inconclusive, do secretin stimulation test.

Treatment

Same as for acute pancreatitis, with emphasis on pain control and abstinence from alcohol and fatty foods. May need pancreatic enzyme supplements. Surgical treatment when conservative measures fail.

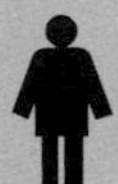

A patient with a history of alcohol abuse presents with severe abdominal pain exacerbated by food. Imaging shows calcifications of pancreas. *Think: Chronic pancreatitis.*

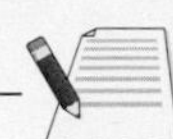

ERCP (endoscopic retrograde cholangiopancreatography): Endoscope inserted through mouth into the duodenum. A smaller scope is then inserted through the ampulla of Vater of the common bile duct allowing visualization (by injecting dye) of the pancreatic duct, hepatic duct, common bile duct, duodenal papilla, and gallbladder. ERCP can be interventional, as well as diagnostic. Stones can be removed, obstructed ducts can be stented, and biopsies can be performed.

DISORDERS OF THE BILIARY TREE

Bile is produced in the liver and stored in the gallbladder where it is acidified and concentrated. The presence of fat and amino acids in the proximal duodenum causes release of cholecystokinin, which stimulates gallbladder contraction.

Cholelithiasis

Gallstones.

Mechanisms of Gallstone Formation

- ↑ secretion of cholesterol in bile.
- ↑ formation of solid cholesterol nuclei.
- ↓ gallbladder emptying.

Signs and Symptoms

- RUQ pain that lasts between 2 and 6 hours.
- About two-thirds of patients will have pain after meals—often worse with fatty foods.
- Nausea and vomiting are common.
- On exam, the patient will be mildly tender in the RUQ *without* guarding or rebound.

Diagnosis

RUQ ultrasound to detect gallstones.

Additional Workup

- Aspartate transaminase (AST)/alanine transaminase (ALT) to evaluate for hepatitis.
- Alkaline phosphatase and bilirubin (direct fraction more elevated than indirect) to evaluate for common duct stones.
- Amylase/lipase for concomitant pancreatitis.

TREATMENT

- Cholecystectomy is definitive; if asymptomatic, do nothing, as only 20% develop symptoms.
- Also can do lithotripsy (extracorporeal shock wave treatment; breaks up stones).
- Low-fat diet for prevention.
- Chenodeoxycholate to dissolve stones (not very effective).

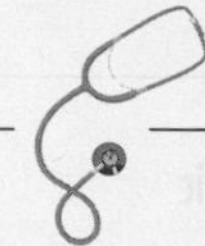

Risk factors for cholelithiasis: 8 Fs
Female
Fat
Fertile
Forty
Fibrosis, cystic
Familial
Fasting
F-Hgb (sickle cell disease)
Also:
Diabetes
Oral contraceptives

Cholecystitis

- Gallbladder inflammation, ischemia, or infection usually due to an obstructing stone.
- *Note*: Infection *is not necessary* to make the diagnosis of acute cholecystitis but may complicate up to 75% of the cases.

ETIOLOGY

- Obstruction with gallstones.
- Infection (*E coli, Klebsiella, Enterococcus, Bacteroides*).
- Abscess.
- Tumor.

SIGNS AND SYMPTOMS

- RUQ pain often longer than the 6 hours' duration.
- Guarding and rebound may occur.
- Fever.
- Tachycardia.
- Murphy's sign (see box).

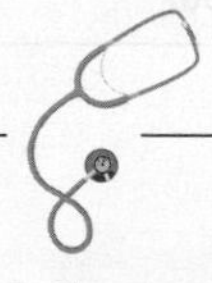

Gallstone composition:
- Cholesterol (70%): Radiolucent (seen in rapid weight loss, oral contraception, ileal disease)
- Pigment (20%): Radiodense (seen in hemolysis)
- Mixed (10%)

DIAGNOSIS

- **HIDA** (the study of choice): For this test, technetium 99m–labeled iminodiacetic acid is injected IV and is taken up by hepatocytes. In normals, the gallbladder is outlined within 1 hour; absence of visible gallbladder on HIDA = cholecystitis.
- **Ultrasound findings:** Presence of gallstones, **thickened gallbladder wall,** pericholecystic fluid (presence of all three has a positive predictive value of > 90%).
- **Other findings:**
  - Elevated white blood cell count with ↑ polymorphonuclear neutrophils (PMNs).
  - Elevated alkaline phosphatase, total bilirubin, gamma-glutamyl transpeptidase (GGT). May see mild elevation of AST/ALT.

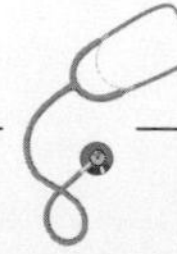

Meperidine (Demerol) is thought to produce less spasm of the sphincter of Oddi than morphine, *although clinical evidence is lacking.*

TREATMENT

- **Cholecystectomy.**
- **Antibiotics** (usually second- or third-generation cephalosporin).
- Pain control.
- Fluids.

COMPLICATIONS

Fistula, gallstone ileus, perforation, pancreatitis, sepsis, gangrenous gallbladder.

Acalculous Cholecystitis

Cholecystitis without stones.

- Makes up 5–10% of cases of cholecystitis.
- Usually occurs in seriously ill patients (eg, trauma, burns).
- Associated with more rapid clinical deterioration and ↑ morbidity and mortality.

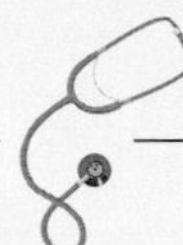

Murphy's sign: The arrest of inspiration while palpating the RUQ. This test is > 95% sensitive for acute cholecystitis, but less sensitive in the elderly.

RISK FACTORS

- ↑ age
- Diabetes mellitus (DM)
- Multiple trauma
- HIV
- Extensive burns
- Major surgery
- Prolonged labor
- Systemic vasculitides
- Gallbladder torsion
- Infections of the biliary tract

Gold standard test for cholecystitis is HIDA scan.

Ascending Cholangitis

Inflammation/infection of the biliary outflow tract usually due to a stone (choledocholelithiasis), a stricture, or tumor.

- The biliary system becomes superinfected (usually with gram-negative bacteria), and without drainage, the patient becomes septic, and may die without immediate intervention.
- Another cause for this is ERCP (iatrogenic), though it is also the treatment (see below).
- Ascending cholangitis is an **emergency.**

SIGNS AND SYMPTOMS

- **Charcot's triad** (RUQ pain, jaundice, fever) occurs in only about 25% of patients and lacks specificity.
- **Reynolds' pentad** (Charcot's triad + shock and altered mental status) carries a worse prognosis.

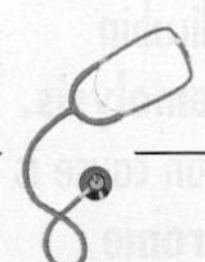

Charcot's triad:

- RUQ pain
- Jaundice
- Fever

For Reynolds' pentad; add:

- Shock (hypotension)
- Altered mental status

DIAGNOSIS

- **Ultrasound** may show stones in the common bile duct.
- Also, intrahepatic **biliary ductal dilatation** is an important finding, as well as **peri-cholecystic fluid.**
- If ultrasound does not give a diagnosis, magnetic resonance cholangiopancreatography (MRCP) is the next diagnostic study.

TREATMENT

Biliary drainage, which can be achieved in several ways:

- ERCP with stone extraction.
- Endoscopic sphincterotomy.
- Percutaneous drain.
- Surgery.
- Also:
  - Fluid resuscitation, vasopressors as needed for hemodynamic support.
  - Broad-spectrum antibiotics to cover *E coli, Klebsiella, Enterococcus,* and *Bacteroides* (gram negative).

Primary Sclerosing Cholangitis

A chronic progressive disorder of unknown etiology characterized by inflammation, fibrosis, and strictures of the medium- and large-diameter intrahepatic and extrahepatic biliary tree.

- Many develop cholangiocarcinoma.
- There is a strong association with **ulcerative colitis.**

TREATMENT

Balloon dilatation of obstructed biliary tree. The only cure is a liver transplant.

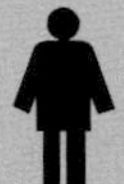

A 34-year-old man with a history of ulcerative colitis presents with jaundice and elevated GGT and alkaline phosphatase. *Think: Primary sclerosing cholangitis.* **Next step:** ERCP showing "string-of-beads" appearance of biliary tree is diagnostic.

DISORDERS OF THE LIVER

Normal Function of the Liver

General rule: When **indirect bilirubin is much higher than direct** bilirubin, it usually means there is an ↑ bilirubin production by **hemolysis.** The other common cause is **Gilbert's syndrome** (harmless, common defect in bilirubin conjugation).

- Carbohydrate metabolism (glucose homeostasis).
- Plasma protein synthesis (albumin).
- Bile acid synthesis.
- Coagulation factor synthesis.
- Lipid synthesis.
- Vitamin storage.
- Detoxification of many endogenous and exogenous substances.
- Hormone metabolism.
- Nitrogenous waste processing (urea cycle).
- See Table 2.3-3 for explanation of liver function tests.

Cirrhosis

Chronic hepatic injury associated with hepatocellular necrosis, fibrosis, and nodular regeneration. There are many causes of cirrhosis (alcohol, hepatitis, etc.) listed below. They all share common clinical picture.

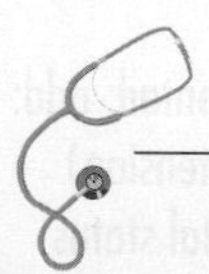

If the transaminases (AST/ALT) stand out as the most abnormal, the defect is usually parenchymal liver damage. If the alkaline phosphatase stands out as most abnormal, it is usually obstructive.

DIAGNOSIS

Can be made by liver biopsy; CT scan can suggest cirrhosis.

SIGNS AND SYMPTOMS

These can be seen with cirrhosis from any cause:

- Loss of appetite, nausea, vomiting.
- Jaundice (from high bilirubin) and pruritis.
- Signs of portal hypertension (varices, spider telangiectasia, ascites, edema, caput madusae).
- Bleeding (from ↓ clotting factors made in liver).

TABLE 2.3-3. A Comparison of Lab Findings in Obstructive and Parenchymal Liver Disease

Test	Obstructive	Parenchymal
AST/ALT	Slight elevation	Very high
Alkaline phosphatase	Very high	Slight elevation
Albumin	Normal	↓
PT	Normal–slight elevation	Very high
Bilirubin: Direct (conjugated)	Normal–very high	Normal–very high
Bilirubin: Indirect (unconjugated)	Normal–slight elevation	Normal–very high
GGT	Very high	Normal–very high

ALT: alanine transaminase; AST: aspartate transaminase; GGT: gamma-glutamyl transpeptidase; PT: prothrombin time.

- Encephalopathy (mental status change possibly due to ↑ NH_3 and ↑ gamma-aminobutyric acid [GABA]).
- Palmar erythema (redness of palms).
- Dupuytren's contractures (contractures of palmar fascia resulting in flexion of fourth digit).
- Gynecomastia and hypogonadism.
- Early in cirrhosis, LFTs are high and there is hepatomegaly; as cirrhosis advances, LFTs begin to normalize (liver is burned out) and liver atrophies (nonpalpable).

Treatment

- Cease alcohol consumption.
- High-protein diet (1 g/kg body weight) and multivitamins.
- Avoid hepatotoxins (eg, acetaminophen, isoniazid).
- Spironolactone (potassium-sparing diuretic) for ascites.
- Lactulose for hepatic encephalopathy (broken down by colonic bacteria and causes NH_3 to convert to NH_4, which cannot cross the blood-brain barrier).

Alcoholic Cirrhosis

Most common cause of cirrhosis in North America.

Etiology

- Caused by chronic alcoholism.
- *Alcoholic fatty liver*, a mostly asymptomatic, reversible form of liver injury, often precedes cirrhosis.
- *Alcoholic hepatitis* initiates the necrosis.

Findings Specific to Alcoholic Cirrhosis/Liver Damage

- AST/ALT ratio > 2.
- GGT is most sensitive serum marker for alcohol bingeing.

NONALCOHOLIC CAUSES OF CIRRHOSIS

- Viral hepatitis.
- Primary biliary cirrhosis.
- Hemochromatosis.
- Cardiac cirrhosis (CHF causing congestive hepatopathy).
- Wilson's disease.
- Alpha-1-antitrypsin deficiency.

Primary Biliary Cirrhosis

Autoimmune disease causing destruction of *intrahepatic* bile ducts.

ETIOLOGY

Unknown, but *antimitochondrial antibodies* are the serologic hallmark, and the pathology results from an autoimmune response to the biliary epithelium.

EPIDEMIOLOGY

More common in middle-aged women, often associated with autoimmune disease (scleroderma, Sjögren's).

SIGNS AND SYMPTOMS

- Pruritus.
- Jaundice.
- Xanthomas (deposits of cholesterol in skin). Presence of an additional (extrahepatic) autoimmune disorder (eg, rheumatoid arthritis or Sjögren's).

Primary biliary cirrhosis: Women, autoimmune diseases vs. **Primary sclerosing cholangitis:** Men, ulcerative colitis

DIAGNOSIS

Presence of antimitochondrial antibodies (90% sensitive).

TREATMENT

- Liver transplant is the only cure.
- Ursodiol (ursodeoxycholate [synthetic bile acid]) may slow progression.

Portal Hypertension

↑ portal vascular resistance caused by cirrhosis, portal vein obstruction, or hepatic vein thrombosis.

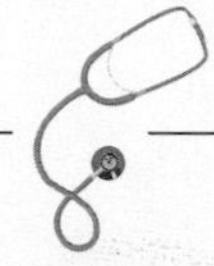

Schistosomiasis is the most common cause of portal hypertension worldwide.

COMPLICATIONS

- Esophageal varices.
- Splenomegaly.
- Ascites.
- Hemorrhoids.
- Caput medusae (periumbilical collateral vessels visible on abdomen).

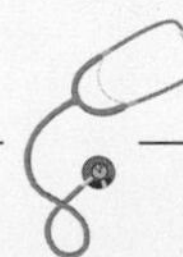

Acute variceal bleeds have a 50% mortality.

TREATMENT

- Creation of shunts to ↓ pressure: Portosystemic shunt surgery.
- Transjugular intrahepatic portocaval shunt (TIPS) between hepatic and portal veins.
- Propranolol reduces portal pressure and reduces chance of variceal bleeds.
- Liver transplant.

Esophageal Variceal Bleeding

- Bleeding from esophageal vessels that have ↑ pressure 2° to portal hypertension.
- **Variceal bleeding** presents as hematemesis or hypotension from blood loss.
- This is a **high-pressure bleed and is an emergency.**

TREATMENT

- **Immediate:** Aggressive hydration (place large-bore catheters and give fluid!) and endoscopic sclerotherapy or banding.
- Balloon tamponade is a last resort.
- **Other therapy:** Somatostatin **(octreotide).**
- Beta blockade.
- Replace clotting factors with fresh frozen plasma if there is a coagulopathy from liver dysfunction.

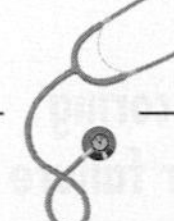

Somatostatin (octreotide)
Inhibits visceral blood flow and that's why it works for upper GI and variceal bleeds.
Inhibits GI motility and that's why it can be used for refractory diarrhea.

A patient presents with bleeding esophageal varices. After stabilizing with IV fluid, what is the next step? *Octreotide* followed by EGD for banding of varices.

Hepatic Encephalopathy

- A reversible (usually) mental status change associated with hepatocellular dysfunction.
- It can happen at any time in a cirrhotic patient, but can be precipitated by infection, GI bleed, or ↑ dietary protein.
- Its cause is unclear, but theorized to be related to ↑ NH_3 and ↑ GABA in the central nervous system (CNS).

SIGNS AND SYMPTOMS

- **Mental status changes,** ranging from mild to marked obtundation/coma.
- **Asterixis** (flapping of hands when arms extended).
- **Fetor hepaticus** (peculiar breath smell) may be present.

DIAGNOSIS

- Mainly clinical grounds, but exclude other causes (acute alcohol intoxication, delirium tremens, metabolic disorders, etc).
- Elevated NH_3 can also help.

TREATMENT

- **Protein restriction.**
- **Lactulose** (involving gut bacteria, it converts ammonia to ammonium ion, which is excreted in stool).
- **Neomycin** (kills urease-producing bacteria in the gut).

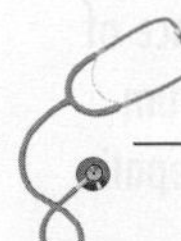

In early liver disease, patients are placed on a high-protein diet because the general state of protein malnutrition puts the body at a disadvantage to fight other stresses such as infection. In end-stage liver disease, the liver cannot break down protein, and the excess accumulation can cause encephalopathy. At this stage, the patient is protein restricted.

Spontaneous Bacterial Peritonitis

- An acute bacterial infection of the peritoneal fluid in patients with ascites.
- Presents with **ascites, fever, and abdominal pain.**

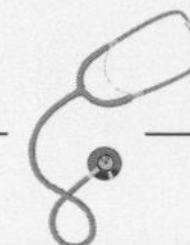

Most common organism in spontaneous bacterial peritonitis: *E coli.*

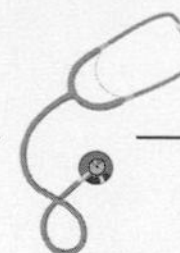

Miscellaneous scoring systems of liver failure (don't memorize, just know about):
MELD scoring: Predicts the survival of a patient with end-stage hepatic disease taking account of International Normalized Ratio (INR), bilirubin, and serum creatinine level.
Child-Turcotte-Pugh score: Used to assess the prognosis of chronic liver disease, mainly cirrhosis, and the necessity of liver transplantation. This scoring system employs bilirubin, presence of ascites, INR, serum albumin, and hepatic encephalopathy.

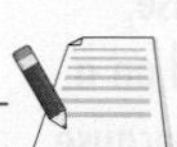

Hepatotoxicity due to acetaminophen (APAP) poisoning can be *prevented* by early determination of APAP levels and administration of *N*-acetylcysteine (NAC).

DIAGNOSIS

Perform **abdominal paracentesis.** Positive results are any of the following: > 250 **polymorphonuclear cells/μL** considered diagnostic (or >100 PMN/μL when patient is receiving peritoneal dialysis) + Gram stain or culture of ascetic fluid.

TREATMENT

Antibiotics with enteric gram negative coverage (eg, cefuroxime).

Hepatorenal Syndrome

- The development of acute renal failure in patients with advanced hepatic disease, characterized by azotemia, renal sodium sparing, and oliguria.
- It is usually seen as worsening renal failure/oliguria and hypotension (from low albumin).
- It can be precipitated by any large fluid shift in a liver-failure patient (eg, diuresis or paracentesis).

DIAGNOSIS

- Urine sodium < 10 mEq/L.
- Hyponatremia

TREATMENT

- None proven effective.
- Infusion of albumin has never proven definitively effective (but it's commonly done).

Hepatitis

Infection or inflammation of the liver due to:

- Viral hepatitis A, B, C, D ("delta"), E, or G; CMV; Epstein-Barr virus (EBV), or herpes virus.
- Alcohol.
- Toxins: Acetaminophen, aflatoxin (found in peanuts).

SIGNS AND SYMPTOMS

- Right upper quadrant pain.
- Nausea, vomiting, malaise, fever.
- Jaundice.

HEPATITIS A VIRUS

- RNA virus.
- Spread by fecal-oral route.
- Incubation period: 15–50 days.
- No chronic carrier or infection state.

DIAGNOSIS

- Anti-HAV IgM: Acute infection.
- Anti-HAV IgG: Immunity from prior infection.

TREATMENT

- Symptomatic.
- **Self-limited, no progression to chronic liver disease.**

PREVENTION

- Safe dietary practices.
- If exposed: Anti-HAV immunoglobulin.
- HAV vaccine is given to all with chronic liver disease (especially hepatitis C), travel to high-risk countries, high-risk behavior, high-risk communities.

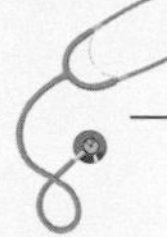

Etiology of viral hepatitis:
Vowels from the bowels (A and E, fecal-oral route)
Consonants from "consumance" (B, C, D, G from sex and blood)

HEPATITIS B VIRUS

- DNA virus.
- Spread by percutaneous or mucous membrane exposure to blood, semen, and saliva.
- Incubation period: 45–160 days.

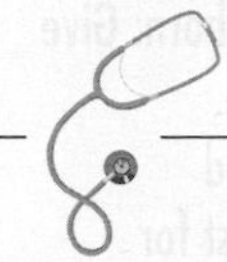

HBV is the *only* DNA hepatic virus.

DIAGNOSIS

See Table 2.3-4 for more complete, but quick rules:

- HbsAg positive: Infection is present.
- Anti-HBc IgM: Acute infection (window period).
- Anti-HBs IgG: Past infection or vaccine (indicates immunity).

TABLE 2.3-4. Hepatitis B Markers

DISEASE STATE	MARKER	APPROXIMATE TIME FROM EXPOSURE TO DETECTION IN SERUM	EXPLANATION
Early infection	HBcAg (hepatitis B core antigen)	Never detectable	Intracellular antigen expressed in infected hepatocytes; not detectable in the serum.
Acute infection	Anti-HBc IgM	1.5–6 months	Window period (there can be a several-week gap between the disappearance of HBsAg and the appearance of anti-HBs in the serum, during this time infection can be detected with anti-HBc IgM).
Active hepatitis or carrier	HBsAg	1–6 months	Viral protein coat.
High infectivity, chronic hepatitis	HBeAg	1–4 months	Indicates ongoing viral replication.
Low infectivity	Anti-HBe	4 months–years	Present in acute phase.
Immunity (past infection or vaccine)	Anti-HBs IgG	6 months–years	In serum after disappearance of HBsAg.
Remote infection	Anti-HBc IgG	6 months–years	Remains detectable longest.

PREVENTION

- Vaccine.
- Hepatitis B immune globulin (HBIG) (if < 7 days of exposure).
- HbsAg positive pregnancy: Infant should receive HBIG and hepatitis B vaccine.

TREATMENT

Lamivudine.

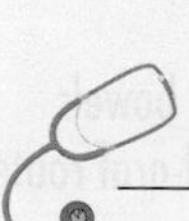

Hepatitis B exposure scenarios:

- Exposed newborn: Give HBIG vaccine.
- Infected blood exposure: Test for hepatitis B and if negative, give HBIG alone.
- Vaccine is okay in pregnancy.

COMPLICATIONS

- One percent will develop fulminant hepatic necrosis.
- Ten percent of adults (90% neonates) will develop chronic carrier state or chronic hepatitis with an ↑ risk of hepatocellular carcinoma (HCC).

HEPATITIS C VIRUS

- RNA virus.
- Spread by blood and body fluid contact (common from past blood transfusions and tattoos, IV drugs).
- Incubation 15–160 days.
- Most common form of hepatitis in the United States.
- Hepatitis G is similar to hepatitis C.

DIAGNOSIS

- Anti-HCV IgG presents 1–6 months after infectivity and indicates chronic or past infection.
- Polymerase chain reaction (PCR) for hepatitis C RNA measures viral load.

TREATMENT

- Interferon and ribavirin (reduce risk of hepatoma).
- Hepatitis C genotype can predict response to therapy.

COMPLICATIONS

Seventy to eighty percent develop chronic hepatitis, and 25% of these develop cirrhosis and/or hepatocellular carcinoma.

HEPATITIS D VIRUS OR "DELTA" AGENT

- Hepatitis D/"delta": "Defective" RNA virus that **requires coinfection with HBV** for replication and expression.
- Spread by blood or body fluid exposure as a *coinfection* (simultaneously with HBV) or a *superinfection* (patient already infected with HBV).
- **Makes hepatitis B more severe.**

DIAGNOSIS

Anti-HDV IgM.

HEPATITIS E VIRUS

- RNA virus.
- Incubation period: 15–60 days.
- Fecal-oral transmission.
- Occurs in India, Asia, Africa, and Central America.

- High rate of fulminant liver failure, especially if pregnant.
- No chronic carrier or infection state.
- Only supportive treatment.

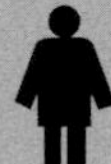

A medical resident develops severe symptoms of fever, jaundice, and *signs of severe liver failure* after returning from a trip to India. *Think: Hepatitis E.* **Next step:** Supportive management.

Liver Transplantation

- Liver transplant is used in selected cases of severe, irreversible liver disease.
- If successful, has a 5-year survival rate of better than 80%.
- Factors to determine eligibility reflect severity of disease: Bilirubin, INR, creatinine.
- Immunosuppression is often required to prevent rejection (cyclophosphamide, tacrolimus, OKT3 (anti–T cell).
- **Acute rejection** is suspected in a patient with RUQ pain, fever, ↑ LFTs. Treat with immunosuppression.
- Donor liver needs to be ABO and size matched, but not HLA matched.
- **Indications for liver transplant** can include select cases of sclerosing cholangitis, primary biliary sclerosis, or specific cases in any cause of liver failure.

DISORDERS OF THE COLON

Carcinoid Tumor

- A neuroendocrine tumor arising from ectodermal stem cells in the gut, usually in the ileum (often in appendix), making up about 30% of gut neoplasms.
- It is generally slow growing and causes symptoms by the aberrant secretion of various neurotransmitters/hormones (most often **serotonin** [5-HT], **bradykinin,** and **histamine**).
- Though slow growing, it can metastasize to lymph nodes, lung, or liver.
- Most are idiopathic, but can be part of **MEN type I.**

Signs and Symptoms

- One or several of the following: flushing (bradykinin); diarrhea (serotonin); wheezing (histamine). Can also get bowel obstruction or appendicitis.
- **Carcinoid syndrome** occurs in 5–10% and consists of severe symptoms of the following triad: cutaneous flushing, diarrhea, and right-sided valvular heart disease (from serotonin).

Diagnosis

Testing for enzyme and hormone levels: Urine levels of 5-hydroxyindoleacetic acid (5-HIAA) and 5-HT (serotonin) + abdominal CT to look for mass.

TREATMENT

- **Surgical excision** or radioablation for local treatment.
- **Somatostatin** (octreotide) has been found to ↓ symptoms (unlikely that it slows progression, but this is controversial).
- Prognosis depends on size of tumor and whether or not there is metastasis.
- The occurrence of carcinoid syndrome usually is associated with worse prognosis.

PROGNOSIS

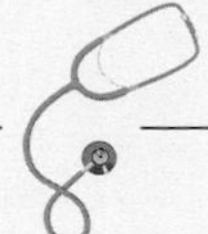
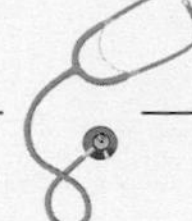

Types of GI cancer differ based on region:
- **Esophagus: Squamous or adenocarcinoma**
- **Stomach, duodenum and jejunum, and colon: Adenocarcinoma**
- **Ileum: Carcinoid, lipoma, and lymphoma**

- Multifactorial. Typically, prognosis can be determined by the size of the primary tumor, the presence or absence of metastases, as well as the anatomic location of the primary tumor.
- Patients with a carcinoid tumor found in the appendix tend to have superior prognoses (probably due to its being found early on, before mets).

Diverticulosis

- An *acquired* condition of the colon in which saclike protrusions of colonic mucosa herniate through a defect in the muscle layer (where nutrient arteries insert) (see Figure 2.3-5).
- Diverticulae are most common in the sigmoid colon, probably because this is the narrowest area of the colon and therefore subject to the highest pressures.
- **Risk factors** are **low-fiber diet** and advanced age.
- Can cause **severe painless bleeding** when there is erosion through a vessel.

TREATMENT

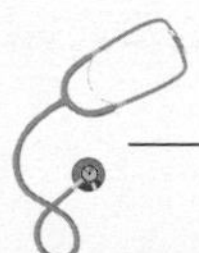

Diverticulosis is the most common cause of massive lower GI bleeding in patients over age 60.

Bleeding scan to localize the vessel and **embolize,** or **colectomy** if refractory.

Diverticulitis

Diverticulitis is inflammation and/or infection of a diverticulum due to impaction of fecal material in the diverticular neck.

SIGNS AND SYMPTOMS

LLQ pain, fever, and may have sigmoid mass on exam.

DIAGNOSIS

Typically done with CT (show inflamed diverticula and pericolic fat).

TREATMENT

- NPO, IV fluids, pain control.
- Antibiotics to cover gram-negative anaerobes, particularly *E coli, Klebsiella, Enterobacter, Bacteroides,* and *Enterococcus* (typically ciprofloxacin and metronidazole [Flagyl] or clindamycin and gentamicin).
- **Never do colonoscopy in a patient with diverticulitis (risk of perforation).**

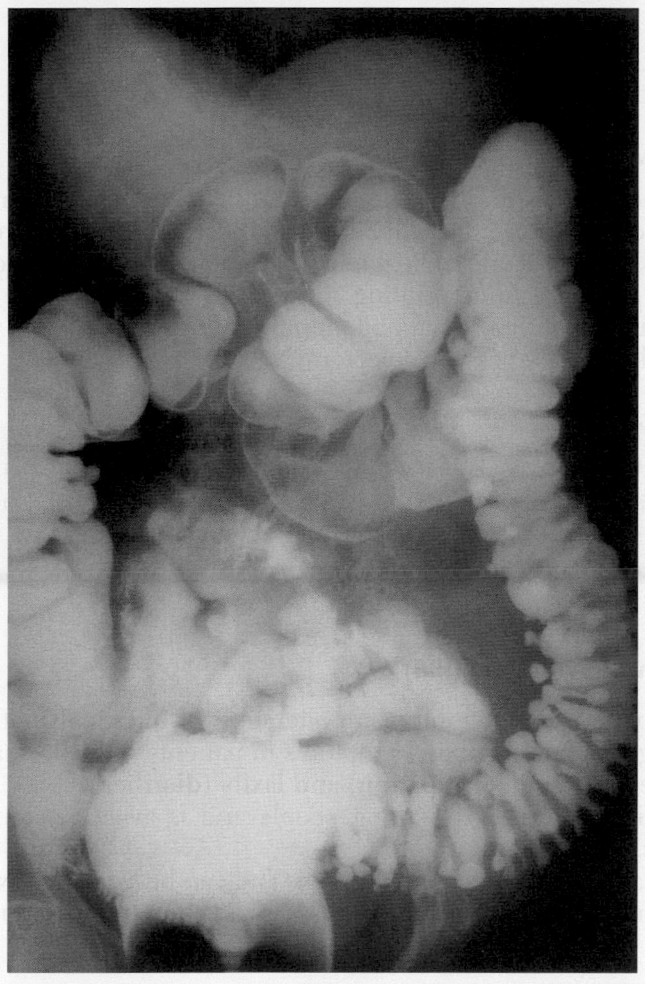

FIGURE 2.3-5. Diverticulosis.

Barium study in a patient with diverticulosis demonstrates many small contrast-filled outpouchings in the sigmoid colon. (Reproduced, with permission, from *Schwartz's Principles of Surgery*, 7th ed. New York: McGraw-Hill, 2000: 1277.)

Pseudomembranous Colitis

- A colonic infection caused by *Clostridium difficile*, a spore-forming anaerobe sometimes found normally in the GI tract. When *C difficile* overgrows, due to eradication of competing gut flora by antibiotics, it may release exotoxins A and B, which damage colonic mucosa.
- Classically associated with **clindamycin**, *but any antibiotic can do it*.

Signs and Symptoms

- Crampy, diffuse abdominal pain and ***foul-smelling diarrhea*** with history of antibiotic use.
- Can have fever.

Diagnosis

- *C difficile* toxin in stool (insensitive).
- Sigmoidoscopy/colonoscopy shows pathognomonic yellowish membranous plaques (pseudomembranes) adherent to colonic mucosa.

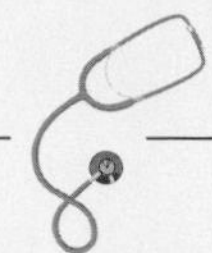

C difficile is the most common cause of nosocomial enteric infection.

TREATMENT

- Stop the offending antibiotic if possible.
- **Metronidazole PO** or **vancomycin PO** (if Flagyl fails).

COMPLICATIONS

Toxic megacolon is a dreaded complication that can occur when inflammation and infection spread through all layers of the colon wall. Severe diarrhea and toxicity develop. Plain radiography may show a long colon loop with diameter > 8 cm and "thumbprinting" (bowel-wall edema)—these patients require careful monitoring, serial abdominal exams, and imaging, as well as a surgical evaluation for possible colectomy.

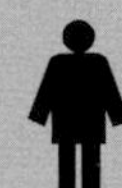

A 68-year-old man in the hospital for 3 weeks for pneumonia returns with new-onset diarrhea. *Think: C difficile*. **Next step:** Send stool for C. diff Toxin A and B from three different samples.

Irritable Bowel Syndrome (IBS)

- Irritable bowel syndrome is an alteration of intestinal motility that → changes in bowel habits. Symptoms in patients with IBS may **fluctuate between spasm (constipation) and laxity (diarrhea)**.
- It typically presents in young people and is twice as common in females.
- It usually has no systemic symptoms and can be **associated with stress**.
- Diagnosis requires that other causes of diarrhea are ruled out.

Giardia infection and lactose intolerance may present similarly to IBS, so they must be ruled out.

TREATMENT

- Reassurance.
- High-fiber and low-fat diet.
- Anxiolytic, antispasmodic, or antidiarrheal in severe cases.

Inflammatory Bowel Disease

- A chronic inflammation affecting the GI tract.
- Two types: Crohn's disease (CD) and ulcerative colitis (UC).

SIGNS AND SYMPTOMS

UC

- Bloody diarrhea (more prominent than in CD)
- Rectal pain
- More acute flares

CD

- Tender RLQ mass
- More indolent, chronic

See Table 2.3-5 for extraintestinal manifestations.

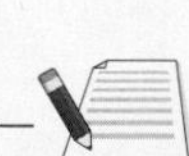

Crohn's: Lower incidence, lower risk of cancer, but more common in men than ulcerative colitis.

EPIDEMIOLOGY

- More common in people of Caucasian and Jewish background.
- Peak incidence in ages 15–35.
- Occurs with familial clustering.

TABLE 2.3-5. Extraintestinal Manifestations of Inflammatory Bowel Disease (occur in 20% of patients)

Eye involvement	▪ Uveitis ▪ Episcleritis	CD > UC Uveitis, erythema nodosum, and colitic arthritis are commonly seen together.
Dermatologic	▪ Erythema nodosum	CD, especially in children > UC Parallels disease course (gets better as IBD improves)
	▪ Pyoderma gangrenosum	UC > CD May or may not follow disease course
	▪ Aphthous ulcers	CD
Arthritis	▪ Colitic arthritis	CD > UC Parallels disease course
	▪ Ankylosing spondylitis	30 times more common in UC Unrelated to disease course
Hematologic	▪ Anemia ▪ Thromboembolism	UC = CD UC = CD
Hepatobiliary	▪ Fatty liver ▪ Hepatitis ▪ Cholelithiasis ▪ Primary sclerosing cholangitis	UC = CD UC = CD UC = CD
Renal	▪ Secondary amyloidosis → renal failure	UC > CD CD Unrelated to disease course

- UC more common in women; CD more common in men.
- Associated **risk of colon cancer is 10–30 times for UC** and 3 times for CD.

Pathology

UC

- Inflammation of the **mucosa only** (exudate of pus, blood, and mucous from the *crypt abscess*).
- Always **starts in rectum** (up to one-third don't progress).
- Primary pathology limited to colon.

CD

- Inflammation involves **all bowel-wall layers**, which is what may → fistulas and abscess.
- Rectal sparing in 50%.
- Granulomas.
- Mouth to anus involvement.

Indications for Colonoscopy

- Primary diagnosis.
- Biopsy of the stricture or filling defects.
- **Surveillance for cancer** if had for > 8 years.

Diagnosis (Colonoscopy Findings)

UC
- **Continuous lesions** (always includes rectum).
- **Aphthous ulcers rare.**
- **Lead pipe colon** appearance due to chronic scarring and subsequent retraction and loss of haustra.

CD
- **Skip lesions:** Interspersed normal and diseased bowel.
- **Aphthous ulcers common.**
- **Cobblestone** appearance (from submucosal thickening interspersed with mucosal ulceration).

Treatment

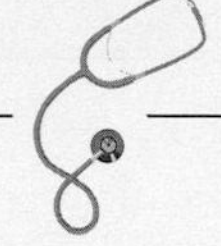

Inflammatory bowel disease symptoms **improve with nicotine (smoking).** Patients can wear dermal patches.

- **Sulfasalazine:**
  - Consists of 5-ASA (active component) and sulfapyridine (toxic effects are due to this moiety).
  - How it works in IBD is unknown (because other NSAIDs do not work). It is activated in the colon by colonic bacteria, so it is ineffective for small bowel.
- **Mesalamine/olsalazine:**
  - Given topically (enema) or orally.
  - Similar to sulfasalazine but active in small bowel if taken orally; active in colon only if given by enema.
- **Corticosteroids:** Given in severe cases; works better in UC than CD.
- **Antibiotics (used for CD):** Metronidazole can be effective.
- **Immunomodulators:**
  - Used in refractory cases, especially in CD on chronic steroids.
  - Include azathioprine and 6-mercaptopurine (both purine analogs) and methotrexate.
  - Infliximab (Remicade) (antibody to TNF-α) is used in refractory CD and in fistulizing forms. It is also used as a steroid-sparing agent for maintenance of remission in the treatment of CD.
- **Surgical treatment:**
  - Surgery in UC can be curative, and is done in intractable disease or complications such as perforation, hemorrhage, or cancer.
  - Surgery in CD is typically not curative (recurrence often seen at anastomosis site) but still done in certain of the above situations.

Complications

UC
- Perforation.
- Stricture (presence may suggest cancer).
- Megacolon.

CD
- Abscess.
- Fistulas.
- Perianal disease (abscess, fistula).

Colorectal Cancer

- The second most common cause of cancer death in the United States.
- Most cases are thought to arise from adenomatous polyps, usually sessile, **villous polyps** ("villains" that cause cancer).
- **Diagnosed with colonoscopy.**

Risk Factors

- Age > 40 years.
- Personal history of adenoma or colon cancer.
- Inflammatory bowel disease.
- Family history.

Signs and Symptoms

- Can be consequence of blood loss (weakness, pallor), constipation (obstructing lesion), frank bleeding, pencil-thin stools, pain, or weight loss.
- **Left colon lesions** usually cause thin stools, rectal bleeding, obstruction.
- **Right colon lesions** usually cause more insidious blood loss (not frank bleeding) and can present with severe anemia.
- **Labs** can demonstrate **Fe-deficient anemia,** elevated carcinoembryonic antigen (CEA)—not recommended for screen or diagnosis, but can be useful to follow disease. Preoperative levels useful in assessing prognosis and follow-up, but otherwise of no diagnostic value. Elevated LFTs may indicate liver metastasis.

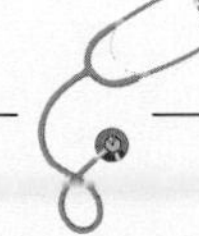

Many colorectal cancers are within reach of the examiner's finger on rectal exam. Many patients with colon cancer have negative FOBT (insensitive).

Screening (American Cancer Society Recommendations)

- Annual digital rectal exam beginning at age 40.
- Annual fecal occult blood test (FOBT) screening beginning at age 50.
- Flexible sigmoidoscopy—every 3–5 years beginning at age 50, if asymptomatic with no risk factors.
- Colonoscopy is recommended for positive FOBT or positive sigmoidoscopy and for patients with inflammatory bowel disease or hereditary colorectal cancer syndromes.
- Colonoscopy generally has been used with ↑ frequency over flexible sigmoidoscopy and may be a better alternative (it views entire colon rather than just sigmoid).
- Diagnosis requires biopsy (see Figure 2.3-6).

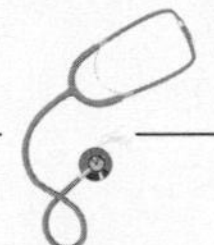

Polyps:

- **Tubular—benign.**
- **Villous or tubulovillous—have malignant potential.**
- **The larger the polyp, the more malignant potential (> 1 cm).**

If a polyp is found on colonoscopy, perform polypectomy/biopsy and repeat colonoscopy in 3 years.

Colon Cancer Staging and Treatment

- Dukes and TNM are both staging systems for colon cancer. TNM is preferred (see Table 2.3-6).
- Radiation is typically used only in rectal cancer.
- Chemotherapy typically consists of 5-fluorouracil (FU) and levimasole with the addition (sometimes) of oxaliplatinum or irinotecan.
- Colonoscopy is needed within 6–12 months postoperatively to exclude synchronous lesions; if negative, then every 3 years.
- Most early-stage cancers are cured.
- TNM staging and treatment made simple:
  - Stage I and II are local lesions confined to colon with no nodes. Usually treat with resection only (5-year survival > 70%).
  - Stage III is node positive. Usually treat with resection + adjuvant chemotherapy (5-year survival 40–60%).
  - Stage IV is metastatic disease. Usually chemotherapy only (can resect lesion if bleeding or obstructed for palliation; 5-year survival < 10%).
- **Duke's staging system for colorectal cancer:**
  - **A:** Mucosal involvement only, above muscularis propria, no lymph node involvement.
  - **B1:** Into muscularis propria but above pericolic fat, no lymph node involvement.
  - **B2:** Into pericolic or perirectal fat, no lymph node involvement.

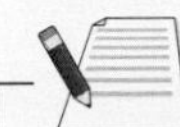

Endocarditis with *Streptococcus bovis* or *Clostridium septicum* is associated with colon cancer.

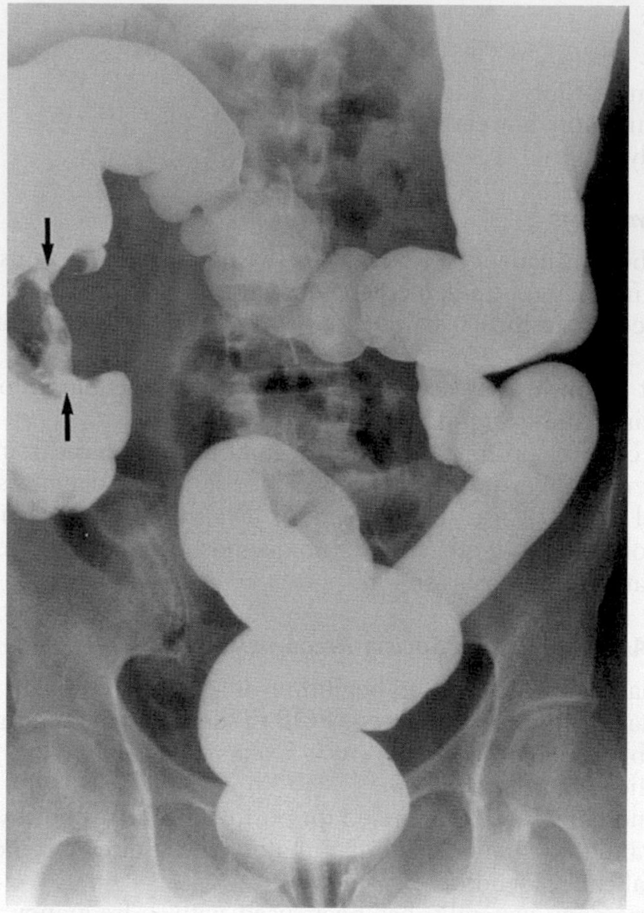

FIGURE 2.3-6. Colon cancer.

Barium study in a patient with colon cancer demonstrates an "apple core"–shaped filling defect at the site of a circumferential neoplasm. (Reproduced, with permission, from Schwartz SI, Fischer JE, Spencer FC, Shires GT, Daly JM. *Schwartz's Principles of Surgery*, 7th ed. New York: McGraw-Hill, 1998: 1347.)

- C1: Same penetration as B1 with nodal metastases.
- C2: Same penetration as B2 with nodal metastases.
- D: Distant metastases.

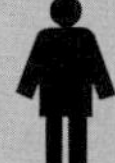

A 70-year-old woman presents with microcytic anemia, weight loss, and a vague abdominal pain that is not related to food or time of day. *Think: Colorectal cancer.* **Next step:** Colonoscopy.

Hereditary Colon Cancer Syndromes

- **Familial polyposis coli** (high risk for colorectal cancer):
  - Autosomal dominant condition in which thousands of adenomatous polyps appear throughout the colon by age 25.
  - Most untreated patients develop colon cancer by age 40.
  - Treatment: Prophylactic *total colectomy.*

TABLE 2.3-6. TNM Staging (Preferred)

Tis	Carcinoma in situ.
T1	Tumor invades submucosa.
T2	Tumor invades muscularis propria.
T3	Tumor invades through the muscularis propria into the subserosa, pericolic or perirectal tissues.
T4	Tumor directly invades other organs or structures.
NX	Regional nodes cannot be assessed.
N0	No positive nodes.
N1	Metastasis in 1–3 regional lymph nodes.
N2	Metastasis in 4 or more regional lymph nodes.
MX	Distant metastasis cannot be assessed.
M0	No distant metastasis.
M1	Distant metastasis.

Stage 0	Tis	N0	M0
Stage I	T1–2	N0	M0
Stage IIA	T3	N0	M0
Stage IIB	T4	N0	M0
Stage IIIA	T1–2	N1	M0
Stage IIIB	T3–4	N1	M0
Stage IIIC	Any T	N2	M0
Stage IV	Any T	Any N	M1

- **Hereditary nonpolyposis colon cancer (HNPCC)** (high risk):
  - Autosomal dominant condition in which three or more relatives of a patient, and at least one first-degree relative, develop colon cancer at an early age.
  - Often multiple other primary cancers in family.
- **Gardner's syndrome** (high risk): Autosomal-dominant disorder characterized by polyposis coli, supernumerary teeth, osteomas, and fibrous dysplasia of the skull.
- **Peutz-Jeghers syndrome** (low to moderate risk):

- Multiple polyposis of small intestine with multiple pigmented melanin macules in oral mucosa.
- Associated with gynecological cancers.

GASTROINTESTINAL BLEEDS

General Approach to Bleeding

- **Resuscitation:**
  - Establish IV access with two large-bore IV catheters and transfuse fluids and blood.
  - Evaluate patient for hemodynamic instability (hypotension, tachycardia, orthostasis).
  - Type and crossmatch, complete blood count (CBC), coagulation studies.
- **Determining the source of bleed** (upper GI [UGI] vs. lower GI [LGI] bleed [UGI bleed anatomically defined as bleeding above the ligament of Treitz]):
  - **History and physical:** Evaluate for localization of abdominal pain or tenderness; significant past medical history of peptic ulcer disease, chronic NSAID use, liver disease, recent vomiting or retching.
  - **Rectal exam** for hemorrhoids, mass, or tenderness.
  - **Stool exam for melana/guaiac.**
  - **Nasogastric lavage** looking for bright red blood or coffee grounds (UGI bleed).
    - **UGI bleed may present as hematemesis** (bloody vomitus), **coffee ground emesis** (dark-colored material representing a mixture of blood and gastric acid), **melena, hematochezia** (bright red blood per rectum), or maroon-colored stools with rapid GI bleeds.
    - **LGI bleeds may present as hematochezia** or **melena** (less common) associated with cecal or right colonic bleeds with slow transit of blood.

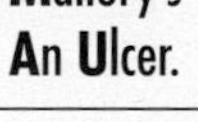

Etiology of UGI bleeds: **M**allory's **V**ices **G**ave (her) **A**n **U**lcer.

Coffee grounds is the term used to describe old, brown, digested blood found on gastric lavage. It usually indicates a source of bleeding proximal to the ligament of Treitz.

UPPER GI BLEEDS

ETIOLOGY

- Mallory-Weiss tear.
- Varices.
- Gastritis/esophagitis.
- Arteriovenous malformation.
- Ulcer: Peptic/duodenal.

SIGNS AND SYMPTOMS

- Hematemesis (bright red or coffee grounds).
- Hypotension.
- Tachycardia.
- Black, tarry stool.
- Very brisk UGI bleeds can be associated with bright red blood per rectum.

Diagnosis

- Gastric lavage severity of bleeding (old vs. new blood).
- Rectal exam with FOBT.
- Endoscopy (also therapeutic): Bleeding scan or arteriography can be done if can not localized bleed.

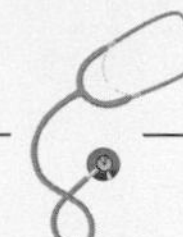

A bleeding scan detects *active* bleeding by infusing a radioactive colloid or radiolabeled autologous RBCs and watching for their collection in the GI tract.

Treatment

Depends on etiology and severity:

- IV fluids and blood.
- Endoscopy with epinephrine injection, cautery or ligation if bleeding ulcers or varices.
- IV proton pump inhibitor.
- Most Mallory–Weiss tears resolve spontaneously.
- For bleeding varices:
  - Somatostatin inhibits gastric, intestinal, and biliary motility, ↓ visceral blood flow.
  - Consider balloon tamponade (rarely used at present).

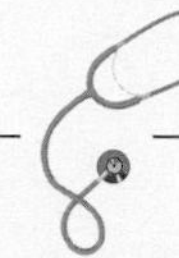

A patient comes in vomiting blood. What do you do?

1. Two large-bore IVs and fluid.
2. Type and crossmatch blood.
3. Endoscopy (for diagnosis and treatment).

Lower GI Bleeds

Etiology

- Cancer or polyps.
- Upper GI bleed (need to rule it out).
- Colitis (infectious, inflammatory bowel disease, ischemic, etc.).
- Angiodysplasia.
- Diverticulosis.
- Hemorrhoids.

Etiology of LGI bleeds: **C**an **U C**ure **A**unt **Di**'s **H**emorrhoids?

Signs and Symptoms

- Hematochezia.
- Melena.
- Signs of blood loss (tachycardia, hypotension).
- Diarrhea (as seen with colitis).

Diagnosis

- Gastric lavage to rule out upper GI source.
- Rectal exam.
- CBC.
- Colonoscopy.
- Bleeding scan or arteriography can be done if colonoscopy cannot be done, or if undiagnostic.

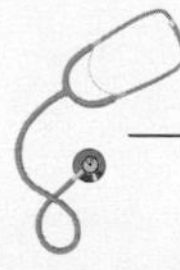

CBC in acute hemorrhage will not reflect the true severity of the bleed for 4–6 hours, as it takes time for the concentrations to change.

Treatment

- IV fluids.
- Blood (RBCs).
- Embolization or surgery.

DIARRHEA

The passage of fluid or semisolid stool with ↑ frequency. Initially, you need to differentiate between infectious versus noninfectious.

History

- **Quantity of diarrhea**: Large-volume (usually small bowel cause) vs. small volume (usually large bowel cause).
- **Quality of stool:** Color, foul odor, blood, mucus, fatty consistency.
- **Length of symptoms: Acute** (< 2 weeks) vs. **persistent** (> 2 weeks) vs. **chronic** (> 4 weeks).
- **Associated symptoms:** Fever, chills, abdominal pain, nausea, vomiting, weight loss.
- **Other questions:** Food intake prior to onset of diarrhea, travel history, presence of predisposing conditions (IBD, small bowel resection, pancreatic disease, immunodeficiency, etc.), medications, recent antibiotic use or hospitalization ↑ risk for *Clostridium difficile* colitis, lactose intolerance, sick contacts.

Exam

General appearance: Does the patient look acutely ill? The presence of one or more of the following will dictate your immediate management of the patient:

- **Vital signs:** Fever, tachycardia, hypotension, orthostatic hypotension.
- **Abdominal exam:** Tenderness, distention, hepatomegaly, ascites.
- **Rectal exam:** Tenderness, mass, stool appearance, occult blood.
- **Skin:** Turgor, rash.

Acute Diarrhea

- Less than 2–4 weeks in duration; usually due to infectious etiology.
- **Workup:**
  - Fecal **leukocytes** (may be suggestive of infectious or inflammatory causes).
  - Stool **culture** for enteric pathogens.
  - Stool test for ***C difficile*** toxins (for pseudomembranous colitis).
  - Stool examination for **ova** and **parasites** (insensitive—must do with three different bowel movements over 3 days).

Common Infectious Pathogens

- **Bacterial:**
  - Noninvasive, all foodborne:
    - Enterotoxigenic *Escherichia coli:* Most common cause of traveler's diarrhea.
    - *Staphylococcus aureus:* Quick onset (3–4 hrs), mostly vomiting, toxin mediated, associated with mayonnaise consumption; patients commonly report having been to a picnic or other such event.
    - *Bacillus cereus:* Associated with reheated rice, commonly from day-old Chinese food.
    - *Clostridium perfringens.*
    - *Vibrio cholerae:* Contaminated water in third-world countries.

- Invasive (bloody):
  - *Campylobacter*: Associated with Guillain-Barré syndrome.
  - *Yersinia*.
  - *Shigella*.
  - *Salmonella*: Raw eggs, uncooked chicken.
  - Enterohemorrhagic *E coli*: Shiga toxin producing *E coli* O157:H7; hemolytic uremic syndrome (HUS).
  - *C difficile*: Pseudomembranous colitis.
- **Viral:** Rotavirus, Norwalk virus, cytomegalovirus (CMV, in the immunocompromised patient).
- **Protozoa** (can also cause chronic diarrhea): *Giardia lamblia* (after hiking trip), *Entamoeba histolytica, Cryptosporidium* (common in AIDS).

Bloody diarrhea—

CASES

C*ampylobacter*
Amoeba (*E. histolytica*)
S*higella*
E *coli*
S*almonella*

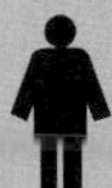

A patient vomits within 6 hours of eating something with mayonnaise (eg, potato salad) at a picnic on a hot day. *Think:* Staphylococcus.

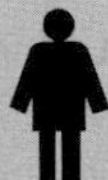

A patient has vomiting/diarrhea after eating reheated rice from leftover Chinese food. *Think:* Bacillus cereus.

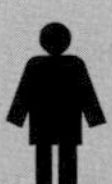

A patient has vomiting and severe watery diarrhea after eating spoiled shellfish. *Think:* Vibrio cholerae.

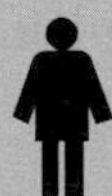

A patient has flatulence and foul-smelling diarrhea after a camping trip. *Think:* Giardia lamblia. **Next step:** Treat with metronidazole.

MANAGEMENT

- Oral or intravenous rehydration and electrolyte replacement.
- Antibiotic therapy when infectious etiology is suspected and patient is moderately to severely ill:
  - If bacterial infections suspected: Empiric treatment with ciprofloxacin or trimethoprim-sulfamethoxazole (TMP-SMX) plus metronidazole for anaerobic coverage. Can also use piperacillin-tazobactam (Zosyn) as monotherapy.
  - If C *difficile* is suspected: PO metronidazole.
  - Treat the underlying disorder (eg, IBD, bacterial overgrowth).
  - Antimotility agents in noninfectious diarrhea (loperamide).

GASTROENTEROLOGY

Chronic Diarrhea

General Classifications and Common Tests

- **Osmotic diarrhea:** Ingestion of nonabsorbable solutes → osmotic water loss in the stool.
  - **Examples:** Magnesium-containing antacids, sodium phosphates, carbohydrates (lactose intolerance).
  - **Test: Fecal electrolytes and calculation of osmotic gap:** Osmotic gap = 290 – 2(Na + K) > 50 mOsm suggestive of an unmeasured solute indicating osmotic component to diarrhea.
- **Secretory diarrhea:** Oversecretion of water by the small and large bowel, which may be caused by bacteria, bacterial toxins, medications, GI hormones (eg, vasoactive intestinal peptide [VIP]), unabsorbed dietary fat.
  - **Examples:** Enteroinvasive bacteria, laxatives, hyperthyroidism, neuroendocrine tumors (eg, carcinoid, VIPoma), irritable bowel syndrome.
- **Inflammatory diarrhea:** Gastrointestinal mucosal irritation and inflammation → an exudative diarrhea.
  - **Examples:** Inflammatory bowel disease (Crohn's, ulcerative colitis).
  - **Tests: Sigmoidoscopy/colonoscopy** in certain cases of colitis will show pseudomembranes or inflammation.
- **Malabsorption diarrhea:** A problem with **either digestion** (ie, lack of digestive enzymes or bile acids) **or transport** (ie, problem with the small bowel mucosa).
  - **Examples:** *Digestive enzyme problems*—chronic pancreatitis, bile acid malabsorption; *transport problems*—celiac sprue, tropical sprue, Whipple's disease.
  - **Tests:**
    - **D-xylose test:** Distinguishes **digestion problem vs. transport problem.** A set amount of D-xylose given PO followed by measuring blood and urine levels to assess for adequate absorption. Xylose requires transport but not digestive enzymes to be absorbed; therefore, adequate amounts in blood/urine demonstrate intact absorption. Low levels of xylose indicate a problem with the small bowel mucosal transport.
    - **Small bowel biopsy:** If a transport problem is suspected in the small bowel, a biopsy will diagnose the cause (eg, Whipple's disease, celiac sprue).
    - **72-hour fecal fat analysis:** Steatorrhea (↑ fecal fat) may be seen in malabsorption due to pancreatic exocrine insufficiency.
- ↓ **transit time:** May → diarrhea by an osmotic mechanism.
  - **Examples**: Dumping syndrome, short gut syndrome.

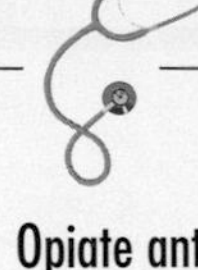

Opiate antidiarrheal agents such as loperamide are generally *contraindicated* in diarrhea due to infectious agents; they promote longer contact time between bacteria and intestinal mucosa.

MAJOR TYPES OF MALABSORPTION

Celiac Sprue

- An **autoimmune condition** affecting the small bowel, triggered by gluten (high-molecular-weight proteins found in wheat, rye, and barley), resulting in malabsorption and diarrhea.
- It is associated with HLA-DR3 and HLA-DQw2.
- Manifestations include vitamin deficiencies, iron deficiency anemia, and malnutrition.

- Diagnosis is made with a small bowel biopsy showing flattened (atrophic) intestinal villi.
- Other tests findings can be the presence of anti-gliadin IgG/IgA, anti-endomysial antibody.
- Treatment is the avoidance of gluten-containing foods (all grains except rice and corn).
- Steroids can be given if severe.

Tropical Sprue

- A malabsorption disease with flattened villi in the **jejunum** similar to celiac sprue—but likely from an infectious etiology.
- It typically occurs to people living in (or visiting) the tropics.
- Symptoms and findings are similar to celiac sprue, but often have megaloblastic anemia due to B_{12} deficiency.
- **Diagnosed by small bowel biopsy demonstrating flattened intestinal villi.**
- Treatment is vitamin B_{12} and folate supplementation in addition to tetracycline.

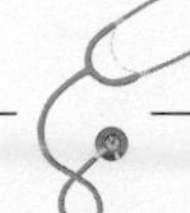

Whipple's Disease vs. Sprue
They can have similar symptoms, but Whipple's is far more severe and has more *constitutional symptoms*, particularly with CNS involvement.

Lactase Deficiency

- Lactase is required to digest lactose, a carbohydrate found in dairy products. Deficiency of lactase results in cramping and diarrhea after ingestion of dairy products.
- Congenital deficiency is rare; a milder late-onset form is commonly found in adults at any time.
- Treat with lactase supplementation and/or the avoidance of dairy products.

Whipple's Disease

- **Whipple's disease** is a severe illness beginning in the GI tract, but spreading systemically, often manifesting with fevers, arthralgias, and CNS symptoms (cranial nerve palsies, memory loss, nystagmus).
- Patients have profound malabsorption syndrome due to destruction of intestinal lamina propria.
- The causative organism is *Tropheryma whippelii.*
- More common in white males.
- **Diagnosis** is made by **PCR testing for *T whippelii*** of the saliva, stool or blood.
- Biopsy demonstrates the replacement of intestinal lamina propria by PAS-positive macrophages.
- **Treatment** is antibiotic therapy with ceftriaxone + TMP-SMX, or tetracycline. Fatal if untreated, curable if treated—a favorite on exams!

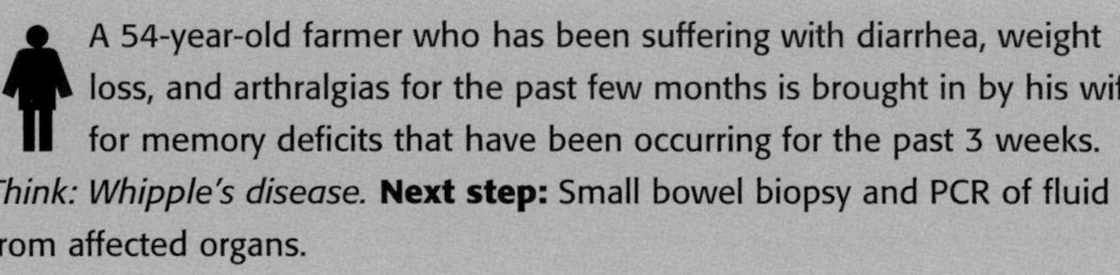

A 54-year-old farmer who has been suffering with diarrhea, weight loss, and arthralgias for the past few months is brought in by his wife for memory deficits that have been occurring for the past 3 weeks. *Think: Whipple's disease.* **Next step:** Small bowel biopsy and PCR of fluid from affected organs.

Protein-Losing Enteropathy

- A condition in which plasma proteins (principally albumin and gamma globulin) fail to be reabsorbed by the gut lumen and are lost in the GI tract; normally they are absorbed by the gut and sent into the portal circulation.
- This occurs due to mucosal injury (inflammatory bowel disease or celiac disease) or ↑ lymphatic pressure (where the proteins are normally absorbed) in gut wall (occurs with neoplasm, CHF).
- Patients get diarrhea and anasarca from protein loss.
- **Diagnose** with alpha-1-antitrypsin levels measured simultaneously in stool and serum.
- **Treatment** is to address underlying cause.

GASTROENTEROLOGY

HIGH-YIELD FACTS IN

Hematology-Oncology

Iron Deficiency Anemia

Anemia from ↓ iron stores, resulting in ↓ hemoglobin synthesis. Most common cause of anemia.

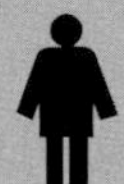

A 47-year-old-man presents with iron deficiency anemia. *Think: Colon cancer unless proven otherwise (up to 20%).* **Next step:** Colonoscopy and endoscopy.

ETIOLOGY

- Blood loss.
- Premenopausal women from menorrhagia.
- Gastrointestinal (GI) blood loss in postmenopausal women and adult men.
- Hookworm in tropical areas.
- Malnutrition/malabsorption (think celiac, etc.).
- Pregnancy.

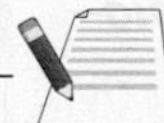

Glossitis means red, beefy (glossy) swollen tongue without papillae, and cheilosis is crusting of angle of mouth.

SIGNS AND SYMPTOMS

- Multigravid woman in her 40s, with tiredness, fatigue, and exertional dyspnea from menorrhagia.
- Pica (ingestion of clay or ice).
- Glossitis and cheilosis (also seen in folate deficiency).
- Spoon nails (koilonychia).

Features of iron deficiency anemia—

Fe KAP

Fe (iron)/**F**atigue
Exercise tolerance ↓
Koilonychia
Angular cheilosis
Pica/**P**allor

DIAGNOSIS

- Microcytic anemia (mean corpuscular volume [MCV] < 80) with ↑ red cell distribution width (RDW; > 15).
- Differential:
  - Thalassemia.
  - Anemia of chronic disease.
  - Sideoroblastic anemia (lead poisoning).
- Low iron, ferritin, and high total iron-binding capacity (TIBC) or transferrin.

Causes of macrocytosis—

FEeD THeM

Folate and vitamin B_{12} deficiency
Ethanol and liver disease
Drugs (AZT, Methotrexate)
Thyroid (hypo)
Hemolysis (Reticulocytosis)
Myelodysplastic syndrome

TREATMENT

Look for the cause, and supplement with oral ferrous sulfate (side effect is lots of constipation—iron is difficult to pass out).

Macrocytic Anemia

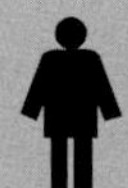

A 38-year-old with HIV on HAART presents with macrocytosis. *Think:* AZT.

There are a variety of causes of macrocytic anemia, including but not limited to folate and vitamin B_{12} deficiency. Other causes include alcohol abuse, certain drugs, metabolic disorders such as hypothyroidism, hemolysis, and bone marrow disorders including myelodysplastic syndrome.

Folate Deficiency Anemia

Anemia from folate deficiency resulting in impaired DNA synthesis.

> ***Causes of folate deficiency anemia—***
>
> ***Pregnant MAN!***
>
> **Pregnancy** and lactation
> **M**alabsorption (celiac and Crohn's)
> **A**lcoholism
> **N**utritional (toast and tea elderly diet)

Etiology

Most common causes of folate deficiency include pregnancy, malabsorption, alcoholism, and malnutrition. Green vegetables are an excellent source of folate and overcooking or lack of adequate intake can lead to deficiencies. In addition, folic acid is absorbed in the upper third of the small intestine, so any disease affecting absorption such as sprue or short gut syndromes will lead to folate deficiency. A thorough history usually reveals the etiology in most cases.

Signs and Symptoms

A typical patient is an elderly, depressed female, living alone and consuming a "tea and toast" diet, presenting with macrocytic anemia, diarrhea, glossitis, and cheilosis. Further questioning reveals that she abuses alcohol daily.

Diagnosis

- High MCV.
- Hypersegmented neutrophils (right shift).
- High homocystiene (also seen in B_{12} deficiency).
- Low red blood cells (RBCs) and serum folate.

> All nutritional anemias (iron, B_{12}, and folate) will have low reticulocytes. Subsequently, reticulocytosis should occur in 3–4 days after replacement.

Treatment

Treat with oral folate.

Vitamin B_{12} Deficiency

Anemia from B_{12} (cobalamin) deficiency resulting in impaired DNA synthesis.

> Folate deficiency can be differentiated from vitamin B_{12} deficiency by the lack of neurologic abnormalities.

Etiology

- Lack of intrinsic factor (pernicious anemia).
- Vegan diet (no dairy).
- Fish tapeworm (*Diphyllobothrium latum*).
- Malabsorption (celiac, Crohn's, bacterial overgrowth, and ileal resection).

Signs and Symptoms

- Anemia (before neurological symptoms).
- Dementia.
- Neurological "megaloblastic madness" symptoms **(not seen in folate deficiency):**
  - Subacute combined degeneration of the dorsal (sensory) and lateral (upper motor neuron) spinal cord columns from myelin deficiency.
  - Symmetrical, affecting the legs and beginning with paresthesias and ataxia (loss of vibration and position sense) and progressing to weakness, spasticity, clonus, and hyperreflexia (upper motor neuron symptoms).

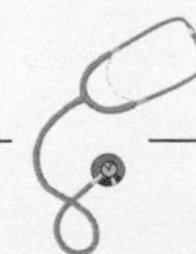

> Anemia precedes neurologic symptoms in vitamin B_{12} deficiency.

DIAGNOSIS

- High MCV.
- Hypersegmented neutrophils (right shift).
- High homocystiene (also seen in folate deficiency).
- **High methylmalonate in urine.**
- Low serum B_{12} level.

TREATMENT

Treat with intramuscular (IM) vitamin B_{12} injections.

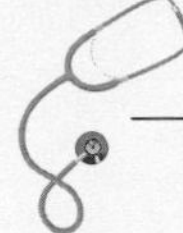

Potassium can drop dramatically during B_{12} replenishment!

Causes of vitamin B_{12} deficiency—VITAMIN B

Vegan diet
Ileal resection
Tapeworm
Autoimmune (pernicious anemia)
Megaloblastic anemia
Inflammation of terminal ileum
Nitrous oxide
Bacterial overgrowth

Pernicious Anemia

PATHOPHYSIOLOGY

- Vitamin B_{12} needs hydrogen ions (gastric acid from parietal cells) to bind to intrinsic factor (IF), which carries it to the terminal ileum where it is absorbed.
- In pernicious anemia, antibodies are made against intrinsic factor and parietal cells, thus impairing the absorption of vitamin B_{12}.
- As parietal cells are destroyed, chronic gastritis and eventually gastric cancer can ensue.
- Other autoimmune processes such as vitiligo are also seen with pernicious anemia.

SIGNS AND SYMPTOMS

- Same as B_{12} deficiency; insidious onset.
- Associated with chronic gastritis, vitiligo, and gastric cancer.

DIAGNOSIS

- Anti-intrinsic factor antibody is the diagnosis of choice (IF-Ab).
- Anti-parietal cell antibody is less sensitive.
- Schilling test (now obsolete): First give IM radioactive vitamin B_{12}. Then give *oral* radioactive iodide. If there is no pernicious anemia, B_{12} will be absorbed and will "spill" in a 24-hour urine specimen (> 10%) as tissue receptors are already saturated.

TREATMENT

Give IM B_{12} shots for life. Newer studies show oral B_{12} in high doses (300–1000 μg/day) is also equally effective.

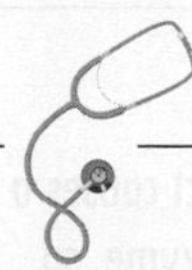

Causes of normocytic normochromic (normal size, normal shape) anemia include:

- Bone marrow problems (aplastic bone marrow, leukemia, myelodysplastic syndromes, etc.)
- ↑ destruction (hemolytic anemias)
- Early nutritional anemias (iron, B_{12}, folate)

Glucose-6-Phosphate Dehydrogenase (G6PD) Deficiency

NORMOCYTIC ANEMIA

There are a myriad of causes of normocytc anemia. Listed below are a few of the more common etiologies encountered in clinical practice.

PATHOPHYSIOLOGY

- An X-linked disease that results from ↓ glutathione in the RBCs.
- G6PD is an enzyme needed to make nicotinamide adenine dinucleotide phosphate (NADPH), which is needed to make glutathione. It helps protect RBCs from the oxidative stress of free radicals.
- In the setting of infections, diabetic ketoacidosis, and medications such as sulfa drugs (trimethoprim-sulfamethoxazole, primaquine), quino-

lones, and also fava beans, hemoglobin (Hb) may precipitate within cells and cause hemolysis. Cells with precipitated Hb have **Heinz bodies,** which are removed by the spleen, resulting in **bite cells.**
- More common in Mediterraneans (Italians, Greeks, Arabs) and African-Americans.

ABCs of G6PD deficiency—

ABCDEFG

Antimalarials
Bactrim/**B**ite cells
Ciprofloxacin
DKA
Inf**E**ction
Fava beans (can be **F**atal without transfusion)
G6PD deficiency

SIGNS AND SYMPTOMS

- Acute hemolysis causing anemia.
- Sudden onset of jaundice (high indirect bilirubin).
- Dark urine (hemoglobinuria).
- Abdominal and back pain.
- Acute tubular necrosis.
- Important cause of neonatal jaundice.

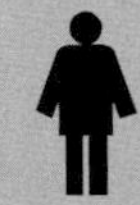

A 31-year-old Italian male with back pain, dark urine, jaundice, and anemia after 2 days of ciprofloxacin. *Think: G6PD deficiency.* **Next step:** Check peripheral smear looking for "bite cells," transfuse if severe anemia, and check renal function.

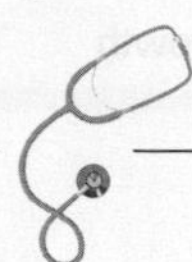

The genetic defect causes a ↓ half-life of enzyme, so older RBCs without G6PD die. Testing after acute attack will show younger RBCs that still have the enzyme, revealing a false-negative test. *Check G6PD assay 3 weeks after acute episode.*

DIAGNOSIS

- Evidence of intravascular hemolysis:
  - Indirect bilirubin elevated.
  - ↓ haptoglobin.
  - Hemoglobinuria.
- Smear will show reticulocytes, **bite cells,** and **Heinz bodies.**
- Negative Coombs' tests (nonautoimmune).
- G6PD assay.

Aplastic Anemia

PATHOPHYSIOLOGY

Marrow failure resulting in **pancytopenia** from stem cell defect, which is usually from immune-mediated injury (idiopathic or after exposure to radiation, drugs, infections, or certain chemicals).

Pure red cell aplasia (anemia only) can be seen in sickle cell patients after parvovirus B19 infection (erythema infectiosum).

ETIOLOGY

- Viral infections (viral hepatitis, **parvovirus** B19).
- Drugs (**chloramphenicol,** benzene, DDT, etc.).

SIGNS AND SYMPTOMS

- Anemia: Weakness, fatigue, and pallor.
- Thrombocytopenia: Mucosal bleeding.
- Neutropenia: Fever and infections.

DIAGNOSIS

- Low reticulocyte count.
- Bone marrow biopsy (hypocellular marrow with lots of white fat cells).
- Normal MCV

TREATMENT

- Immunosuppression (antithymocyte globulin (ATG), cyclosporine, and steroids).
- Young patients: Bone marrow transplant if immunosuppression fails.

Anemia of Chronic Disease

PATHOPHYSIOLOGY

Anemia from chronic diseases (infectious, malignant, and rheumatologic) from impairment in iron mobilization (likely from inflammatory cytokines and an acute phase reactant called hepcidin). These patients have features similar to iron deficiency anemia despite adequate iron stores on lab evaluation.

ETIOLOGY

- Infections (tuberculosis, etc.).
- Malignancies.
- Rheumatologic diseases (systemic lupus erythematosus [SLE], rheumatoid arthritis).

DIAGNOSIS

- ↑ ferritin (acute phase reactant).
- ↓ **TIBC and transferrin** (unlike iron deficiency anemia).
- ↓ serum iron.
- Normocytic to microcytic anemia.
- Normal erythropoietin.

TREATMENT

Treat the underlying cause.

Hemoglobinopathies

Normal electrophoresis pattern in adult:

- Hemoglobin A (96%): α_2/β_2 (normal hemoglobin).
- Hemoglobin F (3%): α_2/γ_2 (fetal hemoglobin, normal till 6 months of age).
- Hemoglobin A_2 (1%): α_2/δ_2.
- There are two α genes and one β gene on each chromosome, making a total of four α genes and two β genes.

α-THALASSEMIA

Genetic defect causing gene deletions of α chains (normal: αα/αα).

EPIDEMIOLOGY

- αα/— thalassemia trait is most common in Asians (hydrops fetalis may result if heterozygotes mate and their offspring lack any alpha genes).
- α–/α– thalassemia trait is most common in Africans.

PATHOPHYSIOLOGY

Ineffective production of α globin chains causes overproduction of β chains that results in unstable soluble tetramers which can precipitate within the cell. Because of this instability, α-thalassemia can cause chronic hemolysis. Severity depends on how many of the four foci get deleted or mutated.

SIGNS AND SYMPTOMS

- 1/4 foci involved = silent thalassemia: Asymptomatic.
- 2/4 foci involved = thalassemia trait: Mild anemia (very low MCV).
- 3/4 foci involved = hemoglobin H (HbH) disease: A significant amount of HbH, consisting of β_4 tetramers in circulation resulting in moderate to severe microcytic, hypochromic, hemolytic anemia with marked splenomegally.
- 4/4 foci involved = hemoglobin Barts, hydrops fetalis (**Bart drops a (α) fetus**): Incompatible with life. Fetal death.
- HbH has extremely high oxygen affinity, and failure to release oxygen in peripheral tissues results in severe CHF and anasarca, termed *hydrops fetalis*.

DIAGNOSIS

- Blood smear: Microcytic anemia, hypochromia, target cells, Heinz bodies.
- HbH precipitates on staining with brilliant **cresyl blue.**

β-THALASSEMIA

Gene defects including deletions, abnormalities of transcription and translation, and instability of mRNA in β globin hemoglobin.

PATHOPHYSIOLOGY

- Ineffective production of β globin chains causes α globin chains to accumulate in the cell.
- The accumulation of α chains form insoluble aggregates that damage cell membranes.
- A partial compensatory ↑ of the δ and γ chains yields elevated levels of HbA_2 ($\alpha_2\delta_2$) or HbF ($\alpha_2\gamma_2$).

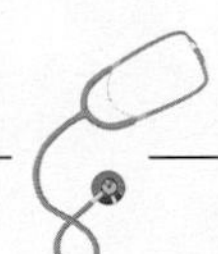

Yersinia enterocolitica is a significant cause of morbidity in patients with thalassemia and other iron overload syndromes (cirrhosis and hereditary hemochromatosis).

SIGNS AND SYMPTOMS

- β-*Thalassemia major* (Cooley's anemia): Associated with jaundice, hepatosplenomegaly, and jaundice.
- β-*Thalassemia minor*: Mild or no anemia.

DIAGNOSIS

Elevated HbF and HbA_2 measurements on hemoglobin electrophoresis.

TREATMENT

- β-*Thalassemia major*: Aggressive transfusions, splenectomy to enhance survival of RBCs, bone marrow transplant.
- β-*Thalassemia minor*: No treatment indicated.

Sickle cell patients should always be on folate! Chronic hemolysis causes folate loss and deficiency.

Sickle Cell Anemia (SCA)

- Autosomal recessive genetic disease characterized by the presence of hemoglobin S in RBCs.
- Hemoglobin S is formed by substitution of valine for glutamic acid in the sixth position of the β-hemoglobin chain.

- This change causes Hb S to polymerize in hypoxic conditions, distorting the red cell into the classic crescent or sickle shape. The ↓ deformability can cause hemolysis and vascular occlusion, causing crisis.
- Sickle cell trait: Heterozygous for sickle gene.
- Sickle cell disease: Homozygous for sickle gene.

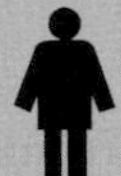

A young African-American man with microcytic hypochromic anemia is found to have a high ferritin and iron with normal RDW. *Think: Sickle cell anemia.* **Next step:** Hemoglobin electrophoresis.

EPIDEMIOLOGY

↑ incidence in African-Americans, and in populations from Africa, the Mediterranean, Middle East, and India.

SIGNS AND SYMPTOMS

Acute Crisis

- Symptoms include arthralgias and pain (back, extremities, chest and abdomen, etc.).
- Caused by vascular sludging and thrombosis. These vaso-occlusive crises may cause organ failure (secondary to infarction), dehydration, fever, and leukocytosis.
- **Acute chest syndrome: Hypoxia, chest pain,** shortness of breath, infiltrates caused by occlusion of pulmonary vasculature by sickled cells and/or infection). It is the most common **cause of death** in sickle patients and is an emergency requiring exchange transfusion with normal red cells. **Treat with exchange transfusion.**
- **Priapism** can occur acutely or chronically. This is a medical emergency, as permanent damage can occur. Genitourinary evaluation is needed.

Chronic Disease Manifestations

- Skeletal: **Aseptic necrosis of femoral head** and *Salmonella* osteomyelitis.
- Biliary disease: Pigmented gallstones (↑ bilirubin).
- Renal: Chronic hematuria, renal papillary necrosis.
- Liver disease: Viral hepatitis (transfusions) and secondary hemochromatosis.
- Pulmonary: Local infection and vascular occlusions (acute chest syndrome), **pulmonary hypertension.**
- Heart: Enlarged, flow murmur, MI.
- Immune: ↑ susceptibility to infections, **functional asplenism** (due to repeated infarction). ↑ **sepsis with encapsulated organisms** (***Streptococcus pneumoniae, Salmonella* osteomyelitis, and *Haemophilus influenzae*).**
- Eye: Ischemic retinopathy.
- Neuro: Cerebrovascular accident (CVA) and transient ischemic attacks (TIAs) (25% risk by age 45).

DIAGNOSIS

- **Hemoglobin electrophoresis will show HbS.**
- Blood smear: Howell-Jolly bodies (cytoplasmic remnants of nuclear chromatin that are normally removed by the spleen), sickled cells.

- Blood tests show anemia and evidence of hemolysis: ↑ reticulocyte count, ↑ indirect bilirubin and leukocytosis.

TREATMENT

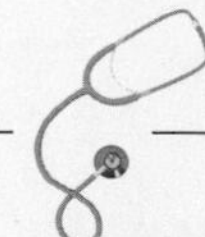

Indications for exchange transfusion in sickle cell disease:

- Stroke/TIA
- Acute chest syndrome
- Priapism
- Third-term pregnancy
- Intractable vaso-occlusive crisis

- **Acute crisis:** Analgesia and hydration (and antibiotics if signs of infection).
- **Acute chest syndrome:** Respiratory support, exchange transfusion, and empiric antibiotics for pneumonia.
- **Long-term treatment:**
  - **Hydroxyurea** acts by increasing amount of fetal hemoglobin; may ↓ frequency of crisis.
  - *H. influenzae* and pneumococcal **vaccines** for prophylaxis.
  - Frequent follow-up.

Hemolytic Anemias

Signs of SCA—SICKLE

Splenomegaly/**S**ludging
Infection
Cholelithiasis/acute **C**hest syndrome
Kidney (hematuria, papillary necrosis)
Liver congestion/**L**eg ulcers
Eye changes

- **Immune-mediated hemolytic anemia:** Presence of autoantibodies to one's RBCs, resulting in hemolysis.
  - Features of hemolysis:
    - Reticulocytosis (bone marrow pushes out immature RBCs).
    - ↑ indirect bilirubin (by-product of lysed cells [globin]).
    - ↑ lactic dehydrogenase (LDH; by-product of lysed cells) and ↓ haptoglobin (binds free hemoglobin released from lysed cells).
    - ⊕ direct Coombs' test (presence of antibody on RBC surface).
    - Splenomegaly (site of clearance).
- **Warm hemolytic anemia:**
  - Most common form of immune-mediated hemolytic anemia.
  - **IgG** antibodies to different RBC antigens (eg, Rh).
  - Do not usually fix complement (IgG).
  - Active at body temperature.
  - **Treat with steroids.** Transfuse if severe anemia. Splenectomy for steroid resistant.
  - Seen with chronic lymphocytic leukemia (CLL), leukemias, SLE, and other autoimmune diseases, and drugs (penicillin, sulfas and antimalarials).
  - Sixty percent of cases are idiopathic.

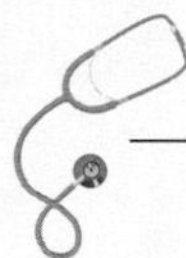

Renal papillary necrosis occurs in SCA because of the very high osmolalities in the renal medulla needed to pull the water from the collecting ducts, causing the RBCs to sickle.

- **Cold hemolytic anemia:**
  - **Immunoglobulin M (IgM)** antibodies.
  - Active at cool temperatures (dissociate at 30°C) such as in distal body parts (blue fingers and toes).
  - **Fixes complement** (IgM).
  - Presence of a high titer of cold agglutinins.
  - Seen acutely with ***Mycoplasma*** and **infectious mononucleosis** (resolve spontaneously) and chronically with **lymphomas** and **Waldenström's macroglobulinemia.**
  - Degree of hemolysis is variable.
  - **Treatment includes keeping warm;** corticosteroids don't work well.
- **Paroxysmal cold hemoglobinuria:**
  - Also called cold hemolysis (hemoglobinuria after exposure to cold).
  - **IgG** antibodies against P group antigen (Donath-Landsteiner Ab).
  - Active at cool temperatures, dissociate at 30°C to cause hemolysis.
  - **Fix complement.**
  - Clinically characterized by **acute intermittent massive hemolysis** and hemoglobinuria following exposure to cold.

A young woman feels weak. Labs show a normocytic, normochromic anemia, with an elevated LDH. Peripheral blood smear shows schistocytes. What is the diagnosis? Microangiopathic hemolytic anemia. When might you see this? TTP or DIC.

TRANSFUSION REACTIONS

Acute Hemolytic Transfusion Reactions

- Life threatening!
- Due to ABO incompatibility.
- These reactions involve naturally occurring host IgM anti-A and anti-B, which fix complement and cause rapid intravascular hemolysis.
- Direct Coombs' test is positive (antibodies on RBCs).
- **Usually due to human error** (improper identification or mislabeling of blood).

Signs and Symptoms

- Begins soon after starting the transfusion.
- **Usually sudden clinical deterioration.**
- Fever +/– chills.
- **Dyspnea** and tachycardia.
- **Back pain,** chest pain, abdominal pain.
- Hypotension.
- Sequelae:
  - Death (40%).
  - Acute renal failure (ATN).
  - Shock.
  - Disseminated intravascular coagulation (DIC).

Treatment

- Discontinue transfusion immediately!
- Hemodynamic support/supportive care/IV fluids.
- Recheck compatibility of blood with blood bank.

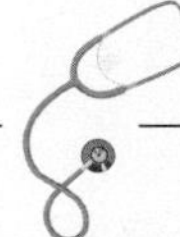

General anesthesia is a frequent setting for blood transfusion. In this setting, immediate hemolytic transfusion reaction should be suspected with:

- Severe hypotension
- Coagulopathic oozing
- Hemoglobinuria/pink serum
- Fevers

A young woman in the hospital was transfused 2 units of red cells after severe bleeding in childbirth. Several hours later, she developed acute shortness of breath, fever, and hypoxia. **Next step:** Chest x-ray. X-ray findings demonstrate diffuse bilateral infiltrates. What is likely diagnosis? Transfusion-related lung injury.

Delayed Hemolytic Transfusion Reactions

- **Mild** and occurs days to weeks after transfusion.
- Patient received a transfusion in the past and is now having immune response after being reexposed to antigen. Due to **anamnestic antibody response to a minor antigen** (Rh or Kidd, not ABO).

- Pretransfusion antibody level low → screening and crossmatch tests usually negative.
- Signs of mild hemolysis: Has high LDH, high total bilirubin, low haptoglobin.

SIGNS AND SYMPTOMS

Commonly: Fever, anemia, or asymptomatic. Rarely, there are serious manifestations that look more like acute transfusion reactions.

TREATMENT

Milder than acute reactions and usually no treatment or just supportive care is required.

Febrile Nonhemolytic Transfusion Reactions

- Common.
- Chills followed by fever within a few hours of transfusion; mild.
- Lasts only a few hours.
- Due to host immune response against transfused leukocytes/platelets or cytokines from donor leukocytes.

TREATMENT

- Discontinue transfusion (can occur after) to rule out acute hemolysis (see Acute Hemolytic Transfusion Reactions).
- Can give Tylenol and Benadryl as prophylaxis, although studies have shown no benefit.
- Not routinely recommended; however, the use of leukocyte-reduced blood products may reduce the incidence of febrile nonhemolytic transfusion reactions.

Allergic Reactions to Plasma

- **Rare.** Usually occurs in patients with congenital IgA deficiency; have anaphylactic reactions to the IgA in donor blood. Anti-IgA antibodies present.
- Can get hives, bronchospasm, anaphylaxis.
- Treatment: Maintain airway and give epinephrine.

Transfusion-Related Acute Lung Injury (TRALI)

- Sudden severe respiratory distress similar to adult respiratory distress syndrome (ARDS).
- Occurs within 6 hours of transfusion.
- Incidence ~ 1 in 5000 transfusions (all types of blood products).
- Caused by donor Ab against recipient granulocytes → agglutination of granulocytes and complement activation in the pulmonary vascular bed → capillary endothelial damage → fluid leak into the alveoli.

SIGNS AND SYMPTOMS

- Chills/fever.
- Chest pain.
- Hypotension.
- Cyanosis, dyspnea, crackles/rales.

- Chest x-ray (CXR) shows diffuse pulmonary edema (diffuse congestion).
- Resolves within 48–96 hours without residual effects (interim ventilatory support often required).
- Treatment is supportive.

COAGULATION

Coagulation Cascade

Common pathway factors: I, II, V, X (see Figure 2.4-1).

Heparin

- ↑ partial thromboplastin time (PTT).
- Affects intrinsic pathway.
- Acts as cofactor to antithrombin III (antithrombin III inhibits factor Xa and thrombin).
- Low-molecular-weight heparins have 10 times activity against factor Xa.
- Safe in pregnancy.
- Adverse effects include bleeding, heparin-induced thrombocytopenia (HIT). Less HIT with low-molecular-weight heparin.

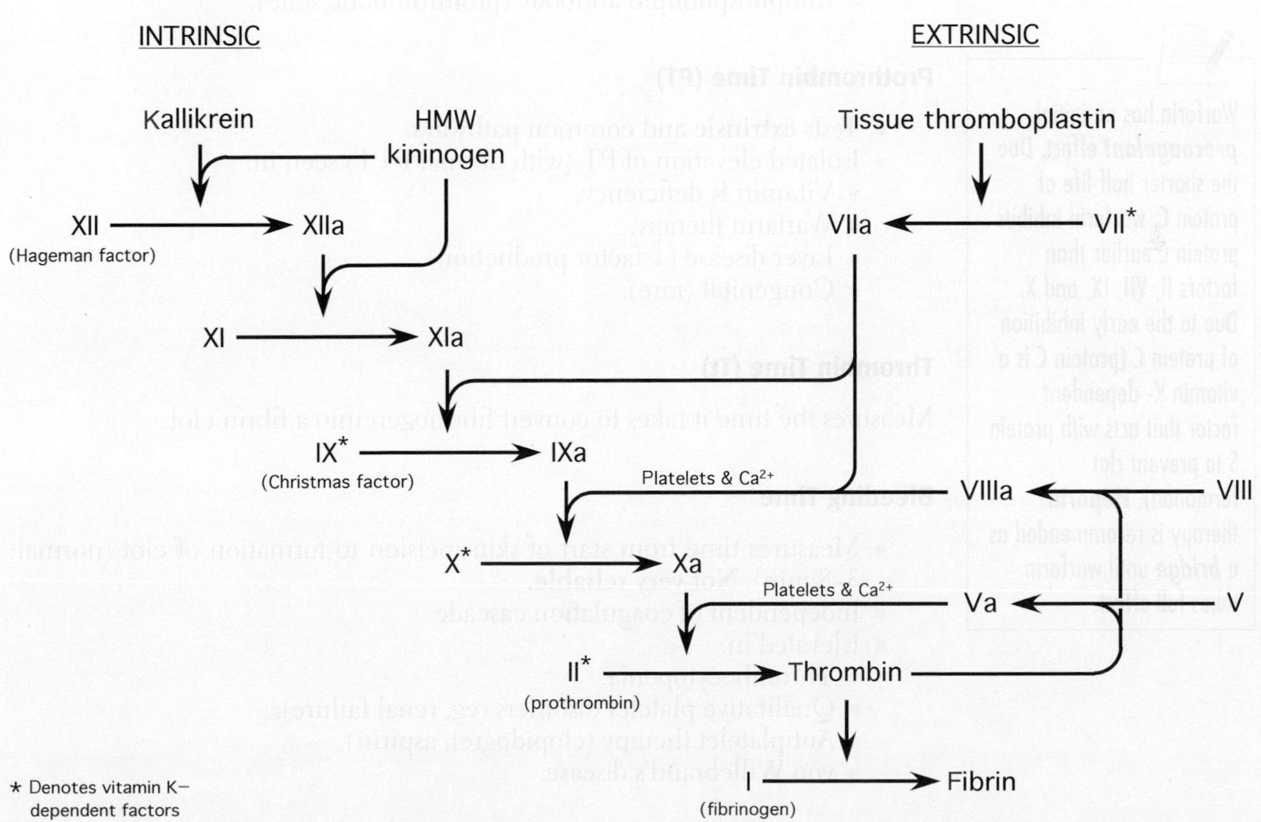

FIGURE 2.4-1. Coagulation cascade.

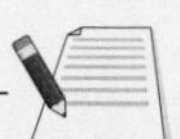

The Three 3's of Heparin:
PTT (3 letters), in**TRI**nsic, AT**III**
Heparin prolongs **PTT.**
PTT measures in**TRI**nsic pathway.
Heparin activates antithrombin **III.**

- **HIT** can be a catastrophic complication of heparin therapy, causing a **paradoxical hypercoagulable state** and high risk of blood clots. Diagnosed with the finding of low platelets and a ⊕ HIT (heparin-platelet factor 4) antibodies. Treated by stopping heparin immediately and anticoagulating with argatroban (a direct thrombin inhibitor). **Suspect this with anyone on heparin and dropping platelets. Assume this diagnosis for anyone on heparin with low platelets and a blood clot.**

Warfarin

- ↑ prothrombin time (PT).
- Affects extrinsic pathway.
- Inhibits vitamin K–dependent factors.
- Primarily affects II, VII, IX, X.
- Teratogenic.

Leafy green vegetables have high vitamin K content, and an ↑ consumption will ↓ the PT (and may go below the therapeutic level) for patients on warfarin.

Activated Partial Thromboplastin Time (aPTT)

- Tests **intrinsic** and common pathways.
- Isolated elevation of PTT (with normal PT) seen in:
  - Heparin therapy.
  - Deficiencies of factors VIII (hemophilia A and von Willebrand's disease), factor IX (hemophilia B), factor XI, and factor XII (asymptomatic).
  - Antiphospholipid antibody (prothrombotic state).

Warfarin has an initial ***procoagulant*** effect. Due the shorter half-life of protein C, warfarin inhibits protein C earlier than factors II, VII, IX, and X. Due to the early inhibition of protein C (protein C is a vitamin K–dependent factor that acts with protein S to prevent clot formation). **Heparin** therapy is recommended as a ***bridge*** until warfarin takes full effect.

Prothrombin Time (PT)

- Tests **extrinsic** and common pathways.
- Isolated elevation of PT (with normal PTT) seen in:
  - Vitamin K deficiency.
  - Warfarin therapy.
  - Liver disease (↓ factor production).
  - Congenital (rare).

Thrombin Time (Tt)

Measures the time it takes to convert fibrinogen into a fibrin clot.

Bleeding Time

- Measures time from start of skin incision to formation of clot (normal: 3–8 min). **Not very reliable.**
- Independent of coagulation cascade.
- Elevated in:
  - Thrombocytopenia.
  - Qualitative platelet disorders (eg, renal failure).
  - Antiplatelet therapy (clopidogrel, aspirin).
  - von Willebrand's disease.

Direct Coombs'

- Tests for antibodies on red blood cells.
- Elevated in:
  - Drug therapy (α-methyldopa, penicillin, tetracyclines, quinidine, insulin).
  - SLE.
  - Autoimmune hemolytic anemia.
  - Transfusion reactions.

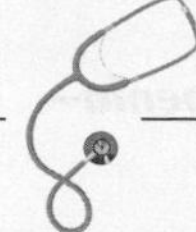

Hypercoagulability and **skin necrosis** are feared complications of warfarin therapy and are easily avoided by using heparin-based therapy at the initiation of warfarin.

Indirect Coombs'

- Tests for antibodies to red blood cells in the serum (not on the cells).
- Elevated in:
  - Acquired hemolytic anemia.
  - Incompatible crossmatched blood.
  - Rh: Women can develop anti-Rh antibodies during pregnancy/delivery of an Rh-⊕ child.
  - Drug therapy (mefenamic acid, α-methyldopa).

Thrombocytopenia

Low platelets can be due to:

- ↓ production (bone marrow problem, as in leukemia).
- ↑ consumption (DIC, TTP, ITP).
- Hypersplenism (sequestration of platelets).
- Lab error: Platelet clumping.

ITP vs. Aplastic Anemia vs. MDS

- **ITP** has **normal RBCs, normal WBCs, only low platelets** with giant (young) platelets on the peripheral smear. Usually don't give platelets—treat with steroids or IVIG.
- **Aplastic anemia** has low RBCs, low WBCs, and low platelets **(all cell lines low)**. No dysmorphic cells on smear.
- **Myelodysplastic syndrome (MDS)** can have **any one or all lineages low**. The smear can show dysplastic neutrophils (hypolobulated), and RBCs with ringed sideroblasts.

Idiopathic Thrombocytopenic Purpura (ITP)

Immune-mediated thrombocytopenia of unknown etiology.

Pathophysiology

Development of antibodies against a platelet surface antigen. The antibody-antigen complexes effectively ↓ platelet count by being removed from circulation.

Signs and Symptoms

- Petechiae and purpura over trunk and limbs.
- Mucosal bleeding.

Diagnosis

- Thrombocytopenia on CBC.
- Absence of other factors to explain thrombocytopenia (diagnosis of exclusion).
- Antiplatelet antibodies **not useful.**

Treatment

- Corticosteroids acutely.
- Intravenous immunoglobulin (IVIG).
- **Platelet transfusion** if significant bleeding present.
- Splenectomy electively to ↓ recurrence.

Causes of thrombocytopenia—

PLATELETS

Platelet disorders: TTP, ITP, DIC
Leukemia
Anemia
Trauma
Enlarged spleen
Liver disease
EtOH
Toxins (benzene, heparins, aspirin, chemotherapy agents, etc.)
Sepsis

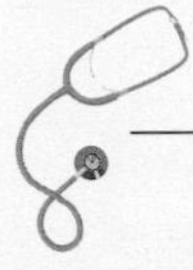

Thrombocytopenia vs. Factor Deficiencies

Thrombocytopenia presents as oozing from mucosal sites (gums) and petechiae. Petechiae = Platelet Problem
Factor deficiencies (eg, hemophilia) present with large bleeds (typically hemarthrosis).

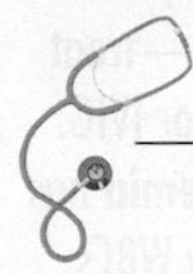

Typically, one transfuses platelets if they drop below 10,000 or if there are signs of bleeding. One unit ↑ platelets by 10,000.

Classic Pentad for TTP—

FAT RN

Fever
Anemia (hemolytic)
Thrombocytopenia
Renal dysfunction
Neurologic dysfunction

Thrombotic Thrombocytopenic Purpura (TTP)

- A microangiopathic hemolytic anemia that results from circulation and deposition of abnormal von Willebrand factor (vWF) multimers (large precursor proteins that are normally cleaved).
- **ADAMTS13** is the protease that normally cleaves these multimers, but is deficient in this condition.
- **This is a life-threatening emergency, with mortality approaching 90% if untreated!**
- Usually caused by an immune process that clears ADAMTS13 after an infection, but some cases are genetic.

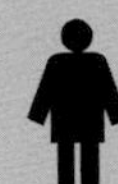

A 37-year-old female presents with fever, confusion, rash, and hematuria. CBC shows low platelets and ↑ creatinine. *Think: TTP.* **Next step:** Plasma exchange, not platelets.

Etiology

- Infection (especially HIV and *E. coli* O157:H7).
- Malignancy.
- Drugs (antiplatelet agents, chemotherapy agents, contraceptives).
- Autoimmune disorders.
- Pregnancy.

Signs and Symptoms

Classic pentad—not all have to be present:

- Fever.
- Altered mental status (waxing and waning).
- Renal dysfunction (hematuria, oliguria).
- Thrombocytopenia—can be mild to severe.
- Microangiopathic hemolytic anemia.

Diagnosis

- Low platelets.
- Evidence of hemolysis: **Schistocytes on peripheral smear,** ↓ haptoglobin, elevated LDH, elevated total bilirubin.
- Renal failure: Elevated blood urea nitrogen (BUN), creatinine.
- Fever.
- Altered mental status.
- **Do not need all;** based on clinical suspicion.

Treatment

- **Plasma exchange** (plasmapheresis) is the **mainstay** of treatment.
- **Do not transfuse platelets!**
- Fresh frozen plasma may help (contains missing ADAMTS13).

Disseminated Intravascular Coagulation (DIC)

Consumptive Coagulopathy

- Acquired coagulation defect that results in consumption of coagulation factors, including **fibrinogen,** causing bleeding and thrombosis.

- Usually secondary to exposure of blood to procoagulants such as tissue factor (fetus, bacteria) and cancer procoagulant resulting in depletion of clotting factors and microangiopathic hemolytic anemia.
- Can be acute and life threatening or can be chronic, as seen with malignancies.

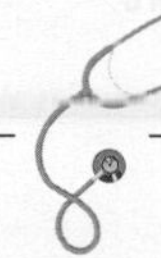

E. coli 0157:H7 is the causative organism in a bloody diarrhea syndrome, which has been associated with the subsequent development of HUS. HUS differs from TTP in severity and lack of neurologic symptoms.

Etiology

- Obstetric problems (retained dead fetus, abruptio placentae, second-trimester abortion, amniotic fluid embolism, preeclampsia).
- Sepsis (particularly with gram-negatives, *Rickettsia*, HUS, malaria).
- Local tissue damage (snake bites, burns, frostbite).
- Extensive trauma.
- Chronic illness: Malignancy (acute myelocytic leukemia [AML]), liver disease.

Signs and Symptoms

- Diffuse, systemic bleeding (not from a single site).
- Usually have some other severe underlying condition also (eg, sepsis).

Transfusing platelets in TTP is thought to "fuel the fire" and exacerbate consumption of platelets and clotting factors, resulting in more thrombi in the microvasculature.

Diagnosis

- ↓ fibrinogen.
- Elevated PT, aPTT, and thrombin time (TT).
- Thrombocytopenia.
- Presence of fibrin split products (elevated D-dimers).
- Evidence of microangiopathic hemolysis (schistocytes) on peripheral smear.

Treatment

- Treat underlying cause.
- Platelets, fresh frozen plasma (FFP), and cryoprecipitate to control bleeding can support until underlying cause is under control.

Etiology of DIC–

How do you "SPELL" DIC?

Sepsis/**S**urgery/**S**nake bite
Pregnancy
Extensive trauma
Liver disease/**L**eukemia
Local tissue damage

A 50-year-old woman who is in the ICU for sepsis has purpura and gingival bleeding on day 2 of her hospital stay, and blood coming from her urinary catheter. PT and PTT are ↑, fibrinogen is ↓. *Think: DIC.* **Next step:** Transfuse FFP and cryoprecipitate.

MISCELLANEOUS BLEEDING DISORDERS

von Willebrand's Disease

Genetic disease, most commonly autosomal dominant, characterized by **lack, or functional defect** of von Willebrand factor (vWF)

Pathophysiology

- Three functions of von Willebrand factor:
  - Forms an adhesive bridge between platelets and endothelium.
  - Also bridges adjacent platelets (aggregation).
  - Acts as a carrier protein for factor VIII.

- Three types of disease:
  - **Type 1** (by far the most common, and will likely be the one on exam): ↓ in amount (quantitative defect) autosomal dominant inheritance.
  - **Type 2: Qualitative defect** of vWF (several subtypes but all with functional defect).
  - **Type 3:** Severely ↓ (**essentially absent**) vWF.

AML type M3 (promyelocytic leukemia) often presents with DIC.

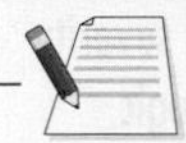

PT and PTT are normal in TTP, whereas they are elevated in DIC.

SIGNS AND SYMPTOMS

- Mostly asymptomatic.
- Often have history of very heavy menstruation, or bleeding with dental procedures, and then might have an episode of severe bleeding during a major surgery.

DIAGNOSIS

Test three parameters: the amount of vWF (vWF antigen); the function of vWF (ristocetin aggregation test, also called ristocetin cofactor assay); and size (multimers). **PTT can also be elevated because vWF carries factor 8.**

- **Type 1:** vWF antigen ↓; ristocetin aggregation test ↓ *in proportion to the ↓ antigen.* Multimers normal size.
- **Type 2:** vWF antigen normal or ↓; *ristocetin test low—out of proportion to any ↓ in the vWF antigen;* multimers usually small (these are abnormal proteins).
- **Type 3:** Both vWF antigen and ristocetin test **very low.**

TREATMENT

- Mild bleeding or minor surgery: DDAVP (desmopressin) ↑ vWF levels by releasing it from endothelium.
- Serious bleeding or major surgery: vWF and factor 8 concentrates.

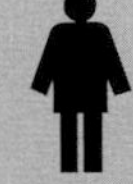

A young man presents with bleeding profusely after having his tooth pulled. Labs demonstrate normal platelets and normal PT, but a prolonged aPTT. What is the likely diagnosis? von Willebrand's disease. First-line treatment? Desmospressin.

Hemophilia

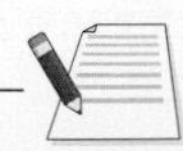

von Willebrand's disease is the most common bleeding disorder.

PATHOPHYSIOLOGY

Sex-linked recessive disease (only males affected) causing a deficiency of factor VIII or IX. Hemophilia A is factor VIII deficiency, and hemophilia B is factor IX deficiency (Christmas disease). They are both X-linked recessive.

SIGNS AND SYMPTOMS

Dependent on amount of active factor (usually measured as a % of normal):

- **5–25% factor VIII or IX activity (mild):** Abnormal bleeding when subjected to surgery or dental procedures, excessive bleeding following **circumcision** of newborns is a clue.
- **1–5% (moderate)** and < 1% **(severe) factor VIII or IX activity: Deep tissue bleeding (muscles)**, typically **intra-articular hemorrhages** or **hemarthrosis** (usually knees).

DIAGNOSIS

- Prolonged aPTT, normal bleeding time.
- Clinical picture, family history, and the factor VIII and IX coagulant activity level.

TREATMENT

- Recombinant factor VIII or IX.
- DDAVP (desmopressin) for patients with mild hemophilia A but not hemophilia B.

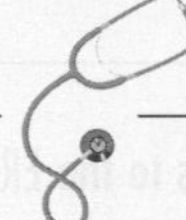

Hemophilia vs. von Willebrand's Disease
Unlike in vWD, bleeding time in hemophilia A is unaffected because no abnormality with platelets is present. More importantly, hemophilia typically has bleeding into a joint (hemarthrosis), and vWF is usually mucosal bleeding or postsurgical procedure bleeding.

HEMATOLOGIC MALIGNANCIES

Hemolytic malignancies include any cancer of blood cells. In the context of malignancies, the term *clone* or *clonal* refers to a process in which the abnormal cells or process have **arisen from a single precursor.** This is the basic concept of cancer. When there is an abnormal growth of a specific cell, it is important to determine if they are clonal (cancer or precancer) or **polyclonal** (from multiple parent cells, and usually a **reaction** to another process). For example, if the lymphocytes in a patient with a lymphocytosis are clonal, then the patient has leukemia; if they are polyclonal, these cells are likely reacting to an infection.

Glanzmann's thrombasthenia is a *qualitative* disorder of platelets with a defect in GP IIb/IIIa. Normal number of platelets, but don't work. If bleeding, give platelets!

Acute Leukemias

- Acute leukemia is a disease in which patients present with a relatively sudden acute illness, which can be manifested by bleeding or extreme weakness or infection. This is in contrast to chronic leukemias, in which the patients can be asymptomatic for months or years, and are often picked up on routine blood tests. Any leukemia is a cancer of the blood.
- **Two basic types: lymphocytic and myeloid.** Each has subsets within: acute lymphocytic leukemia (ALL) and acute myelocytic leukemia (AML), discussed in detail below.

PATHOPHYSIOLOGY

- The clonal progenitor cells (*lympho**blast*** or *myelo**blast***) proliferate, eventually taking over the bone marrow and inhibiting the growth of normal cells.
- Clinical manifestations occur because of the loss of normal bone marrow elements and by infiltration of the body's tissues by malignant cells.

A 22-year-old woman recently received her first dose of chemotherapy for acute lymphocytic leukemia (or could be lymphoma). She has extreme fatigue and a fever. Labs reveal a high LDH with low calcium and high phosphate. What is likely diagnosis? Tumor lysis syndrome. Next step: Aggressive hydration. What are you worried about? Renal failure.

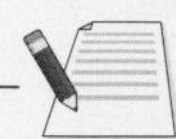

A patient presents to the ER feeling extremely weak. CBC shows Hgb 7.2 g, platelets of 9, and WBCs of 49,000. **Next step:** Check coags, correct coagulopathy emergently (platelets and blood products), then bone marrow biopsy.

Signs and Symptoms

- **Acutely ill!**
- Anemia: Weakness, fatigue, pallor, cardiopulmonary compromise.
- Neutropenia: Infections, fever.
- Thrombocytopenia: Petechiae, purpura, hemorrhages.
- Marrow infiltration: Bone pain.

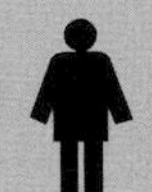

A 25-year-old man presented to the clinic with ↑ night sweats, fever, and weight loss. On laboratory testing, leukemoid reaction was detected, with ↓ LAP score. Peripheral smear showed ↑ blast cells with intracytoplasmic rods. What would you do to confirm the diagnosis? Bone marrow aspiration and biopsy. (LAP score - Leukocyte Alkaline Phosphatase score, typically low in malignancy.)

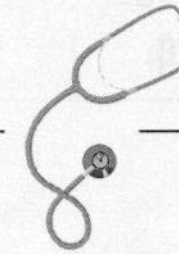

Tumor lysis syndrome is seen in leukemias (especially after initiation of chemo) and other aggressive hematological malignancies. Rapid cell breakdown → high uric acid, hyperkalemia, hyperphosphatemia, hypocalcemia, acute renal failure, and ↑ LDH. **Treated with fluids, correcting electrolyte imbalance, and allopurinol.**

Diagnosis

- **Initial finding:** Numerous and monotonous **blasts** found on the peripheral smear (large, immature cells with large nuclei, unclumped chromatin). Other cells are ↓.
- **Bone marrow biopsy** showing > 30% infiltration with blasts (usually almost entirely made of blasts).
- **Other tests** (used for leukemias and lymphomas):
  - **Flow cytometry:** Evaluates which proteins are expressed on the cell surface; expression of different proteins is associated with different stages of development (ie, blasts), and specific constellations of proteins are associated with different lymphomas.
  - **Fluorescent in situ hybridization (FISH):** A sensitive method to look for specific cytogenetic lesions associated with different leukemias and lymphomas.

Treatment

Please see Table 2.4-3 for complete list of the various chemotherapies available for selected malignancies.

- Three steps of chemotherapy:
  - *Induction:* High doses of chemotherapy are used to induce remission.
  - *Consolidation:* Chemotherapy is then administered to eradicate residual, undetectable malignant cells.
  - *Maintenance:* Ongoing chemotherapy to keep the number of malignant cells low.
- Complete remission is the goal in cancer patients. This is achieved if normal marrow elements are being produced and less than 5% residual blasts are present in the bone marrow.

Signs of LEUKEMIA

Light skin (pallor)
Energy ↓
Underweight
Kidney failure
Excess heat (fever)
Mottled skin (hemorrhages)
Infections
Anemia

Acute Myelocytic Leukemia (AML)

Epidemiology

- More common in **adults.**
- Association with history of benzene exposure.
- Eight subtypes: M0–M7:
  - M1–M3 have granulocytic differentiation.
  - M4 and M5 are monocytic precursors.

- M6 have predominance of erythroblasts.
- M7 is mainly megakaryocytic.

SIGNS AND SYMPTOMS

- Fatigue, hemorrhage, or bruising (30%).
- Infection of lung, skin (25%).
- Splenomegaly is rare (25%) compared to other types of leukemia.

DIAGNOSIS

Specific characteristics:

- M3—acute promyelocytic leukemia: Associated with DIC, Auer rods, t(15;17); in which there is a defect in the vitamin A receptor, treatment is different than others: all-trans retinoic acid (ATRA—vitamin A) + chemotherapy. Prognosis is better than other AMLs.
- **AML** related to **prior exposure to chemotherapy** (for a previous cancer) has a poor prognosis. Likewise, AML that evolves from **underlying myelodysplasia (MDS)** (often seen in elderly) has a **poor prognosis.**
- M5: Associated with gingival hyperplasia.
- M4, M5: Central nervous system (CNS) manifestations.
- t(8;21) seen in M2 and t(15;17) seen in M3 have better prognosis.

TREATMENT

- **Induction:** Cytarabine + an anthracycline (daunorubicin)—50–80% receive remission.
- **Consolidation:** Same chemotherapy as induction.
- **Maintenance:** Clinical trials determining best drugs.
- Stem cell transplantation is also potentially curative, usually for relapsing or high-risk patients.
- M3 treated with ATRA in addition to chemotherapy.

ACUTE LYMPHOCYTIC LEUKEMIA (ALL)

EPIDEMIOLOGY

- Primarily a disease of children, but accounts for 20% of adult leukemias.
- Generally, prognosis is inversely related to age. Younger patients (kids to young adults) have good prognosis, but older have a poor prognosis.
- Three subtypes:
  - **L1** occurs in 80% of ALL cases in **children.**
  - **L2** most **adult cases.**
  - **L3** cell is leukemic manifestation of Burkitt's lymphoma t(8;14) involving c-myk gene.

A 27-year-old woman presents to your office with night sweats, weakness, and weight loss. Laboratory work reveals anemia, thrombocytopenia, and a WBC of 47,000. Peripheral smear demonstrates blasts with intracytoplasmic rods. How do you confirm the diagnosis? Bone marrow aspiration and biopsy. What is likely diagnosis? Acute promyelocytic leukemia (M3). What translocation would you find on cytogenetic studies? t(15;17).

SIGNS AND SYMPTOMS

- Acute onset.
- Malaise, fever, lethargy, weight loss, bone pain, infection, and hemorrhage.
- **Lymphadenopathy**, can have mediastinal mass.
- CNS involvement.
- Testicular involvement.
- Splenomegaly and hepatomegaly can be seen.

DIAGNOSIS

- Blasts in peripheral blood.
- Blasts taking over bone marrow on bone marrow biopsy; other cells ↓.
- 25–30%: Philadelphia chromosome (chromosome 22) arising from t(9;22)—poorer prognosis.

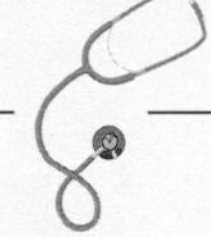

ATRA → maturation of immature cells in M3 and reduces the life-threatening DIC that can worsen with chemotherapy.

TREATMENT

- **Various regimens—you don't have to know details of chemo types.**
- General concept is that there is an induction, consolidation, and maintenance, as with AML (AML maintenance is only in specific patients).
- ALL treatment goes on for about 2 years, as opposed to AML treatment, which is shorter.
- The other difference is that ALL patients typically require CNS prophylaxis/treatment (intrathecal chemotherapy, usually given through lumbar puncture).
- *Induction:* Four or five drugs such as vincristine, prednisone, daunorubicin, L-asparaginase, and cyclophosphamide are used.
- *Consolidation:* Cell-cycle phase-specific antimetabolites.
- *Maintenance:* Low-dose chemotherapy is standard.
- Specific case: Patients with Philadelphia chromosome often need to go straight to bone marrow transplantation because their prognosis is so poor.

M3 = Acute promyelocytic anemia or APL: **DIC** (main cause of death), t(15;17) treated with ATRA, better prognosis.
M5 = gingival hyperplasia.

Chronic Leukemias

Chronic leukemias—chronic myelogenous (or myelocytic leukemia and chronic lymphocytic leukemia)—differ from acute leukemias in that these patients are often **asymptomatic for years** before having clinical problems. Though ultimately life threatening, they are rarely an emergency on presentation. **Patients generally look clinically well—not acutely ill.**

CHRONIC MYELOCYTIC LEUKEMIA (CML)

- A clonal proliferation (cancer) of cells in the myeloid lineage.
- One of several myeloproliferative disorders (others are polycythemia vera, essential thrombocythemia and general myeloproliferative disease).
- It has 25% risk/year of transforming to acute leukemia (blastic transformation).

PATHOPHYSIOLOGY

- Philadelphia chromosome t(9;22) causes fusion of Bcr and Abl, forming a protein (a tyrosine kinase) that constantly sends cell proliferation signals.
- Phases:
  - **Chronic phase** (most common presentation): High peripheral white counts (can be several hundred thousand **myeloid cells of varying stages of maturation—most not blasts**), big spleen (can cause early satiety and abdominal fullness). **These patients are often asymptomatic!** (You will likely be tested on chronic phase, so focus on this!)
  - **Accelerated phase:** More than 15% blasts in peripheral blood. RBCs and platelets begin to ↓. Symptoms of bone pain and weakness start.
  - **Blastic phase:** Looks like an **acute leukemia** with many blasts (> 30% in the peripheral blood and marrow). Sick patient—severe **fatigue and weakness!**

Philadelphia chromosome t(9;22) represents a poor prognosis in ALL, but in the setting of a myeloid disorder, it is diagnostic for CML which has a good prognosis.

> A 60-year-old male presenting with fever, **petechiae, bleeding gums,** and fatigue for 2 weeks is found to have hemoglobin of 6, platelets of 30,000, WBC of 80,000 comprised of 80% blasts with Auer rods.
> *Think: APL.* ***Next step:*** Stabilize patient, treat infection, and give blood products as needed, then bone marrow biopsy (check cytogenetics for targeting therapy because t(15;17) will benefit from ATRA).

DIAGNOSIS

- Examining the peripheral blood smear shows leukocytosis with **immature myeloid cells of varying stages of maturation** (some totally mature neutrophils, too). This is in contrast with any acute leukemia in which there are monotonous immature cells (blasts).
- Bone marrow biopsy and cytogenetics showing Philadelphia chromosome t(9;22) are diagnostic.
- Leukocyte alkaline phosphatase is *low* in CML cells (*high* in infectious causes of leukocytosis).

TREATMENT

- **Imatinib** (Gleevec) is a tyrosine kinase inhibitor that inhibits Philadelphia chromosome and induces indefinite remission (a revolutionary breakthrough!). It is the treatment of choice. Side effects include bone marrow suppression and cardiac toxicity.
- **Allogenic bone marrow transplant** may still have a role for younger or refractory patients.

Better prognosis of CML is associated with:
- Young age (< 40)
- No thrombocytopenia
- Early stage
- Low percentage of blasts

CHRONIC LYMPHOCYTIC LEUKEMIA (CLL)

- Most common type of leukemia in the Western world and is **often asymptomatic.**
- Malignant clonal disorder of **mature B lymphocytes** (rarely T cells) that **can but does not always** progress to cause lymphadenopathy, splenomegaly, and bone marrow failure.
- Generally a chronic disorder that can last for years.
- Identical to small lymphocytic lymphoma (SLL)—which is the term when the disease is confined only to lymph nodes.

Ninety percent of patients with CML have the Philadelphia chromosome t(9;22).

- Some patients have immune dysfunction that → infection or autoimmune processes.
- **Richter's transformation** is the rare transformation to an aggressive large cell lymphoma. Typically very refractory to treatment.

Signs and Symptoms

- Many are asymptomatic, and a routine CBC shows a lymphocytosis.
- Lymphadenopathy, splenomegaly, and cytopenias in later stages.
- At later stages of disease, patient may have classic "B" symptoms of fever, night sweats, and weight loss.
- Can have infections, **hemolytic anemia (classic complication)**, or ITP from a dysfunctional immune system.

A 32-year-old male presents to his doctor with fullness after only eating a small portion of food. Otherwise, he feels fine. His CBC is normal except for a WBC count of 120,000. Peripheral smear shows myeloid cells in varying stages of maturation. Likely diagnosis? CML. What would you likely find? t(9;22) on cytogenetics. What would you treat with? Imatinib.

Diagnosis

- Often suspected or found incidentally on routine CBC (↑ lymphocytes, > 5000 needed to make diagnosis but often > 100,000). Diagnosis is made with flow cytometry of peripheral blood demonstrating CLL clone.
- Peripheral smear will reveal **numerous mature-appearing lymphocytes** (small cells with dense nuclei and scant cytoplasm).
- Lymph node biopsy can also be used for diagnosis.

Stage/Survival

	Rai Stage	Survival
0	Lymphocytosis only	> 10 yrs
I	Adenopathy	6–7 yrs
II	Splenomegaly	6–7 yrs
III	Hgb < 10	2–3 yrs
IV	Thrombocytopenia	2–3 yrs

Treatment

- **Observation only for early asymptomatic patients in early stages.**
- There is no cure, but many therapies and combinations are effective, including fludarabine (purine analog), rituximab (antibody to CD20), chlorambucil (alkylating agent).
- Autoimmune hemolytic anemia can be treated with steroids.

- Frequent infections with hypogammaglobulinemia can be treated with intravenous immunoglobulin.

A 72-year-old man presents for a normal checkup. He feels great, and exam is entirely normal except for some palpable small axillary lymph nodes. Laboratory revealed a normal CBC except a WBC of 80,000 made up of primarlily lymphocytes. What is your most likely recommendation? *Observation.*

A 75-year-old man has had CLL for 8 years and has never required treatment. Over the past 2 weeks he has had dramatic weakness, night sweats, and rapidly enlarging nodes, and he has lost 10 pounds. What do you suspect? Richter's tranformation.

Myeloproliferative Disorders

- Myeloproliferative diseases are a group of disorders originating from clones of different granulocyte cell lines: neutrophils (CML), RBC (polycythemia vera), or platelets (essential thrombocytosis).
  - General myeloproliferative disease (neutrophils, RBCs, and platelets all elevated) and primary myelofibrosis are other types of myeloproliferative diseases.
- In any of these disorders, there may be a mixed picture, with more than just the primary cells being elevated (eg, patients with polycythemia vera may have elevated neutrophils as well as RBCs).
- Patients with any of these disorders are at risk for progression to AML or myelofibrosis (ultimately resulting from the cytokine secretion of myeloid cells). CML is discussed in the chronic leukemias section.

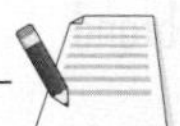

Why is a lymphocyte count of 200,000 an emergency in a patient with acute leukemia, but not so in a patient with CLL? CLL cells are small and nonsticky mature cells that have little risk of hyperviscosity. Acute leukemic cells are large, sticky blasts that can cause sludging in the CNS or pulmonary vasculature.

Polycythemia Vera (PV)

A myeloproliferative disease that results in ↑ red blood cells.

Etiology

- **Primary PV:** A primary bone marrow cause (*low* erythropoietin). This is a clonal process.
- **Secondary PV** (other causes that result in ↑ erythropoietin); nonclonal.
- Hypoxia (high altitudes, lung disease).
- Smoking (due to carboxyhemoglobin).
- Paraneoplastic (usually renal cell carcinoma and hepatoma aberrantly producing erythropoietin).

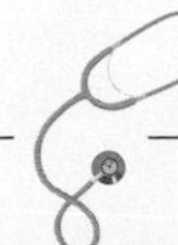

CLL patients can commonly have either de novo hemolytic anemia, or treatement-associated hemolytic anemia after receiving a purine analog (fludarabine).

Epidemiology

- Males are more commonly affected.
- More common in people > 60.

SIGNS AND SYMPTOMS

- Ruddy complexion.
- Pruritus after shower.
- Abdominal fullness (from splenomegaly).

RISKS

- Thrombosis (deep venous thrombosis [DVT], stroke, myocardial infarction [MI]).
- Bleeding.
- Transformation to AML or to myelofibrosis.

DIAGNOSIS

- Hemoglobin usually > 16.5 g/dL (females) and > 18.5 g/dL (males) and low erythropoietin in primary (must rule out secondary causes).
- Ninety percent of patients with PV have a JAK2 mutation.

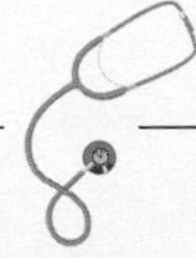

Why do patients with essential thrombocytosis bleed? The excess platelets consume von Willebrand factor and deplete it—thereby causing an acquired form of von Willebrand's disease.

TREATMENT

- Serial phlebotomy to keep Hct down and aspirin.
- Add hydroxyurea in elderly or history of thrombosis.

ESSENTIAL THROMBOCYTOSIS

- Elevation of platelets—the most benign of the myeloproliferative diseases.
- Often, patients are **asymptomatic**. They are at **risk for thrombosis or bleeding.**
- One must rule out secondary causes of thrombocytosis to make the diagnosis. Examples of secondary: iron deficiency (classically associated with high platelets) and reactive (platelets can go up in response to any inflammatory process).
- **Treat with aspirin + either hydroxyurea or anagrelide** (used to suppress platelet production).

PRIMARY MYELOFIBROSIS

- Also called agnogenic myeloid metaplasia.
- Can occur either de novo or as a progressive manifestation of other myeloproliferative diseases.
- Other causes of bone marrow fibrosis are M7 AML and hairy cell leukemia, among other conditions.
- Often presents with weakness from severe anemia and symptoms from splenomegaly or hepatomegaly (both caused by extramedullary hematopoiesis).
- Peripheral smear shows teardrop cells and immature cells (cells forced out of the marrow).
- Treatment is steroids or thalidomide—and neither work well.

MYELODYSPLASTIC SYNDROME (MDS)

- A clonal myeloid disorder (not usually classified as a myeloproliferative disorder) in which abnormal myeloid precursors give rise to dysplastic and ineffective myeloid cells.
- Can manifest in multiple ways and levels of severity.

- Patients can have a single cell line affected (ie, **anemia**) or be pancytopenic.
- It is typically a disease of the **elderly,** but can also result from prior chemotherapy ("treatment-induced MDS").
- Peripheral smear often shows nucleated red blood cells (pushed out from bone marrow) or **dysmorphic neutrophils.**
- There are various treatments with moderate efficacy, though no cure.
- Demethylating agents (decitabine or 5-azacitadine) are recent advancements, but often transfusion support is the only treatment used.
- Complications include infection, transformation to AML or myelofibrosis.

Lymphomas and Multiple Myeloma

HODGKIN'S LYMPHOMA

PATHOPHYSIOLOGY

- Follicular B cells undergo a transformation to malignant cells.
- The malignant cell in Hodgkin's lymphoma is called the **Reed-Sternberg cell.**
- Often, biopsies reveal few Reed-Sternberg cells surrounded by numerous immune and inflammatory cells.
- Two major types of Hodgkin's lymphoma exist:
  - **Classical,** composed of subtypes nodular sclerosing (most common), mixed cellularity, lymphocyte depleted, and lymphocyte rich. Reed-Sternberg cells have very little similarity to their normal B-cell counterpart in this group.
  - **Nonclassical** has only one subgroup, which is the lymphocyte predominant.

EPIDEMIOLOGY

- Bimodal distribution having peaks in 30s and 70s.
- Some cases have an association with Epstein-Barr virus (EBV).

CLINICAL PRESENTATION

- Typically presents with cervical lymph node enlargement or a mediastinal mass.
- "B" symptoms: Fever, night sweats, weight loss without trying.
- Pruritus is another classic symptom of Hodgkin's lymphoma.

DIAGNOSIS

- Lymph node biopsy (excisional) demonstrating the presence of Reed-Sternberg cells.
- Staging:
  - **Stage I:** One lymph node enlarged.
  - **Stage II:** More than one node, on same side of the diaphragm.
  - **Stage III:** Nodes on both sides of diaphragm.
  - **Stage IV:** Extranodal involvement (eg, bone marrow).
  - If there are "B" symptoms, add a "B" to any stage (ie, one node + "B" symptoms = stage IB).

TREATMENT

- Usually a good prognosis, particularly in young patients.
- Numerous regimens exist but currently ABVD (Adriamycin, Bleomycin, Vinblastine, and Dacarbazine) is the treatment of choice.
- Occasionally, radiation has a role in bulky lymph nodes, or when there is only one site of disease.
- New biologic chemotherapy agents (see Table 2.4-1)

NON-HODGKIN'S LYMPHOMA

Non-Hodgkin's lymphoma can arise from B or T lymphocytes, but B-cell lymphomas are far more common. They can be divided into **aggressive or indolent types:**

- **Aggressive or high-grade lymphomas** (eg, large B-cell lymphoma, Burkitt's, lymphoblastic lymphoma) are often symptomatic with "B" symptoms. Untreated survival is short, but many cases are highly curable with treatment.
- **Indolent or low-grade lymphomas** (eg, follicular lymphoma, marginal zone lymphoma) are often asymptomatic and slow growing, but with time can cause symptoms and clinical deterioration. Untreated patients can survive for years, but even with treatment, these diseases are usually *not* curable. Typically treated only if symptomatic.

TABLE 2.4-1. Biologic Chemotherapeutics

DRUG	TARGET	USES
Biologics: all ending with **-Mab** are **M**onoclonal antibodies:		
Rituximab	Antibody to CD20 of B cells	B-cell non-Hodgkin's lymphomas
Infliximab	Antibody to TNF	Crohn's, rheumatoid arthritis
Bevacizumab	Antibody to VEGF	Lung, colon, kidney cancers
Abciximab	Gp IIb/IIIa of platelets	MI, angioplasty
Trastuzumab	Her2/neu	Breast cancer
Those ending with **-NIB** are small molecule tyrosine kinase i**N**(h)**IB**itors:		
Imatinib (Gleevec)	bcr/abl	CML, ALL
Erlotinib	EGF receptor	Lung/pancreas cancer
Sorafenib/Sunitinib	VEGF inhibitors	Kidney and liver cancer

ALL, acute lymphocytic leukemia; CML, chronic myelocytic leukemia; EGF, endothelial growth factor; MI, myocardial infarction; TNF, tumor necrosis factor; VEGF, vascular endothelial growth factor.

SIGNS AND SYMPTOMS

These symptoms can occur in any lymphoma, even in advanced stages of indolent lymphomas:

- "B" symptoms (fatigue, fever, night sweats, weight loss, infections).
- Lymphadenopathy.
- Cytopenias from bone marrow involvement.

DIAGNOSIS

- Lymph node biopsy: This is critical to evaluate the tissue architecture.
- Flow cytometry—this evaluates which proteins are expressed on the cell surface; specific constellations of proteins are associated with different lymphomas (this method is also important in any leukemia diagnosis).
- **FISH** is a sensitive method to look for specific cytogenetic lesions associated with different leukemias and lymphomas.
- Unlike Hodgkin's disease, histology of the nodes is a major predictor of prognosis.

TREATMENT

- Add rituximab to chemotherapy for all B-cell lymphomas.
- Do no treat asymptomatic indolent lymphomas.

SPECIFIC TYPES

- **Follicular lymphoma:**
  - Typically a low-grade lymphoma seen in middle aged or elderly.
- Commonly asymptomatic, painless, diffuse, long-standing lymphadenopathy in a middle-aged individual.
- Bone marrow involvement and disseminated disease is present in the majority of patients.
- Classic cytogenetic lesion is t(14;18) involving BCL-2 (anti-apoptosis protein).
- Divided into low, intermediate, and high grades; high-grade behaves like an aggressive lymphoma.
- **Treat only if symptomatic.** Among many acceptable treatments/combinations are alkylating agents (cyclophosphamide), monoclonal antibodies (rituximab), and corticosteroids.
- **Diffuse large cell lymphoma:**
  - Most common intermediate/high grade lymphoma.
  - May present in a variety of extranodal sites, particularly the gastrointestinal tract and the head and neck.
  - **Often curable.** Treat with chemotherapy—R-CHOP (**R**ituximab, **C**yclophosphamide, Doxorubicin [**H**ydroxydaunomycin], Vincristine [**O**ncovin], **P**rednisone).
- **Lymphoblastic lymphoma:**
  - Very high-grade lymphoma often seen in children; behaves like an acute leukemia.
  - Derived from thymic T-cells and often presents with large mediastinal mass.
  - Often seen in children.
  - Associated with testicular, CNS, and marrow involvement.

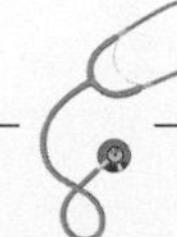

Why are there lytic lesions and hypercalcemia in multiple myeloma patients? Myeloma cells overproduce osteoclast activating factor that causes ↑ bone turnover.

- **Adult T-cell leukemia/lymphoma:**
  - **Associated with HLTV-1 virus,** seen in patients from Japan and the Caribbean.
  - Often presents with hypercalcemia.
  - Although high grade, not typically curable.
- **Burkitt's lymphoma:**
  - **High-grade lymphoma** more common in children than adults.
  - **Endemic type (African)** associated with EBV and jaw lesions.
  - **Nonendemic type:** Diffuse lymphadenopathy.
  - Classic cytogenetic lesion is t(8;14) involving the **c-myc gene.**
  - Bone marrow can have a "starry sky" appearance (from macrophages eating away the necrotic cells and leaving spaces between cells).
  - Treatment includes high-dose cyclophosphamide, methotrexate, and cytarabine and intensive CNS prophylaxis.
- **Mantle cell lymphoma:**
  - Has both high- and low-grade features.
  - Can be very aggressive (high-grade feature) but usually relapses after treatment (low-grade feature).

MULTIPLE MYELOMA

- Plasma cells normally produce antibodies to fight infections. Multiple myeloma is the clonal proliferation of plasma cells usually characterized by the **presence of monoclonal immunoglobulin** or **immunoglobulin fragments (light chains)** in the serum and urine.
- Other manifestations include bone destruction **(lytic lesions)** and **hypercalcemia.**
- Patients also can get renal failure, usually from protein damage.

EPIDEMIOLOGY

Typically elderly; twice as common in African-Americans than whites.

SIGNS AND SYMPTOMS

Patients can present with a pathologic fracture (where a lytic lesion was), hypercalcemia, renal failure, weakness, infection, hyperviscosity from high protein, anemia from bone marrow failure.

DIAGNOSIS

- **Serum and urine electrophoresis (SPEP/UPEP):** These will detect the presence of a monoclonal protein in the serum or urine. Light chains (without the rest of the immunoglobulin) are referred to as **Bence Jones proteins.**
- **Immunofixation** is another method to detect monoclonal proteins.
- **Bone marrow biopsy** shows elevated plasma cells (normal is < 5%).
- Other possible findings:
  - Peripheral blood smear: **Rouleaux formation.**
  - Radiography: **Lytic lesions** on x-ray (needs whole body skeletal survey or x-rays, *not* bone scan).
  - **Elevated total protein** on chemistry.

Why are there lytic lesions and hypercalcemia in multiple myeloma patients? Myeloma cells overproduce osteoclast activating factor that causes ↑ bone turnover

TREATMENT

- There is no cure.
- Multiple effective therapies exist, including older chemotherapies (melphalan) and newer (bortezomib and lenalidomide). Steroids are effective.

- Autologous bone marrow transplant (use the person's own stem cells) is also used.
- Bisphosphonates may delay or prevent lytic lesions, and ↓ hypercalcemia.

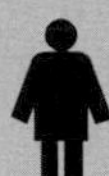

A 60-year-old man with punched out lytic lesions in the skull and mild anemia. *Think: Multiple myeloma.* **Next step:** Check serum and urine protein electrophoresis (SPEP and UPEP).

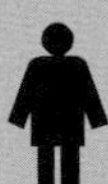

A 68-year-old man presents with low back pain, hypercalcemia, anemia, and azotemia. *Think: Multiple myeloma* (common triad of back pain, anemia, and renal insufficiency).

SOLID TUMOR MALIGNANCIES

Breast Cancer

Epidemiology

- Second most common cause of **cancer death** in women in the United States (most common is lung cancer, as in men). One in eight lifetime risk.
- One percent of all breast cancer occurs in men.
- Ten percent caused by mutations in one or more of the following genes: p53 (tumor suppressor), BRCA-1, BRCA-2, erbB2 (HER-2/neu).

Risk Factors

- Age, prior breast cancer, family history, previous benign biopsy, ↑ estrogen exposure.
- **Causes of ↑ estrogen exposure:** Early menarche, late menopause, nulliparity/late pregnancy, no breast-feeding.
- Oral contraceptives **do not** ↑ risk; but hormone replacement therapy **does** ↑ risk.
- BRCA-1 and BRCA-2 have ↑ risk of breast (50–85%) and ovarian cancer (50%). Prophylactic bilateral mastectomy and oophorectomy should be considered.
- Ductal carcinoma in situ (DCIS) and lobular carcinoma in situ (LCIS).

Screening

- **Breast exams:**
  - Annually by physician (starting at age 20).
  - Monthly self-exam (best time is 3–5 days after onset of menses) does not ↓ mortality.
- **Mammograms:**
  - Not done if < **35 years** because of a dense breast.
  - **40–49 years:** q1–2y is controversial but recommended by most.
  - 50+: Annually until age 70, then only if life expectancy is > 10 years.

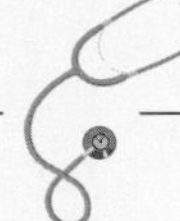

Adverse effects of chemotherapy agents:
Cisplatin: Nephrotoxicity
Bleomycin and **Meth**otrexate: Pulmonary fibrosis (**bleo**mycin blasts the lungs with **METH**ane)
Vin**cristine** = neurotoxic, palsies (**Kristine** lost her **nerves)**
Doxo**rubi**cin = cardiotoxic (**Rubi** lost his heart)
Tamoxifen = uterine cancer (selective estrogen antagonist at breast is an agonist at uterus causing uterine hyperplasia/cancer)
Asparaginase = pancreatitis
CYclophosphamide = hemorrhagic **CY**stitis

- **Evaluation of breast masses:**
  - Cancer is usually painless.
  - Sonography—differentiate cystic from solid masses.
  - Fine-needle aspiration (FNA).
  - **Excisional/open biopsy**—definitive diagnosis.
  - **Diffusely inflamed and indurated breast** (**peau d'orange**—looks like the skin of an orange): Signifies inflammatory breast cancer in which the cancer has infiltrated the dermal lymphatics. Typically very aggressive with poor prognosis.

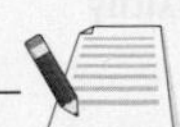

Most cases of breast cancer are *not* associated with known gene mutations.

Prognosis

Prognosis depends on staging, tumor grade, and hormone receptor status (estrogen/progesterone positive is better).

One in eight women who live to age 80 will develop breast cancer.

Treatment

- For **nonmetastatic disease:** Surgical resection.
  - Breast conservation (lumpectomy) is usually possible, but mastectomy is required for very large tumors (> 7 cm) and other specific situation.
  - If lumpectomy only, adding radiation reduces the risk of local recurrence (but not mortality).
  - Adjuvant systemic (chemo) treatment is needed if tumor > 2 cm or there are ⊕ axillary lymph nodes.
  - Special cases:
    - In estrogen/progestin receptor-⊕ patients, tamoxifen (an estrogen/progesterone receptor blocker) is used in premenopausal women and an aromatase inhibitor should be used for postmenopausal women.
    - Trastuzumab (herceptin) is used for HER-2/neu-⊕ patients.
    - Chemotherapy typically used includes adriamycin, cyclophosphamide, and taxanes, or a combination of two of the three.
- For **metastatic disease:** Chemotherapy, hormonal therapy, and/or trastuzumab can be used, depending on receptor status.

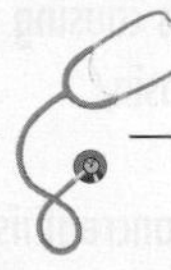

The breasts of young women contain a high proportion of fibrous tissue, rendering mammograms uninterpretable. As women age, the fiber is replaced by fat, which mammograms can evaluate effectively. At age 35 a woman is still at low risk for breast cancer, yet has undergone fatty replacement of a substantial amount of the fiber, making it a good time for the baseline mammogram.

Ovarian Cancer

Epidemiology

- Ovarian cancer is the fourth most common cause of death from cancer among women of all ages in the United States.
- Most patients present in advanced stages.

Signs and Symptoms

Abdominal bloating, **enlarging pants size,** ascites.

Risk Factors

- ↑ **risk:** Older age at first pregnancy/nulliparous; family history/BRCA1 and 2.
- ↓ **risk** (by prolonging periods of anovulation): Childbearing and breastfeeding, oral contraceptives, tubal sterilization.

FIGO Staging

- **Stage I:** Ovary only.
- **Stage II:** Ovary + pelvic extension.

- **Stage III**: Ovary + peritoneal carcinomatosis with ascites (70% of patients)—but confined to abdominal cavity.
- **Stage IV**: Metastasis outside of abdominal cavity.

SCREENING

Not recommended.

PROGNOSIS

Forty percent 5-year survival depending on stage and presentation.

TREATMENT

- Surgery alone for stages IA and IB.
- Surgery (debulking) followed by chemo (paclitaxel + platinum agent) for more advanced stages (**surgical debulking is done even when there are metastases**).

Cervical Cancer

Cervical cancer is a consequence of sexually transmitted infection of human papillomavirus (HPV) types 16 & 18 accounting for 70%.

RISK FACTORS

- HPV.
- Human immunodeficiency virus (HIV).
- Smoking.
- Early age at first intercourse.
- Large number of sexual partners.

SIGNS AND SYMPTOMS

- Foul-smelling vaginal discharge.
- **Postcoital** and irregular vaginal bleeding.
- Pelvic pain.
- Dyspareunia.

SCREENING

- Yearly Papanicolaou (Pap) smear test starting at age 21 in virgins or age at first sexual intercourse until age 65. Perform every 2–3 years if three consecutive negative Pap smears.
- Counsel patients about protective effect of barrier contraceptives.

FIGO STAGING

- **Stage I**: Confined to cervix.
- **Stage II**: Cervix + uterus but not to pelvic wall or lower third of vagina.
- **Stage III**: Invades pelvic wall or lower third of vagina.
- **Stage IV**: Invades other organs in pelvis (bladder) or distant mets.

TREATMENT

- Colposcopic-directed cervical or cone biopsy for carcinoma in situ (stage 0).
- Radical hysterectomy for disease invading cervix (**stage I**). Fertility preservation, if desired, may be possible in limited disease.

- Radiation therapy (usually with cisplatinum chemotherapy) for disease that invades beyond cervix (**stages II–IV**) but without distant metastasis.
- Recurrent or distant metastasis: Radiation for palliation and/or chemotherapy.

Prognosis

Depends on nodal status and stage:

- **Stages I and II:** 5-year survival is 80%.
- **Stage III:** 5-year survival is 40%.

Prostate Cancer

- Prostate cancer is an adenocarcinoma that is the most common cancer in men and third most common cause of cancer death in men in the United States.
- Incidence ↑ with age, with most in men older than 50 years.
- There is a higher incidence in African-Americans.

Signs and Symptoms

- Usually asymptomatic, diagnosed by elevated prostate-specific antigen (PSA).
- Dysuria and urinary hesitancy (more common with benign prostatic hyperplasia [BPH] than prostate cancer) or hematuria.
- New-onset erectile dysfunction.
- Back pain—when presenting with bone mets to spine.

Screening

- Screening (PSA) begins at age 50 until age 75 (or when life expectancy < 10 years); start at age 40 for African-American men or those with BRCA-1 or family history.
- Yearly digital rectal exam to look for nodules.
- Yearly PSA (controversial).
- For PSA > 4.1, transrectal ultrasonography (TRUS) with biopsy of suspicious areas.

Staging and Treatment

- In addition to staging, factors that define high risk are high PSA score and high Gleason score.
- Generally, treatment is surgery or radiation for local disease.
- Prostate cancer typically grows in response to testosterone, so blocking testosterone is an important part of treatment in advanced stages.
- Those with high risk (as defined by a high Gleason score or high PSA) but local disease may benefit from adjuvant hormonal deprivation ("hormonal therapy").
- Metastatic disease can be treated with hormonal therapy alone.
- Commonly used hormonal therapies are anti-androgen agents (eg, flutamide), gonadotropin-releasing hormone (GnRH) agonists (paradoxically, this can ↓ testosterone production), and orchiectomy.
- **T1 (nonpalpable) and T2 (palpable) disease:**
  - Prostatectomy or radiotherapy.
  - Consider both or adding anti-androgen therapy if pathologically high Gleason score or high PSA.
- **T3 disease (extracapsular extension):**

- Radical prostatectomy or radiation.
- Consider hormonal therapy.
- **Metastasis:**
  - Hormonal therapy.
  - Consider chemotherapy if refractory to hormonal therapy.

PROGNOSIS

Ten-year survival rates are 75% when the cancer is confined to the prostate, 55% for those with regional extension, and 15% for those with distant metastases.

Testicular Cancer

- A common cancer in men age 20–40, and is seen more frequently in whites.
- Though other types exist, 95% are germ cell tumors.

CLASSIFICATION

- Germ cell tumors are divided into **seminomas (50%)** and **nonseminomas (50%).**
- Nonseminomas have the following subtypes: choriocarcinoma (secretes human chorionic gonadotropin [hCG]); endodermal sinus tumor (yolk sac tumor; secretes alpha-fetoprotein [AFP]); embryonal carcinoma (secretes hCG and AFP); teratoma (cell types from more than one layer—ecto-, meso-, or endoderm).

FINDINGS

- Painless testicular mass or persistent swelling is cancer unless proven otherwise.
- Metastases may present as back pain (retroperitoneal), para-aortic/supraclavicular nodes, or dyspnea (lung mets).

DIAGNOSIS

- **Do not perform scrotal biopsy** (risk of seeding retroperitoneum by disruption of fascial planes).
- **Orchiectomy from inguinal approach.** Ultrasound should be done prior to surgery to rule out infections or benign conditions such as varicoceles.
- Tumor markers: **LDH for seminoma** (if β-hCG or AFP is elevated, it is automatically considered a nonseminoma regardless of LDH), **β-hCG for choriocarcinoma,** and **AFP for yolk sac tumor.**

TREATMENT

- Cure rates are high, even in advanced stages due to the chemosensitivity of nonseminomas and the radiation sensitivity of seminomas.
- **Nonseminoma:** Orchiectomy, retroperitoneal lymph node dissection (RPLND), and chemotherapy for lymph node involvement or metastasis. Patients without lymph node involvement or metastases have a 95% cure rate.
- **Seminoma:** Orchiectomy and retroperitoneal radiation has 98% cure rate for nonmetastasized seminomas; chemotherapy for metastases.

A 23-year-old man presents with gynecomastia and substernal pain, and physical exam reveals painless testicular mass. *Think: Malignancy.* **Next step?** CXR. Finding? Mediastinal mass = germ cell tumor. Young men with mediastinal mass. *Think:* Lymphoma or germ cell tumor.

Renal Cell Carcinoma

Presentation

- Triad of flank mass, hematuria, and abdominal pain. Diagnosed with abdominal CT scan.
- Paraneoplastic syndromes: Hypercalcemia, polycythemia.
- **Renal vein thrombosis** and **IVC thrombus** are classic findings (see Table 2.4-2).

Treatment

- Early stages (within kidney): Radical nephrectomy.
- Advanced stages (mets or invading the capsule): Interleukin-2 (IL-2) may → remission in 10% of patients who can tolerate it; vascular endothelial growth factor (VEGF) inhibitors (sunitinib or sorafenib).

Bladder Cancer

Usually, cell type is transitional cell carcinoma. Rarely can be "small cell" (neuroendocrine tumor).

Risk Factors

Smoking and occupational (dye) exposure.

TABLE 2.4-2. Paraneoplastic and Distant Effects of Tumors

Effect	Molecule	Associated Neoplasm
Cushing's syndrome	ACTH or ACTH-like peptide.	Small cell lung carcinoma.
SIADH	ADH or ANP.	Small cell lung carcinoma and intracranial neoplasms.
Hypercalcemia	PTH-related peptide, TGF-α, TNF-α, IL-2.	Squamous cell lung carcinoma, renal carcinoma, breast carcinoma, multiple myeloma, and bone metastasis (lysed bone).
Polycythemia	Erythropoietin.	Renal cell carcinoma (hypernephroma).
Lambert-Eaton syndrome	Antibodies against presynaptic Ca^{2+} channels at NMJ.	Thymoma, bronchogenic carcinoma.
Gout	Hyperuricemia due to excess nucleic acid turnover (ie, cytotoxic therapy).	

ACTH, adrenocorticotropic hormone; ADH, antidiuretic hormone; ANP, atrial natriuretic peptide; IL-2, interleukin-2; NMJ, neuromuscular junction; PTH, parathyroid hormone; TGF, transforming growth factor; TNF-α, tumor necrosis factor-α.

Presentation

Painless hematuria.

Diagnosis

CT urogram and cystoscopy. Urine for cytology (10% yield).

Treatment

- Localized (not invading bladder muscle): Surgery + intravesical chemo or bacillus Calmette-Guerin (BCG).
- Advanced: Chemotherapy.

Hepatocellular Carcinoma

Epidemiology

- More common in Asia.
- Seen in patients with cirrhosis, especially hepatitis B and hemochromatosis.

Screening

- Liver ultrasound +/– **AFP (tumor marker)** every 6 months in patients with cirrhosis or chronic hepatitis B.
- MRI for more definitive diagnosis.

Treatment

- Depends on the degree of cirrhosis and the size of the tumor.
- For local disease, options include surgery, radiofrequency ablation, and chemoembolization.
- For metastatic disease, VEGF inhibitors (sunitinib or sorafenib) can be given.

MISCELLANEOUS METASTATIC DISEASE

- **Liver metastasis:**
  - Liver and lung are the most common sites for metastatic disease.
  - Primary tumors that metastasize to the liver: **Colon** > **Stomach** > **Pancreas** (all three GI from portal circulation) > **Breast** > **Lung.**
- **Bone metastasis:**
  - Breast and prostate are the most common.
  - Kidney, thyroid, testes, lung, prostate, breast.
    - Lung = Lytic
    - Breast = Both lytic and blastic
    - Prostate = blastic
  - **Brain metastasis:**
  - Fifty percent of brain tumors are metastatic lesions.
  - Primary tumors metastasizing to the brain: **Lung, Breast, Skin** (melanoma), **Kidney** (renal cell carcinoma), **GI.**

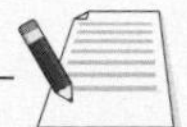

Lots of Bad Stuff Kills Glia (Origin of brain mets: Lung, Breast, Skin, Kidney, GI)

ONCOLOGIC EMERGENCIES

Hypercalcemia

- The most common metabolic emergency of malignancy.
- Symptoms and signs include confusion, nausea, fatigue, ↓ PO intake, polyuria, depression, psychosis/confusion, nephrolithiasis (**BONES, STONES, GROANS, and PSYCHIATRIC OVERTONES**).
- Can progress to severe confusion and coma.
- Electrocardiogram (ECG) may show QT interval shortening.
- Usual cancers: Multiple myeloma, breast cancer, squamous cell (lung cancer, head and neck), renal cell cancer, lymphomas.
- Either from bone mets, PTH related peptide or 1-25 vitamin D (lymphomas).
- **Treatment: Aggressive rehydration with normal saline**, furosemide if patient is fluid overloaded, **bisphosphonates (takes 2–3 days).** Calcitonin as a temporizing measure has limited role due to tachyphylaxis.

Febrile Neutropenia

Fever in the setting of clinically significant neutropenia (absolute neutrophil count < 500).

Workup

- Careful history and physical.
- Chest x-ray.
- Pan-culture.

Treatment

- Antibiotics should be started empirically (usually cefepime +/– aminoglycoside); add vancomycin if the person has hypotension, history of methicillin-resistant *Staphylococcus aureus* (MRSA), or an **infusaport** (access device for transfusions or chemotherapy) or a skin source).
- If vancomycin is not added initially, then add vanco at day 3 if patient continues to have fever and neutropenia. Add antifungals (voriconazole) on day 5 if no improvement.

Tumor Lysis Syndrome

- Cell breakdown causes release of intracellular ions (potassium and phosphorus) and DNA breakdown causing **hyperuricemia.**
- Seen in leukemias, lymphomas, and after chemotherapy in bulky tumors.
- Uric acid can cause acute renal failure and gout.
- Electrolyte disturbances: Hyperkalemia, hyperphosphatemia and hypocalcemia (from binding to phosphorus). **High LDH**.
- Treat with IV fluids, allopurinol.
- Severe cases require urine alkalinization and IV therapy with rasburicase (an enzyme that degrades uric acid).

Superior Vena Cava (SVC) Syndrome

Caused by obstruction of the superior vena cava by external compression, tumor invasion, or thrombus formation in the SVC lumen.

SIGNS/SYMPTOMS

Dyspnea, facial edema and plethora, cough, neck and arm edema.

DIAGNOSIS

CT chest, chest x-ray.

TREATMENT

- Chemotherapy, **radiation.**
- Intubation/tracheal stent if airway compromise.
- Steroids (controversial).

Spinal Cord Compression

- Compression of spinal cord secondary to vertebral collapse or extension of tumor from vertebra.
- Most commonly affects the thoracic spine.
- Back pain in cancer patient with neurological symptoms = cord compression.

SIGNS/SYMPTOMS

- Back pain.
- Loss of bowel or bladder function.
- Muscle weakness.
- Saddle anesthesia.

DIAGNOSIS

- Thorough neurologic exam, including rectal exam for evaluation of sphincter tone.
- MRI spine with gadolinium.

TREATMENT

High-dose steroids + radiation therapy or surgical decompression.

TABLE 2.4-3 Common Classes of Chemotherapies

Specific Drugs (Examples)	Indications	Specific Toxicity
Drug Class: Alkylating agents	**Mechanism:** Formation of DNA cross-links and hence inhibition of DNA function and synthesis.	**General Toxicities:** Myelosuppression, mucosal toxicity-mucosal ulceration, diarrhea, nausea and vomiting.
Cyclophosphamide/ Ifosfamide	HL, NHL, ALL/CLL, Multiple myeloma, breast/ lung/ovary/ testicular cancer.	Hemorrhagic cystitis.
Melphalan	Multiple myeloma, ovarian cancer.	Myelosuppression, hypersensitivity.
Chlorambucil	CLL, HL/NHL.	Myelosuppression, bone marrow failure.
Bendamustine	CLL, NHL.	Pancytopenia, hyperbilirubinemia.
Temozolomide	Brain cancer, malignant melanoma.	Myelosuppression, elevated LFTs.
Procarbazine	HL, NHL.	Myelosuppression, reproductive dysfunction, hemolysis (in G6PD deficiency).
Dacarbazine	HL, malignant melanoma.	Myelosuppression, metallic taste, rash.
Drug Class: Platinum compounds	**Mechanism:** Form intrastrand and interstrand DNA cross-links; bind to nuclear and cytoplasmic proteins.	
Cisplatin	NSCLC, breast cancer, bladder cancer, head and neck cancer, ovarian cancer.	**Nephrotoxicity,** peripheral **neuropathy,** myelosuppression, ototoxicity.
Carboplatin	NSCLC, breast cancer, bladder cancer, head and neck cancer, ovarian cancer.	Myelosuppression.
Oxaliplatin	Colorectal cancer, pancreatic cancer.	Myelosuppression, peripheral neuropathy.

Drug	Mechanism of Action	Indications	Toxicity
Drug Class: Antimetabolites			
Subclass: Folic acid analogs			
Methotrexate	Inhibits dihydrofolate reductase, inhibits thymidylate synthetase.	NHL, bladder cancer, head and neck cancer.	Mucositis, diarrhea, myelosuppression. **Don't give if any effusions (drug will stay there).**

TABLE 2.4-3 Common Classes of Chemotherapies *(continued)*

DRUG	MECHANISM OF ACTION	INDICATIONS	TOXICITY
Subclass: Pyrimidine analogs			
Cytarabine	Inhibits DNA synthesis and repair.	Acute leukemias (AML and ALL).	Myelosuppression, **cerebellar toxicity.**
5-Fluorouracil (5-FU)	Interferes with DNA synthesis, Inhibits thymidylate synthetase, incorporates into RNA.	Colorectal cancer, stomach cancer, head and neck cancer, breast cancer.	Mucositis, bone marrow suppression.
Capecitabine	Oral version of 5-FU. Interferes with DNA synthesis, inhibits thymidylate synthetase, incorporates into RNA.	Colorectal cancer, gastroesophageal cancer, pancreatic cancer, breast cancer.	Hand-foot syndrome, myelosuppression.
Gemcitabine	Inhibits DNA synthesis, inhibits ribonucleotide reductase.	Pancreatic cancer, NSCLC, breast cancer.	Myelosuppression, edema, hepatotoxicity.
Subclass: Purine analogs			
6-mercaptopurine (6-MP)	Inhibits purine nucleotide synthesis, inhibits DNA/RNA synthesis.	ALL, AML.	Myelosuppression, hepatotoxicity.
Cladribine	Incorporates into DNA, inhibits DNA synthesis and repair.	**Hairy cell leukemia.**	Myelosuppression.
Fludarabine	Incorporates into DNA, inhibits DNA synthesis and repair.	NHL, **CLL.**	Myelosuppression, myalgias, arthralgias.
Hydroxyurea	Interferes DNA synthesis (antimetabolite), **↑Hb F level in sickle cell anemia.**	CML, polycythemia vera, essential thrombosis, **sickle cell disease.**	
Drug Class (sort of): Natural products			
Subtype: Vinca alkaloids (from plant)			
Vinblastine	Inhibits microtubule formation and mitosis.	**HL,** NHL, breast cancer, testicular cancer, Kaposi's sarcoma.	Myelosuppression, hypertension.
Vincristine	Inhibits microtubule formation and mitosis.	Leukemias, HL, NHL.	**Neuropathy**, myelosuppression.

(continued)

TABLE 2.4-3 Common Classes of Chemotherapies *(continued)*

DRUG	MECHANISM OF ACTION	INDICATIONS	TOXICITY
Subtype: Taxanes (from plant)			
Docetaxel	Interfere with microtubules, inhibit mitosis.	Breast cancer, metastatic prostate cancer, NSCLC.	**Fluid retention**, neurotoxicity, myelosuppression.
Paclitaxel	Interfere with microtubules, inhibit mitosis.	Breast cancer, NSCLS, ovarian cancer.	**Neuropathy,** myelosuppression.
Subtype: Camptothecins (topoisomerase I inhibitors) (from plant)			
Topotecan	Inhibits topoisomerase I.	Ovarian cancer, small cell lung cancer.	Myelosuppression.
Irinotecan	Inhibits topoisomerase I.	Lung cancer, colorectal cancer.	Diarrhea, nausea, myelosuppression.
Subtype: Epipodophyllotoxins (topoisomerase II inhibitors) (Podophyllotoxin derivative)			
Etoposide	Inhibits topoisomerase II.	NHL, NSCLC, gastric cancer.	Mucositis, myelosuppression, alopecia.
Teniposide	Inhibits topoisomerase II.	ALL.	Mucositis, myelosuppression.
Miscellaneous			
Arsenic	DNA fragmentation, induces apoptosis, degrades PML/RAR alpha protein.	Acute promyelocytic leukemia (M3).	
Asparaginase (enzyme)	Hydrolyzes asparagine and hence inhibits protein synthesis.	ALL.	**Pancreatitis**, coagulation abnormalities—bleeding and clotting
ATRA (tretinoin)	**Induces differentiation of promyelocytes, thereby reducing DIC when chemo starts.**	Acute promyelocytic leukemia **(M3).**	**ATRA syndrome:** Severe fluid retention that can cause respiratory failure. Treat with steroids.
Drug Class: Antibiotics			
Bleomycin	Binds to DNA, causing DNA breaking.	HL, NHL, germ cell cancer, squamous cell cancer.	**Pulmonary fibrosis,** mucositis, dermatotoxicity.
Daunorubicin/Doxorubicin (adriamycin)	Binds to DNA causing DNA breaking, inhibits toposiomerase II.	ALL, lymphomas, breast cancer.	**Cardiotoxicity,** myelosuppression.

TABLE 2.4-3 Common Classes of Chemotherapies *(continued)*

DRUG	MECHANISM OF ACTION	INDICATIONS	TOXICITY
Small molecules (usually inhibit a tyrosine kinase in the cell signaling)			
Erlotinib	Inhibits EGFR tyrosine kinase.	**NSCLC**, pancreatic cancer.	**Skin rash,** interstitial lung disease.
Imatinib	**Inhibits Bcr-Abl tyrosine kinase.**	**CML (revolutionary breakthrough with great results),** GIST.	Fluid retention and edema, myalgias.
Sorafenib and sunitinib	Inhibits multiple kinase receptors involved with VEGF.	Unresectable hepatocellular cancer, renal cell carcinoma.	Skin rash, fatigue, ↑ INR.

ALL, acute lymphocytic leukemia; ATRA: all-trans retinoic acid; CML, chronic myelocytic leukemia; CLL, chronic lymphocytic lymphoma; EGFR, endothelial growth factor; HL, Hodgkin's lymphoma; GIST, gastrointestinal stromal tumor; G6PD, glucose-6-phosphate dehydrogenase; INR, International Normalized Ratio; NHL, non-Hodgkin's lymphoma; NSCLC, non–small cell lung cancer; PML, promyelocytic leukemia; RAR, retinoic acid receptor; VEGF, vascular endothelial growth factor.

HIGH-YIELD FACTS IN

Infectious Disease

DEFINITIONS

- **Infection:** Microbial process characterized by an inflammatory response.
- **Bacteremia:** Invasion of and presence of bacteria in the blood.
- **Systemic inflammatory response syndrome (SIRS):** Characterized by two or more of the following:
  - Temperature > 38°C or < 36°C
  - Heart rate > 90
  - Respiratory rate > 20 per minute or $PaCO_2 < 32$
  - White blood cell count > 12 or < 4 or greater than 10% immature neutrophils
- **Sepsis:** SIRS and a nidus of infection.
- **Severe sepsis:** Sepsis with evidence of organ hypoperfusion.
- **Septic shock:** Severe sepsis with hypotension despite adequate fluid resuscitation requiring vasopressors to maintain blood pressure.

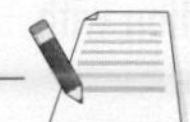

Always treat a pregnant woman for a UTI, even if it's asymptomatic. First-line treatments are nitrofurantoin or a beta-lactam (penicillin or cephalosporin).

- Asymptomatic bacteremia should **not** be treated in the following populations: women (premenopausal, nonpregnant), diabetics, elderly, nursing home residents or patients with spinal cord injury or indwelling urethral catheters. These patients tend to have colonized or contaminated specimens.
- Asymptomatic bacteremia **always** should be treated in pregnant women.
- Asymptomatic pyuria (WBCs in urine) should **not** be treated in most cases.

GENITOURINARY INFECTIONS

Urinary Tract Infection (UTI), Cystitis, and Pyelonephritis

DEFINITIONS

- A **urinary tract infection** (UTI) is a general term encompassing infection anywhere from the urethral meatus to the kidneys. **An uncomplicated UTI** is one that occurs in healthy, nonpregnant females, all others are generally **complicated UTIs.**
- **Cystitis** is infection of the bladder.
- **Pyelonephritis** is infection involving the renal parenchyma.
- **Bacteriuria** is the presence of bacteria in the urine, which may or may not be symptomatic.
- **Pyuria** is the presence of WBCs in the urine, usually associated with bacteriuria.
- **Hematuria** is the presence of RBCs in the urine, often seen with cystitis.

EPIDEMIOLOGY

- More common in women by a ratio of 30:1 from age 1 through 50; beyond age 50 the ratio is 2:1.
- UTI is the most common infectious complication of pregnancy.
- In the elderly, UTI is the most frequently documented infection, the most common cause of sepsis, and the most common nosocomial infection.

RISK FACTORS

- Men:
  - Uncircumcised males.
  - Prostatic hypertrophy.
  - Phimosis.
  - Anal intercourse or vaginal intercourse with urinary tract infected partner.

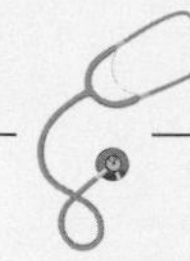

Men with cystitis should be investigated for an underlying cause such as prostatitis or urinary retention.

- **Women:**
  - Recent sexual intercourse.
  - History of prior UTI.
  - Use of spermicide.
  - Postmenopausal state.
- **Both:**
  - Instrumentation/catheterization (see Table 2.5-1 for common procedures).
  - Immunocompromise.
  - Genitourinary tract abnormalities.

Etiology

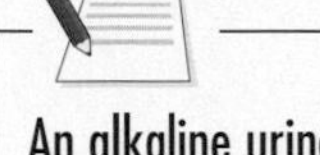

An alkaline urine is suggestive of infection with *Proteus mirabilis* or *Ureaplasma urealyticum.*

- *Escherichia coli* is by far the most common pathogen, accounting for 80–85% of community-acquired UTIs and 50% of nosocomial ones.

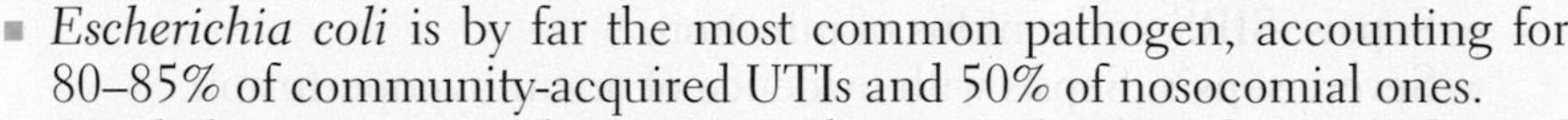

- *Staphylococcus saprophyticus* contributes to 5–15% of uncomplicated cases, mostly in young women.
- *Klebsiella, Proteus, Pseudomonas,* and enterococci account for most of the remainder of cases.
- Group B strep accounts for only ~ 1% of cases but is a clinically important pathogen in the pregnant patient at term—**always test third-trimester pregnant patients for this.**

TABLE 2.5-1. Common Genitourinary Procedures

Test	Description	Uses
Intravenous pyelography	Contrast is injected into a peripheral vein, followed by radiographs, allowing visualization of the renal parenchyma and the ureters.	Basically anytime you want to visualize the ureters and kidneys. Examples: suspicion of infection, tumor, renal damage of any sort (e,g., pyelonephritis).
Voiding cystourethrogram	Contrast medium is placed into the bladder via catheter and visualized with x-ray during active micturition.	Investigation of abnormalities of bladder and ureters. Examples: **structural abnormality** (congenital, ectopic drainage, strictures, vesicoureteral reflux, ureteroceles) or **functional abnormality** (neurogenic bladder, stress incontinence) of ureters.
Cystometry	Bladder is filled with water via catheter. Bladder is emptied into a measuring device. The pressure is recorded during this process.	Investigation of bladder function in the setting of incontinence or urgency (eg, is benign prostatic hypertrophy obstructing bladder outflow? Is there outflow obstruction, or is bladder not contracting for other reasons?)
Cystoscopy	Introduction of either a flexible or rigid scope into the urethra.	Visualize inside of bladder. For example, investigate hematuria—is there tumor there (can biopsy also)? Bladder stone? Also therapeutic—can crush bladder stones.
Renal ultrasound	Advantage is that it is noninvasive.	Visualize kidneys. First step in investigating kidney failure. "Atrophic kidneys" suggest kidney damage. Also can see tumors, hydronephrosis, thrombus.

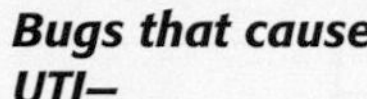

SIGNS AND SYMPTOMS

- **General UTI:** Dysuria, frequency, urgency, nocturia, suprapubic pain, cloudy, malodorous urine, or bloody urine.
- **Pyelonephritis:** Spiking fever, shaking chills, costovertebral angle tenderness, nausea, vomiting, anorexia.

DIAGNOSIS

- **Urine dipstick** can detect **leukocyte esterase** (correlates to pyuria—or leukocytes in the urine) and **nitrites** (made by certain common UTI bugs, eg, Enterobacteriaceae); the most widely available and cost-effective test; fairly sensitive and specific.
- The presence of leukocyte esterase and nitrites usually indicate a UTI.
- **Urine analysis** involves spinning down and directly visualizing the presence of WBCs (pyuria) (> 5 WBCs is ⊕).
- **Interpretation of all tests must take into account the presence or absence of symptoms.**
  - **Nitrites:** May have false ⊖ if bacteria that do not produce nitrite, or if already on antibiotics or if voided urine not in bladder long; may have **false** ⊕ due to meds altering dipstick color, or if not fresh urine.
  - **Leukocyte esterase:** False-⊕ leukocyte esterase results are seen with fecal contamination; false ⊖—patient already on antibiotics.
- **Pyuria** is present in nearly all UTIs; its absence suggests another diagnosis. Greater than 5 WBC per high power field is definitively ⊕ (2–5 is a gray area); this is around > 8 WBC/µL or 8000 WBC/mL.
- **Urine culture** is the definitive test. A ⊕ result is defined as > 10,000 colony-forming units (CFUs) per milliliter with a single organism in symptomatic patients, and > 100,000 CFU/mL in an asymptomatic patient. Urine cultures should always be obtained for complicated UTIs, due to high rate of bacterial resistance.
- **Imaging** is not indicated for uncomplicated UTI. CT scan or renal ultrasound can demonstrate perinephric/intrarenal abscesses, nephrolithiasis, or obstruction. If pyelonephritis does not improve after 48–72 hours, these causes should be sought.

TREATMENT

- Most uncomplicated UTIs are treated with a short course (3–5 days) of oral antibiotics on an outpatient basis. Complicated UTI requires a longer duration of antibiotics.
- Bacteriuria in pregnancy is *always* treated, regardless of the presence of symptoms, due to high rate of progression to pyelonephritis. Empiric category B antibiotics are nitrofurantoin and ampicillin.
- Consider hospitalization and intravenous antibiotics for high-risk patients: elderly, immunocompromised, those with indwelling catheters, sepsis, and patients who are unable to tolerate oral intake.

Bugs that cause UTI–

SEEKS PP

S. *saprophyticus*
E. *coli*
E*nterobacter*
K*lebsiella*
S*erratia*
P*roteus*
P*seudomonas* (especially with GU instrumentation)

INFECTIOUS DISEASE

Vaginitis

The normal flora of the vagina creates an acidic environment (pH 3.5–4.5) in large part through the colonization of lactobacilli. This protects the vagina from pathogenic organisms. When this environment is disturbed, infections become possible.

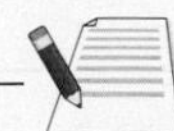

Lactobacilli are used to make yogurt. A Yoplait a day keeps vaginitis away.

INFECTIOUS DISEASE

The "whiff" test: Application of KOH to the wet mount will enhance the odor of both *Gardnerella* and *Trichomonas.* **On wet mount:** "Clue cells" = bacterial vaginosis; motile flagellated organisms = trichomoniasis.

CAUSES

- Bacterial vaginosis (BV)—*Gardnerella.*
- *Trichomonas vaginalis* (sexually transmitted).
- Yeast—*Candida albicans.*

SIGNS AND SYMPTOMS

- Vaginal itch and burning sensation.
- Abnormal odor.
- Discharge:
  - BV: Fishy odor of discharge.
  - *Trichomonas:* Fishy odor of discharge, strawberry cervix.
  - **Yeast:** Cottage cheese–like discharge.

DIAGNOSIS

Wet mount:

- BV: Clue cells (epithelial cells coated with bacteria).
- *Trichomonas:* Motile trichomonads.
- Yeast: Pseudohyphae.

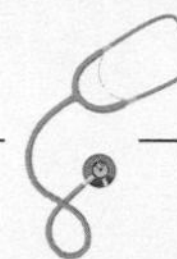

Metronidazole is contraindicated in first-trimester pregnancy. Use clotrimazole instead.

TREATMENT

- Metronidazole for BV and *Trichomonas.*
- Treat sexual partners as well in *Trichomonas* (sexually transmitted).
- Azole antifungals or nystatin for yeast infection.

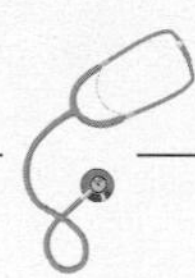

Warn patients against having any alcohol while on metronidazole. It can cause a disulfiram-like reaction when co-ingested with alcohol.

SEXUALLY TRANSMITTED DISEASES (STDS)

Syphilis

- A sexually transmitted or congenital disease with variable clinical manifestations, depending on stage of the disease.
- Transmitted primarily through sexual contact but can be spread through any mucosal or epithelial abrasion.
- The causative organism is *Treponema pallidum,* a spirochete.
- Once the spirochete has entered the body, it spreads throughout most organ systems and the disease then progresses through three active stages.

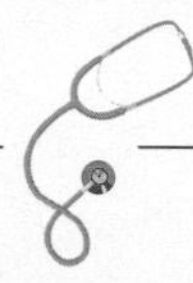

De Musset's sign (head bobbing seen in aortic insufficiency) was first described in prostitutes with syphilitic aortitis.

SIGNS AND SYMPTOMS

All patients develop a *painless* chancre at inoculation site. If untreated, some patients progress to a disseminated (2°) stage, during which the organism is spread throughout the entire body and is highly infectious.

- 1° syphilis:
  - A **painless "buttonlike" chancre** with indurated borders develops at inoculation site within 2–6 weeks after exposure.
  - Accompanied by regional lymphadenopathy ("**bubo**") within 1 week.
  - Chancre can last up to 6 weeks if untreated.
- 2° syphilis:
  - Appears 4–6 weeks after 1° syphilis resolves, lasts for 6–8 weeks.
  - Maculopapular rash (multiple, discrete, firm, "ham-colored" papules scattered symmetrically over trunk, **palms and soles,** and genitals).

Argyll Robertson (syphilitic) pupil is like a prostitute: It accommodates but doesn't react.

- **Condylomata lata:** Soft, flat-topped pink papules on anogenital region that are painless, wartlike lesions.
- Flulike symptoms: Fever, malaise, arthralgia, generalized lymphadenopathy, and splenomegaly.

- **Latent phase:**
  - This stage can last for several years.
  - Patients are asymptomatic but remain seropositive.
- **3° syphilis:**
  - Develops at any time during the latent phase and continues indefinitely if not treated.
  - **Gummas:** Rubbery granulomatous lesions in subcutaneous tissues of central nervous system (CNS), heart, aorta.
  - Cardiovascular: Vasa vasorum vasculitis, aortic insufficiency.
  - Neurosyphilis: Seizures, personality changes, psychosis, **tabes dorsalis** (posterior column degeneration).
  - The syphilitic pupil is also known as **Argyll Robertson pupil.**

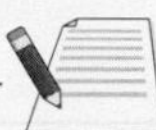

Rapid plasma reagin (RPR) syphilis screening is part of dementia workup.

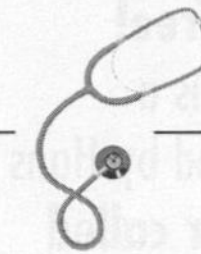

VDRL/RPR false ⊕ are seen in:

- Systemic lupus erythematosus (SLE)
- Infectious mononucleosis
- Hepatitis C

Laboratory

- **Venereal Disease Research Laboratory (VDRL) and rapid plasma reagin (RPR):** Good screening tests but nonspecific.
- **Fluorescent treponemal antibody-absorption test (FTA-ABS):** Done when VDRL or RPR is ⊕. Good sensitivity and specificity. Remains ⊕ for life, regardless of treatment.
- **Darkfield microscopy:** Smear of exudate from primary chancre or secondary papular lesions reveal a 5- to 20-µm-long spirochete, with kinking and contractile movements but without locomotion.
- *T. pallidum* does not grow in regular blood cultures.
- If neurosyphilis is suspected, cerebrospinal fluid (CSF) should be sent for WBC count, protein, glucose, and VDRL.

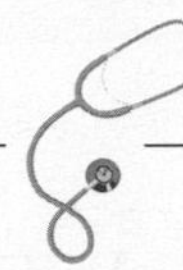

Jarisch-Herxheimer reaction: Fever, fatigue, and transient worsening of mucocutaneous symptoms, typically seen in treatment of 2° syphilis with penicillin. ***It is not a drug allergy!***

Treatment

Penicillin G; can consider tetracycline for nonpregnant patients with severe penicillin allergies; however, desensitization therapy is preferred in these cases whenever possible.

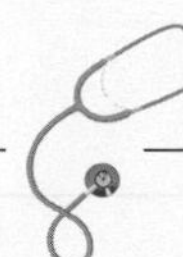

If maternal syphilis infection is untreated by 16 weeks' gestation, child may be born with congenital syphilis and is at risk of stillbirth.

Balanitis

Inflammation of the glans penis.

Causes

- *Candida albicans*, other infectious agents.
- Allergic reaction (often to latex condoms).
- Reactive arthritis (formerly known as Reiter's syndrome).

Treatment

Treat underlying cause: Candidal infections are treated with nystatin/topical azoles. Reactive arthritis is treated with NSAIDs.

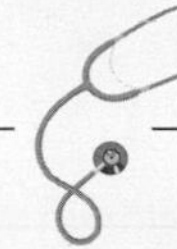

Any patient who presents with balanitis should be screened for diabetes (candidal infections are common in diabetics and uncommon in normal men).

Genital Herpes

Infection with herpes simplex virus. Type 1 usually associated with oral lesions, and type 2 with genital lesions, but not always.

SIGNS AND SYMPTOMS

- **Painful** vesicular lesions on erythematous base.
- Local lymphadenopathy.
- Neuralgia often precedes an outbreak.

LABORATORY

- Tzanck smear test and culture.
- Herpes serology.

TREATMENT

Antiviral agents acyclovir, famciclovir, and valacyclovir are not curative but effective in reducing the severity and frequency of outbreaks, as well as the degree of viral shedding.

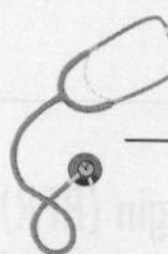

Reactive Arthritis: Can't See, Can't Pee, Can't Climb a Tree!
Reactive arthritis is a condition described by Hans Reiter (**no longer called Reiter's syndrome** secondary to his involvement with the Nazis in WWII) with the classic triad of nongonococcal urethritis, conjuctivitis, and arthritis.

Human Papillomavirus (HPV)

STD caused by the human papillomavirus, of which there are many subtypes.

EPIDEMIOLOGY

- Most common sexually transmitted disease.
- Commonly asymptomatic in men.
- Certain serotypes have been implicated as causative agent in cervical cancer (16, 18, 31 most common).

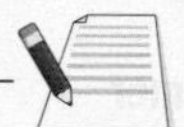

Infections can remain dormant for years, but the herpesvirus is continuously shed and can be transmitted during latent phases.

SIGNS AND SYMPTOMS

- Bowenoid papules on penis.
- Condyloma acuminata (papillomatous growths with a soft, macerated surface).
- Warts grow on mucous membrane of penis, perineum, vulva, vagina, and vaginal canal.

DIAGNOSIS

Most HPV warts are flat and invisible to the unaided eye. Coating them with 1% acetic acid turns them white. All white lesions on colposcopy are biopsied for HPV.

HSV meningitis presents with fever, confusion, and photophobia, and MRI usually shows a temporal lobe lesion. Give: IV acyclovir.

TREATMENT

- Lesions are removed via cryosurgery, laser ablation, or chemical ablation (podophyllin).
- **Gardasil (HPV vaccine)** is used to prevent infection with cervical cancer-associated serotypes.

Urethritis

Neisseria gonorrhoeae and *Chlamydia trachomatis* are the two most common organisms:

- ***N. gonorrhoeae*** (gonococcus [GC]) can cause cervicitis, urethritis, epididymitis, conjunctivitis, PID, pneumonia, and lymphogranuloma venereum.
- ***C. trachomatis*** can cause cervicitis, urethritis, epididymitis, conjunctivitis, pelvic inflammatory disease (PID), pneumonia, and lymphogranuloma venereum.

HPV types 16, 18, 31, 45, 51, 52, and 53 are associated with cervical cancer.

DIAGNOSIS

Polymerase chain reaction (PCR) analysis of vaginal or penile swab, or urine culture.

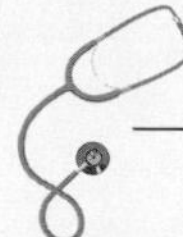

HPV: Mother may infect newborn during delivery, causing **laryngeal papillomatosis.**

TREATMENT

- Single-dose therapy:
  - **For GC:** 125 mg ceftriaxone IM.
  - **For *Chlamydia*:** 1 g azithromycin PO.
- Above combination often given empirically, thereby avoiding compliance issues.
- Multiple 7-day combinations exist, if above regimen is not chosen.
- Sexual partners should be treated concurrently; if the partner is not present, the patient is often given an extra prescription to be taken by their partner.

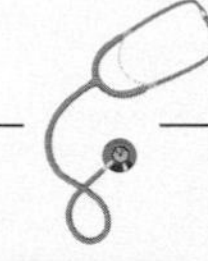

Always treat *Chlamydia* and GC concurrently because coinfection is often present.

Pelvic Inflammatory Disease (PID)

- Infection of the upper genital structures in women (uterus, oviducts, ovaries), often with involvement of neighboring organs.
- Usually, this is GC or *Chlamydia* untreated and progressing (see urethritis).
- Both, particularly *Chlamydia*, can be chronic and cause scarring of the fallopian tubes and infertility.

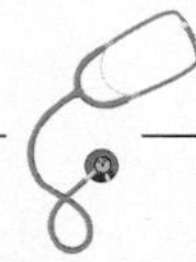

The discharge of GC is purulent, whereas that of *Chlamydia* is nonpurulent.

RISK FACTORS

- Younger age at first sexual contact.
- Multiple sexual partners.
- Use of intrauterine device (IUD).
- Prior history of PID.
- Recent intrauterine instrumentation.

SIGNS AND SYMPTOMS

- Lower abdominal pain.
- Tenderness to pelvic exam.

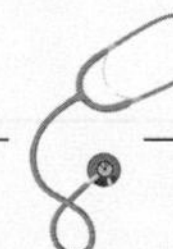

Chlamydia is the leading infectious cause of blindness worldwide (trachoma).

DIAGNOSTIC CRITERIA

Cervical motion and adnexal tenderness *plus* one or more of the following:

- Fever > 101°F.
- Abnormal vaginal/cervical discharge.
- Lab evidence of GC or *C. trachomatis.*
- Elevated erythrocyte sedimentation rate (ESR) or C-reactive protein.

TREATMENT

- **Outpatient:**
  - Treat for GC and *C. trachomatis,* major causative organisms.
  - Offer HIV testing.
  - Remove any infected foreign body.
  - Treat all sexual partners.
- **Inpatient:** Hospital admission and IV antibiotics (ceftriaxone and azithromycin) is warranted if any of the following: high fever, uncertain diagnosis, pregnancy, can't take PO, immunosuppression, first episode in nulligravida, can't follow up in 48 hours, failure of outpatient therapy.

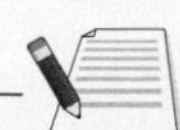

C. trachomatis is a major cause of PID and infertility (fallopian tube scarring causes infertility).

Prostatitis

Two types—bacterial and nonbacterial.

> A 19-year-old sexually active female presents with left lower quadrant crampy pelvic pain for 1 week. Physical exam reveals a temperature of 101°F, cervical motion tenderness, and a mucopurulent vaginal discharge. Laboratory results reveal ESR 65 and WBC 16. *Think: Pelvic inflammatory disease.* Check for GC and chlamydia. **Next step:** Give IV antibiotics (ceftriaxone and azithromycin).

Bacterial Prostatitis

Inflammation of the prostate due to bacteria ascending the urethra and then passing into the prostate through the prostatic ducts.

Causes

- *E. coli.*
- *Pseudomonas*

Signs and Symptoms

- Perineal and suprapubic pain.
- Dysuria and urinary frequency.
- Fever.
- Tender, boggy prostate on physical exam.
- Chronic bacterial prostatitis is uncommon and presents as recurrent UTI.

Laboratory Findings

- Leukocytosis with neutrophil predominance.
- Urinalysis (U/A) shows bacteriuria and pyuria.

Treatment

- Outpatient therapy consists of TMP-SMZ or ciprofloxacin (flouroquinolone is preferred) for 21 days.
- Indications for hospitalization include severe comorbidities, poor patient compliance, or sepsis.

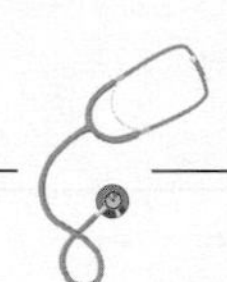

Care must be taken during the rectal exam on a prostatis patient. Vigorously massaging the prostate can → bacteremia.

Nonbacterial Prostatitis

- An inflammatory process in the prostate from an unknown etiology.
- Viral agents or an autoimmune reaction are possible causes.
- This is the most common cause of chronic prostatitis.

Signs and Symptoms

- Urinary frequency and dysuria.
- Nontender, enlarged prostate on physical exam.

Laboratory

- U/A and urine culture are ⊖.
- Leukocytes can be seen in prostatic secretions.

Treatment

- A trial of antibiotics is often given.
- Anti-inflammatories for symptomatic relief.

PNEUMONIA AND UPPER RESPIRATORY TRACT INFECTIONS

Community-Acquired Pneumonias (CAPs)

Top five bacterial etiologies of CAP:

1. *Streptococcus pneumoniae* (most common).
2. *Staphylococcus aureus* (methicillin-resistant [MRSA] becoming more common in the community).
3. *Legionella.*
4. *Haemophilus influenzae.*
5. Atypicals: *Chlamydia pneumoniae* and *Mycoplasma pneumoniae.*

Treatment

Treatment is almost always initiated with an empirically selected antibiotic: macrolide in simple cases; respiratory flouroquinolone (levofloxacin, moxifloxacin) or beta-lactam plus a macrolide for patients with significant comorbidities.

Typical Pneumonias

- ***S. pneumoniae:***
  - Most common CAP; typically has lobar consolidation with "rusty-colored" sputum.
  - Gram-⊕ cocci, grows in chains.
  - Causes multiple infections, including acute sinusitis, otitis media, meningitis, septic arthritis, pneumonia, cellulitis, erysipelas, bacteremia, and others.
  - People with defective complement/antibody function, prior hospitalization, splenectomy, renal insufficiency, diabetes, and other conditions are predisposed to community-acquired *S. pneumoniae.*
  - Treat with beta-lactam antibiotics; most also susceptible to flouroquinolones, macrolides.
  - Prophylaxis against common serotypes is available with polysaccharide vaccine (especially adults age 65 and over) or conjugate vaccine (infants and small children).

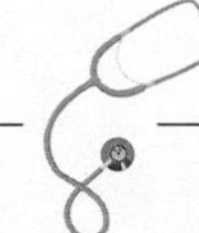

Austrian syndrome is the triad of pneumococcal endocarditis, pneumonia, and meningitis. Rare, but seen in alcoholics and IV drug users.

- ***Staphylococcus aureus* pneumonia:**
  - Consider this in a patient with viral infection ~ 2 weeks before. "Salmon pink" sputum and cavitary lesions.
  - Gram-⊕ cocci in clusters.
  - Treat with beta-lactams or vancomycin if MRSA is suspected.
- ***Klebsiella pneumoniae:***
  - "Currant jelly" sputum, "bulging fissure" on chest x-ray (CXR).
  - "Friedlander's bacillus."
  - May cause biliary or urinary tract infections in hospitalized patients.
  - Treat with cephalosporin +/– aminoglycoside.
- ***Haemophilus influenzae:***
  - Gram-⊖ coccobacilli.

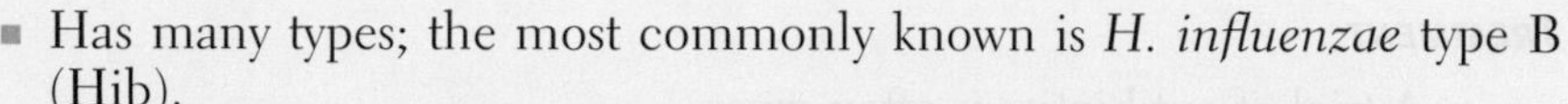

- Has many types; the most commonly known is *H. influenzae* type B (Hib).
- Nontypable *H. influenzae* is responsible for sinusitis, otitis media, and CAP, especially in chronic obstructive pulmonary disease (COPD) patients.
- Infection with Hib causes meningitis, especially in children < 3 years of age; currently, there is an Hib vaccine to protect against this.
- Treat with third-generation cephalosporin, quinolone, doxycycline.

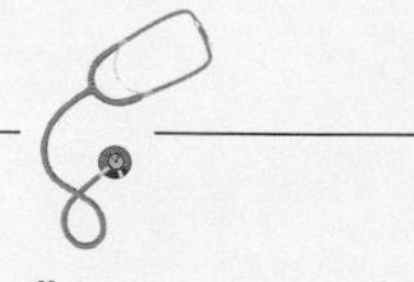

All HIV-⊕ patients should receive the pneumococcal and *H. flu* vaccines.

- ***Moraxella catarrhalis:***
  - Gram-⊖ coccus.
  - Mostly in COPD and immunocompromised patients; causes upper respiratory infections and pneumonia.
  - Susceptible to penicillin/clavulanic acid, macrolides, and trimethoprim-sulfamethoxazole (TMP-SMZ).

Atypical Pneumonias

- ***Mycoplasma pneumoniae:***
  - One of the most common community-acquired pathogens causing pneumonia in healthy persons under age 40; most common in ages 5–20.
  - Causes atypical pneumonia ("walking" pneumonia).
  - Insidious onset with an incubation period of up to 3 weeks.
  - Patients present with fever, pharyngitis, headaches, chills, tonsillitis, arthritis, hemolytic anemia, change in mental status, or erythema multiforme.
- ***Chlamydia pneumoniae:***
  - Common cause of CAP in children and young adults.
  - Transmission is person to person.
  - Patients often present with fever, nonproductive cough.
  - CXR shows segmental infiltrates.
  - Treat with quinolone or cephalosporin and macrolide.

A patient who works in a pet store presents with diffuse, bilateral infiltrate. *Think*: Chlamydia psittaci.

- ***Chlamydia psittaci:***
  - Obligate intracellular parasite.
  - Host is avian species **(think prior exposure to bird)**.
  - Transmitted via the respiratory route.
  - Patient presents with fever, headache, chills, cough, myalgias, abdominal pain, nausea, vomiting.
  - On physical exam ~ 70% of patients will have splenomegaly.
  - Can be treated with tetracyclines.
- ***Legionella pneumophila:***
  - Gram-⊖ rod, anaerobic.
  - Source is typically bodies of water; can be spread through air conditioning systems.
  - Causes Legionnaire's disease, which consists of **pneumonia,** change in mental status, headaches, **diarrhea,** abdominal pain, nausea, vomiting, high fever, hyponatremia **(think Legionnaire's anytime you hear pneumonia + GI symptoms).**
  - Elderly and those with chronic lung diseases are at greatest risk.
  - Diagnose with direct immunofluorescent antigen or urinary antigen.
  - Treat with macrolides, quinolones, doxycycline.

A 21-year-old woman who complains of dry cough, malaise, and low-grade fevers for 2 weeks has a CXR with hazy infiltrates. *Think:* Mycoplasma pneumoniae. **Next step:** Treat with macrolide if no comorbidities.

A patient presents with confusion and diarrhea and is found to have a large infiltrate on CXR with a pleural effusion. *Think:* Legionella pneumophila. **Next step:** Check *Legionella* antigen in the urine and serum PCR for *Legionella* antigen; start macrolide therapy and third-generation cephalosporin empirically until results become available.

INFECTIOUS DISEASE

Hospital-Acquired Pneumonias

- **HAP**: Fever, leukocytosis, and infiltrate on CXR in any patient receiving care within the hospital for 48 hours or more.
- *Pseudomonas, Enterobacter, Klebsiella pneumoniae, E coli, H influenzae, S aureus.*
- **Must always cover for *Pseudomonas;*** use fourth-generation cephalosporin, carbapenem, or piperacillin/tazobactam.
- Cover for MRSA with vancomycin in high-risk cases.
- ***Pseudomonas aeruginosa:***
  - Gram-⊖ bacillus.
  - Usually acquired in the hospital.
  - Most common organism in ventilator-associated pneumonia.
  - Cystic fibrosis patients can be colonized by *P. aeruginosa*, which correlates with severity of airway disease.
  - Common infectious agent associated with exacerbations of bronchiectasis.
- ***Acinetobacter baumanii:***
  - Small gram-⊖ coccobacilli.
  - Often colonize respiratory secretions and endotracheal tubes but also causes nosocomial infections, **particularly ventilator-associated pneumonia.**
  - Often multidrug resistant.
  - Treat with a third-generation cephalosporin and an aminoglycoside.

An elderly patient hospitalized for 3 weeks following an episode of decompensated heart failure now has fever, elevated WBC, and infiltrate on CXR. *Think: Hospital-acquired pneumonia.* **Next step:** Start pipercillin-tazobactam + vancomycin to cover *Pseudomonas aeruginosa,* resistant *S. pneumoniae,* and MRSA.

Health Care–Associated Pneumonias

- Patients from the community who received acute hospital care for more than 48 hours within the past 90 days, reside in a long-term care or other health care facility, or frequent facilities such as dialysis centers.
- Microbiology and management are similar to **hospital-acquired pneumonia.**

Aspiration Pneumonias

- Patients with a history of losing consciousness (eg, alcoholic binge, seizures, etc.) or with neurologic impairment (cerebrovascular accident [CVA], multiple sclerosis, etc.) presenting with a right middle lobe or right lower lobe infiltrate.
- Typical organisms include **anaerobes** such as *Bacteroides, Fusobacterium nucleatum, Peptostreptococcus,* along with gram negatives like *E coli, Pseudomonas,* and *Klebsiella.*
- Must provide broad-spectrum coverage for gram-⊖ and anaerobic organisms, with agents such as piperacillin-tazobactam or carbapenems.

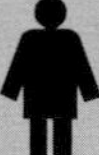

One week following a CVA, a 78-year-old patient develops fever and a right lower lobe infiltrate. *Think: Aspiration pneumonia.* **Next step:** Start imipenem empirically and obtain induced sputum cultures.

Other Respiratory Infections

- **Adenovirus:**
  - DNA virus.
  - Infections occur primarily during the fall and spring seasons.
  - Causes upper respiratory tract infection.
  - Supportive treatment.
- **Epstein-Barr virus (EBV):**
  - DNA virus.
  - Causes **infectious mononucleosis,** which is characterized by pharyngitis, fever, tender cervical **lymphadenopathy, +/– splenomegaly.**
  - Patients with mononucleosis should not engage in contact sports due to the risk of splenic rupture.
  - Laboratory studies will show abnormal liver function tests (LFTs) and lymphocytosis.
  - **Diagnose with heterophile antibody titers or, serum IgG/IgM for EBV.**
  - May be associated with hairy leukoplakia.
  - Supportive treatment.
- **Influenza virus:**
  - RNA virus.
  - Three types: A and B constitute one genus, and C makes up the other.
  - Influenza A periodically undergoes major antigenic changes, known as **antigenic shifts,** causing epidemics.
  - Transmission is via areosolized particles.
  - Patients present with fever, headache, malaise, myalgias, cough, pharyngitis, arthralgias, or lymphadenopathy.

- Influenza may be complicated by a primary viral pneumonia or a 2° bacterial pneumonia caused by *S aureus, S. pneumoniae,* or *H. influenzae.*
- Prophylaxis is with yearly flu vaccinations.
- May treat with amantadine/rimantadine or oseltamavir; however, treatment is largely supportive.

- **Parvovirus B19:**
  - DNA virus.
  - Causes **erythema infectiosum, also known as "fifth disease,"** in children.
  - Spread through respiratory secretions in people who appear to have the common cold.
  - In adults, parvovirus B19 presents as acute, symmetric **arthritis of the hands,** wrists, and knees.
  - Can also cause an aplastic anemia syndrome, particularly in sickle cell patients.
  - Treat supportively; may treat arthritis with nonsteroidals.

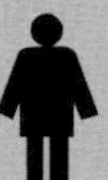

A day care worker presents with fever and arthritis of the hands. *Think: Parvovirus B19.* **Next step:** Check serum parvovirus B19 antigen, IgG, and IgM.

- **Rhinovirus:**
  - RNA virus.
  - Causes the common cold, which presents as nasal congestion, rhinorrhea, sneezing, headache, and malaise.
  - Self-limited.
  - Treatment is supportive.
- ***Corynebacterium diphtheriae*:**
  - Gram-⊕ bacillus.
  - Diphtheria presents as upper respiratory infection (not pneumonia) with low-grade fevers, sore throat, nausea, vomiting.
  - On exam, may find **grayish exudates in oropharynx that can coalesce to become a pseudomembrane.**
  - Treat with macrolide or penicillin, diphtheria antitoxin (IV infusion).
  - Prevent with TDaP (tetanus, diphtheria, pertussis) vaccine for kids and boosters for adults.

COMMON SKIN INFECTIONS

Staphylococcus aureus

- Gram ⊕, coagulase ⊕.
- Commonly causes infections of skin, septic arthritis, catheter infections, and endocarditis. **See *S aureus* syndromes below.**

Toxic Shock Syndrome

- Seen in menstruating women using "super-absorbent" tampons.
- Exotoxin mediated, produced by strains of *Staph* A and some group A strep species.

- Consists of fever, rash, desquamation of skin, nausea, along with evidence of organ failure (kidney, liver, respiratory, cardiovascular).
- Treat by removing foreign body and supportive care (antibiotics are controversial, but clindamycin may ↓ toxin; beta-lactams and vancomycin are also sometimes used in conjunction with clindamycin).

Scalded Skin Syndrome

- The most severe form is toxic epidermal necrolysis (TEN).
- Starts as periorbital or perioral erythematous rash and progresses to limbs.
- In days, the skin sloughs off.
- Must treat as burn, with careful monitoring and aggressive fluid administration depending on the extent of skin involvement.
- Also, meticulous skin care must be provided to prevent super-infection.

Streptococcus pyogenes

- Gram-⊕ cocci, group A beta-hemolytic.
- Causes soft tissue infections such as cellulitis, impetigo, and necrotizing fasciitis.
- Also causes pharyngitis, pneumonia, toxic shock–like syndrome.
- Treat with penicillin.
- **Postinfection sequelae:**
  - **Scarlet fever:** Presents as pharyngitis, strawberry tongue, and a rash that begins on the trunk and spreads to the extremities. Palms and soles have no rash but undergo desquamation.
  - **Poststreptococcal glomerulonephritis:** Glomerulonephritis ~ 2 weeks after strep infection.
  - **Streptococcal toxic shock syndrome:** Similar to staphylococcal type.

IMMUNITY

Humoral Immunity

- Branch of immune system composed of circulating or cell-bound proteins.
- Facilitates and directs cell destruction.
- Inactivates toxins.
- Two main components:
  1. **Immunoglobulins:** Produced by B lymphocytes and plasma cells (see Table 2.5-2).
  2. **Complement:** Produced by the liver.

Cellular Immunity

- Branch of immune system composed of ***cells*** (as opposed to immunoglobulins/proteins).
- T lymphocytes:
  - Cytotoxic T cells: Kill cells expressing foreign antigens, CD8+.
  - Helper T cells: Enhance activity of other T cells, B cells, and macrophages, CD4+.
  - Suppressor T cells: Inhibit cellular immune response, CD8+.

TABLE 2.5-2. Immunoglobulins and Their Functions

IgG	■ ~ 70% of total immunoglobulins. ■ Predominant antibody in secondary immune response. ■ Fixes complement (sometimes). ■ Crosses placenta. ■ Four subtypes. ■ **Long lasting, evidence of previous exposure to antigen.**
IgA	■ ~ 20% of total immunoglobulins. ■ Present in serum, colostrum, saliva, tears, and respiratory and intestinal mucosa **(think of it as the first line of defense in mucosa—defects result in lots of mucosal infections).**
IgM	■ ~ 10% of total immunoglobulins. ■ **Fixes complement strongly!** ■ Predominant antibody in primary immune response **(it is the first responder to infection before IgG is made).** ■ Is a pentamer (huge protein). ■ **Indicates acute infections.**
IgD	■ ~ 1% of total immunoglobulins. ■ B cell surface receptor.
IgE	■ 0.01% of total immunoglobulins. ■ Triggers histamine release from mast cells: Immediate hypersensitivity reactions (allergy, anaphylaxis, asthma). ■ Also rises in parasitic infections. ■ **When elevated think: allergy/hypersensitivity or parasite!**

- Neutrophils.
- Eosinophils.
- Mast cells.
- Reticuloendothelial system (monocytes, macrophages, histiocytes, Langerhans' cells, Kupffer cells, etc.).
- Natural killer cells.

IMMUNODEFICIENCY

Cell-Mediated Immunodeficiency (CMI)

- Major diseases causing cell-mediated immunodeficiency (CMI):
  - AIDS.
  - Leukemias and lymphomas.
  - Diabetes mellitus (**test questions: diabetics are prone to *Mucor* and *Rhizopus* infections.**).
  - Sarcoidosis.
  - **Iatrogenic CMI:**
    - High-dose corticosteroids.
    - Chemotherapy.
    - Radiation therapy.

Mucor—who gets it? Diabetics and immunosuppressed. How do you treat it? Surgery (actual resection of the fungus) and amphotericin.

- **CMI-associated infections** (think about classic infections AIDS patients get):
  - **Viruses:** Herpesviruses, cytomegalovirus (CMV), human papillomavirus (HPV), human herpes virus (HHV)-6.
  - **Fungi:** *Cryptococcus, Candida, Histoplasma, Coccidioides, Aspergillus, Pneumocystis jiroveci* (PCP).
  - **Protozoa:** *Toxoplasma, Cryptosporidium, Giardia lamblia.*
  - **Helminths:** *Strongyloides stercoralis.*
  - **Bacteria:** *Listeria, Nocardia,* ***Mycobacterium tuberculosis*** **reactivation,** nontuberculous mycobacteria, *Legionella, Salmonella.*

Humoral Immune Deficiency Disorders

- Patients with humoral immune deficiency disorders are commonly infected with encapsulated bacteria (similar to asplenic patients).
- **Common variable hypogammaglobulinemia:**
  - Can be acquired at any age.
  - Low levels of IgG, IgA, and IgM.
  - Normal numbers of B cells, but are defective.
  - Patients usually well until 15–30 years of age.
  - Classically get sinopulmonary infections with ***Streptococcus pneumoniae, Haemophilus influenzae, Klebsiella pneumoniae,*** and ***Mycoplasma;*** also autoimmune diseases.
- **Selective IgA deficiency:**
  - Most common of the selective immunoglobulin deficiencies.
  - Present with mucous membrane infections (URI, UTI, GI).
  - Low-molecular-weight IgM ↑ in partial compensation.
  - Serum may contain anti-IgA, IgE.
  - IgA replacement may cause **anaphylaxis** (don't do it).
  - Patients who are transfused with blood products and get anaphylaxis—think: **IgA deficiency responding to the IgA in donor's blood.**
- **Other:** CLL, multiple myeloma (these conditions leave people with abnormal antibody production). They also get sinopulmonary infections similar to common variable hypogammaglobulinemia (above).

Major Causes of Fever in the Immunocompromised

- **Cancer patients:** Certain types of cancer can create an immune abnormality. Leukemias, lymphomas, and multiple myeloma are examples. Although leukocytosis may be present, these white cells are dysfunctional and immunity is impaired.
  - Fever of unknown origin; often tumor related.
  - Bacteria: Gram-positive or gram-negative aerobes, anaerobes at site of mixed infection.
  - Viruses: Respiratory syncytial virus (RSV), parainfluenza, adenoviruses, herpes simplex virus (HSV), CMV.
  - Fungi: *Candida, Aspergillus, Cryptococcus, Trichosporon, Mucor, Pneumocystis jirovecii* and *Toxoplasma* also seen.
  - **Classic test examples** are **shingles in a multiple myeloma** patient, ***Listeria*** **meningitis in a CLL** patient.
  - Any cancer that is **treated with chemotherapy** is at risk for both cellular and humoral deficiencies.

- Neutropenia typically occurs 7–10 days after the last chemotherapy, when the "nadir" of all cell lines occurs. If a patient presents with fever any time during chemotherapy, neutropenia must be suspected and counts must be checked.
- If the patient is neutropenic, they must be treated empirically with IV antibiotics covering for bacterial (especially gram-⊖/*Pseudomonas*) infections (see below).
- Fevers of unknown causes in cancer patients are often due to the tumor itself.

- **Transplant patients:** These patients are extremely immunosuppressed around the transplant procedure (whichever type) itself, and less so later on, due to the use of ongoing immunosuppressive agents (usually steroids or a T-cell suppressive agent such as temsirolimus or cyclosporine) that prevent rejection of the transplanted organ or bone marrow.
- **Bone marrow transplant:**
  - There are basically two types: allogeneic (utilizes donor marrow from someone else) and autologous (uses stem cells harvested from the patient's own bone marrow).
  - Whereas both these types of patients are severely immunosuppressed soon after the transplant, this is far greater in allogeneic transplant patients.
  - Allogeneic patients also have longer suppression due to the common ongoing requirement of immunosuppressive agents to prevent host-versus-graft rejection.
  - **Classic infections** include the following:
    - **Early (1–4 weeks) infections:** HSV, bacteria, *Candida*, *Aspergillus*.
    - **Mid (4–26 weeks):** HSV, CMV, varicella-zoster, *Aspergillus*, PCP.
    - **Late:** Encapsulated bacteria (*S. pneumoniae*, *Neisseria meningitidis*, and *H. influenzae)*, aspergillosis, HSV, CMV.
- **Solid organ transplant:** Influenced by time since transplant, and type of transplant.
- **Organisms include:**
  - **Bacteria:** Includes gram positive and negative.
  - **Viruses:** CMV, EBV, HBV, hepatitis C virus (HCV), adenovirus.
  - **Fungi:** *Aspergillus*, *Pneumocystis jiroveci*.
- **Splenectomy patients:** Encapsulated organisms (*S. pneumoniae*, *N. meningitidis*, and *H. influenzae*); **parasites:** malaria, *Babesia*.

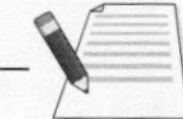

Functionally asplenic patients (sickle cell disease) or postsplenectomy patients are at ↑ risk for infection with encapsulated organisms even if they are not neutropenic. Asplenic patients require vaccinations against *S. pneumoniae*, *N. meningitidis*, and *H. influenzae*.

Sickle cell patients can commonly get osteomyelitis caused by *Staphylococcus*.

INFECTIOUS DISEASE

General Principles of Evaluation and Management of Fever in Immmunocompromised Patients

Diagnostic Studies

- Complete blood count (CBC) with manual differential and coagulation studies.
- Culture urine and blood.
- CXR regardless of physical exam findings.
- Culture sputum with cough or if CXR warrants.
- Culture stool and CSF in AIDS patients, look for cryptococcal antigen.
- In AIDS and transplant patients, obtain CMV antigen.
- **If neutropenic:**
  - Immediately start broad-spectrum therapy (eg, piperacillin/tazobactam, third-/fourth-generation cephalosporin, or carbapenem).
  - If patient has an indwelling catheter (eg, central line or chemotherapy port), add vancomycin to cover MRSA.

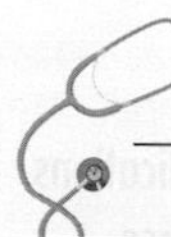

Neutropenic patients are vulnerable to more than one infection at a time. More than one organism may emerge during a single febrile episode. Be aggressive with broad-spectrum antibiotics.

- Adjust therapy based on culture results.
- If still febrile in 3 days, add antifungal (eg, voriconizole, amphotericin).
- **If pulmonary infiltrate on CXR**: Immediately begin with broad-spectrum therapy (eg, piperacillin/tazobactam, third-/fourth-generation cephalosporin, or carbapenem) and adjust according to culture (similar to neutropenic patients).

HUMAN IMMUNODEFICIENCY VIRUS (HIV) AND ACQUIRED IMMUNODEFICIENCY SYNDROME (AIDS)

AIDS Definition

Any HIV-infected individual with:

- A CD4 count of < 200/μL, regardless of the presence of symptoms or opportunistic diseases.
- An AIDS-defining clinical condition, regardless of CD4 count.

Major AIDS-Defining Conditions

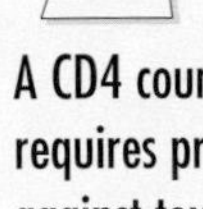

A CD4 count of < 100 requires prophylaxis against toxoplasmosis.

- Candidiasis (pulmonary or esophageal).
- Cervical cancer (invasive).
- *Cryptococcus* (extrapulmonary).
- CMV retinitis with vision loss.
- Encephalopathy, HIV-related.
- Herpes simplex (chronic ulcers, pulmonary, or esophageal).
- Kaposi's sarcoma.
- Lymphoma (Burkitt's or 1° brain).
- *Mycobacterium avium* complex.
- *Mycobacterium tuberculosis.*
- Atypical mycobacteriosis.
- PCP.
- Recurrent pneumonias.
- CNS toxoplasmosis.
- Wasting syndrome due to HIV.

Life Cycle of HIV

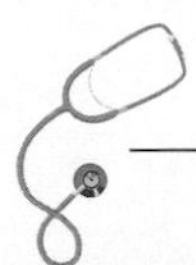

Antiretroviral medications work against reverse transcriptase and proteases that cleave the newly formed viral proteins after translation. Newer targets are cell-entry mechanisms and integrase.

- HIV is an **RNA virus** that binds CD4 molecule on a CD4+ human leukocytes.
- HIV RNA internalized into host cell.
- **HIV reverse transcriptase transcribes HIV RNA into dsDNA** (step inhibited by therapy).
- DNA translocates to nucleus and integrates into host genome.
- Translated into long HIV polypeptides.
- **Virally encoded protease** cleaves polypeptides at specific sites to generate functional proteins (step inhibited by therapy).
- New infective virus particle (proteins plus genomic viral RNA) assembles at host cell membrane.
- Budding of new virus particle.

Transmission of HIV

- **Sexual contact:**
  - Worldwide, HIV is predominantly transmitted by heterosexual sex.
  - One-half of U.S. cases are still among homosexual men.
  - Incidence of heterosexual transmission in the United States is increasing, mainly among women and minorities.
  - HIV is present in infective quantities in seminal fluid and vaginal and cervical secretions.
  - Strong association of HIV transmission with receptive anal intercourse.
  - Vaginal intercourse: 20-fold greater chance of transmission from man to a woman than woman to a man.
  - Oral sex: Much less efficient mode of transmission.
  - Genital ulceration ↑ chances of transmission (both infectivity and susceptibility to infection).
  - Lack of circumcision is associated with higher risk of infection.
- **Blood products:**
  - Sharing contaminated injection drug syringes.
  - Transfusion of contaminated blood products.
  - An estimated 10,000 individuals in the United States were infected by contaminated blood products (many hemophilia patients, for example) before spring 1985; currently minimal risk of HIV from transfusions due to sensitive screen procedures.
  - **Occupational transmission:**
    - Transmission risk after skin puncture from blood contaminated sharp object from person with documented HIV infection is 0.3%.
    - Transmission for hepatitis B following similar exposure is 20–30%.
    - The higher the viral load of the infected patient, the greater the chances of transmission.
    - Postexposure prophylaxis and wound cleansing after exposure ↓ rate of HIV seroconversion by 79% (to 0.06% for HIV).
- **HIV-⊕ mothers to infants intrapartum, perinatally, or via breast milk:**
  - HIV can be transmitted from mother to fetus during pregnancy, delivery, or through infected breast milk.
  - Transmission rate from untreated mother to newborn is approximately 25% in the United States.
  - Zidovudine treatment of HIV-infected pregnant women from the beginning of the third trimester through delivery, with treatment of the infant for 6 weeks after birth, ↓ transmission rate to 8%.
  - Breast milk transmission (7–22%) is most important in developing countries where other means of infant nutrition are not readily available.
- **Transmission by other body fluids:** HIV can be identified in almost any body fluid but transmission risk via saliva, sweat, tears, and urine is very small.
- There is **no evidence** that HIV can be transmitted by insects.

Centers for Disease Control and Prevention (CDC) recommendations for HIV post-exposure prophylaxis (ie, a needle stick): Zidovudine, lamivudine, and indinavir for 4 weeks.

AIDS Epidemiology

- **Worldwide:**
  - Approximately 33 million people were living with HIV infection worldwide as of December 2007.
  - Sixty-eight percent live in sub-Saharan African countries.

- **United States:**
  - AIDS was the sixth leading cause of death in Americans aged 25–44 years in 2006.
  - Among new infections diagnosed in 2006, 26% were women, 53% were men who have sex with men. Nearly half were African-American.
  - The overall incidence of AIDS has remained stable since the late 1990s.
  - African-Americans and Hispanic-Americans constitute a disproportionately high number of HIV cases.

HIV Disease Course (Without Therapy)

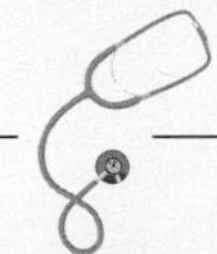

Measures of AIDS progression (2 parameters looked at):

- Status of disease: CD4 count
- Rate of activity/ progression: Viral load (measure of HIV RNA)

0–12 Weeks (Acute HIV syndrome; see below)

- Virus enters bloodstream and is cleared by lymphoid organs or spleen.
- Virus replicates to critical level in lymphoid organs (lymphadenopathy).
- Burst of viremia occurs, disseminating virus throughout body.
- Eventually partial immunologic control of virus replication occurs.
- **Acute HIV syndrome:**
  - Approximately 60% experience acute viral syndrome within 3–6 weeks of primary infection.
  - Symptoms (usually last ~ 1 week):
    - **General:** Fever, pharyngitis, lymphadenopathy, headache, lethargy, nausea, vomiting, diarrhea.
    - **Neuro:** Meningitis, encephalitis, peripheral neuropathy.
    - **Dermatologic:** Erythematous maculopapular rash and mucocutaneous ulceration.
  - Ten percent have fulminant course—clinical and immune deterioration immediately after the initial viral syndrome subsides.
  - Ninety percent become asymptomatic (clinically latent phase).

12 Weeks to 8–10 Years

- HIV evades immune system by:
  - Killing off most of the HIV-specific cytotoxic T cells with an overwhelming burst of HIV antigen.
  - Saturating the antigen presenting cells in lymphoid tissue with HIV antigen (these cells would otherwise help create more virus specific cytotoxic T cells).
- Clinical latency is the disease-free state when opportunistic infections do not occur, but continued decline of CD4 T cells occurs due to viral cytotoxicity.
- CD4 counts fall approximately 50 cells/μL/year.

> 10 Years

- CD4 count falls below critical level (usually about 200 cells/μL).
- Patient becomes highly susceptible to opportunistic diseases (see Table 2.5-3).
- CD4 counts may drop to < 10 cells/μL, yet patients can survive for months.
- Patient eventually succumbs to opportunistic infection or neoplasm.

TABLE 2.5-3. Diseases Associated with CD4 Thresholds in AIDS

CD4 Counts			
350	**200**	**100**	**50**
▪ Pneumococcal pneumonia	▪ Kaposi's sarcoma	▪ Toxoplasmosis	▪ MAC
	▪ Tuberculosis	▪ Disseminated *Candida*	▪ Cytomegalovirus
	▪ Oral thrush	▪ Cryptococcosis	▪ PML
	▪ Oral hairy leukoplakia		
	▪ PCP		
	▪ Lymphoma		

MAC, *Mycobacterium avium* complex; PCP, *Pneumocystis jiroveci* pneumonia; PML, progressive multifocal leukoencephalopathy (JC virus)

Treatment of HIV Infection

General Patient Management

- Disease necessitates patient education about complications, transmission, and prognosis.
- All patients with HIV (especially those with CD4 counts < 200) should designate an individual with durable power of attorney.

Initial and Follow-up Studies

- Routine chemistry, CBC, and CXR.
- CD4 counts.
- Two separate HIV RNA levels.
- VDRL.
- Anti-*Toxoplasma* Ab titer.
- Purified protein derivative (PPD) skin test.
- Mini mental status exam.

Antiretroviral Therapy

Major drug classes for HIV therapy are reverse transcriptase inhibitors (nucleoside analogs and non-nucleoside), protease inhibitors, fusion inhibitors, and integrase inhibitors.

- **Nucleoside analog reverse transcriptase inhibitors (NRTIs):** Act as DNA chain terminator.
- **Zidovudine (AZT):**
  - First drug approved for HIV treatment.
  - Most appropriately used as part of combination retroviral therapy.
  - Also used as monotherapy for prevention of maternal-fetal transmission of HIV.
  - **Side effects:** Headache, malaise, nausea, fatigue (often subside with extended therapy), macrocytic anemia secondary to low erythropoietin (can be managed with recombinant erythropoietin injections), proximal myopathy.

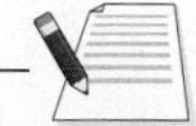

Generally you will not be required to know the specific drug names, however you should familiarize yourself with the classes of drugs available and their mechanisms of action.

  - **Lamivudine (3TC):**
    - Only for use in combination with AZT.
    - Strains of HIV that are resistant to lamivudine are sensitive to zidovudine.
    - **Toxicities: Pancreatitis, peripheral neuropathies.**
  - Others include **didanosine, stavudine, abacavir, emtricitabine,** and **tenofovir** (nucleotide analog).
- **Non-nucleoside reverse transcriptase inhibitors (NNRTIs):**
  - **Nevirapine, delavirdine** (rarely used), **efavirenz,** and **etravirine.**
  - Bind to reverse transcriptase outside the active site and cause conformational changes that ↓ enzyme activity.
  - Monotherapy causes rapid resistance.
  - Main toxicity is maculopapular rash.
- **Protease inhibitors:**
  - **Saquinavir, ritonavir, indinavir, nelfinavir, lopinavir, atazanavir** inhibit the activity of HIV protease.
  - Less toxic than the reverse transcriptase inhibitors.
  - Monotherapy results in rapid emergence of drug-resistant strains.
  - Indinavir: Main side effects are nephrolithiasis and asymptomatic indirect hyperbilirubinemia. Potent and well tolerated compared to saquinavir and ritonavir.
  - Ritonavir: Mainly used in low doses to boost other protease inhibitors.
- **Fusion inhibitors:**
  - **Maraviroc** prevents HIV binding and entry into cells by binding CCR5.
  - **Enfuvirtide** prevents HIV virion fusion with cells by binding gp41; available only as injection.
  - Used in combination therapy regimens for patients with drug-resistant virus.
- **Integrase inhibitor:**
  - Single agent approved—raltegravir.
  - Prevents the insertion of viral genome into host DNA (integration).
  - Used in salvage therapy regimens.

TREATMENT RECOMMENDATIONS

- Initiate therapy with two nucleoside reverse transcriptase inhibitors (eg, AZT, 3TC) and a boosted protease inhibitor (eg, indinavir/ritonavir) or a non-nucleoside reverse transcriptase inhibitor (eg, efavirenz) in any one of these conditions:
  - Symptomatic/history of AIDS-defining illness.
  - CD4 count < 200–350.
  - HIV-associated nephropathy.
  - Pregnancy.
  - Co-infection with HBV requiring treatment.
- Recent studies have shown no benefit in treating asymptomatic individuals with CD4 counts > 500. In fact, due to emergence of resistant strains, deferring antiretroviral therapy until necessary is recommended.
- Newer regimens use combination pills which can be taken daily, making patient compliance less of a factor in disease control.

Opportunistic Infections in AIDS and Other Immunocompromised States

Pneumocystis jiroveci Pneumonia (PCP)

- Formerly known as *Pneumocystis carinii.*
- PCP is declining, but remains the most common initial AIDS-defining illness in the United States.
- Seen largely in patients who are not aware of their HIV status or are not receiving treatment.
- PCP is most common in those with a previous episode of PCP.

Clinical Findings

- Patients often appear nontoxic and have clear lungs but low oxygen saturation.
- Often have dyspnea on exertion and weight loss.
- Spontaneous pneumothorax complicates PCP in 2% of cases.

Diagnosis

- **Definitive:** Bronchoalveolar lavage/or transbronchial biopsy.
- **Other findings:**
  - ↓ oxygen saturation.
  - CXR usually normal or shows faint, bilateral interstitial infiltrate.
  - Lactate dehydrogenase (LDH) is often elevated.

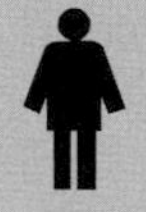

A 34-year-old patient with unknown HIV status presents with weight loss, dry cough, dyspnea, **hypoxemia,** and vague bilateral infiltrates on chest x-ray. *Think: PCP.* **Next step:** Provide supplemental oxygen and start TMP-SMZ.

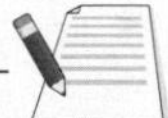

An HIV patient presents with dry cough for 1 week. He denies fever, night sweats, and chills. His WBC is normal. *Likely diagnosis?* Mycoplasma pneumoniae (Lesson: community-acquired pneumonias are still most common, even in AIDS patients.) Always treat for CAP also until any suspected opportunistic organisms are confirmed.

Treatment

- **TMP-SMZ:**
  - Fifty to sixty percent have side effects including rash, fever, leukopenia, thrombocytopenia, and hepatitis.
  - Twenty-one-day course.
  - Patients get worse before they get better and will not improve until the end of the first week of treatment.
  - May give pentamidine for patients intolerant of TMP-SMZ.
- **Glucocorticoids:**
  - Initiate in any AIDS patient with PCP if $PaO_2 < 70$ mmHg or a-A gradient > 35 mmHg.
  - Start no later than 36–72 hours after starting TMP-SMZ.
  - Twenty-one-day course (with subsequent taper).
  - ↓ mortality by approximately 50%.
- **Prophylaxis in patients with CD4 < 200 or previous PCP:** Give TMP-SMZ (three times/week instead of daily), or dapsone in sulfa-allergic patients or aerosolized pentamidine for those unable to take systemic prophylaxis (see Table 2.5-4).

TABLE 2.5-4. Prophylaxis in AIDS

INFECTION	PROPHYLAXIS	INDICATION
Pneumocystis jiroveci pneumonia	Bactrim or dapsone in patients with sulfa allergies	CD4 < 200
Toxoplasmosis	Bactrim or dapsone in patients with sulfa allergies	CD4 < 100
Tuberculosis	Isoniazid	PPD > 5-mm induration (not erythema)
Mycobacterium avium complex	Azithromycin or clarithromycin	CD4 < 100

TOXOPLASMOSIS

- Most common cause of secondary CNS infection in AIDS.
- Seroprevalence in United States is 15%; toxoplasmic encephalitis occurs in one-third of all seropositive AIDS patients without prophylaxis.
- Late complication.

CLINICAL PRESENTATION

- Fever, headache, and focal neurological deficits (90%).
- Seizure, hemiparesis, and aphasia also occur.
- **AIDS patient with meningitis:**
  - Sensation of smell and behavior changes: *Think HSV (temporal lobe involvement).*
  - India ink stain with round organisms: *Think Cryptococcus.*

DIAGNOSIS

- Magnetic resonance imaging (MRI) or head computed tomography (CT) with contrast shows **multiple ring-enhancing lesions** (see Figure 2.5-1).
- IgG antibodies to *Toxoplasma.*

TREATMENT

- Pyrimethamine and sulfadiazine: Leukopenia is the major side effect (treat leukopenia with folinic acid).
- Lifelong treatment for toxoplasmosis is necessary, due to relapse rate of 50% within 6 months.
- TMP-SMZ given for PCP prophylaxis is also effective as prophylaxis against toxoplasmic encephalitis. Patients with CD4 count < 100 should receive prophylaxis against *Toxoplasma.*
- **AIDS patient with brain lesion:**
  - Ring-enhancing lesion with mass effect: Toxo
  - Periventricular ring: CMV
  - Other: CNS lymphoma (associated with EBV)

PROTOZOAL DIARRHEA IN AIDS

ETIOLOGY

Cryptosporidia, microsporidia, and *Isospora belli* are the most common bugs.

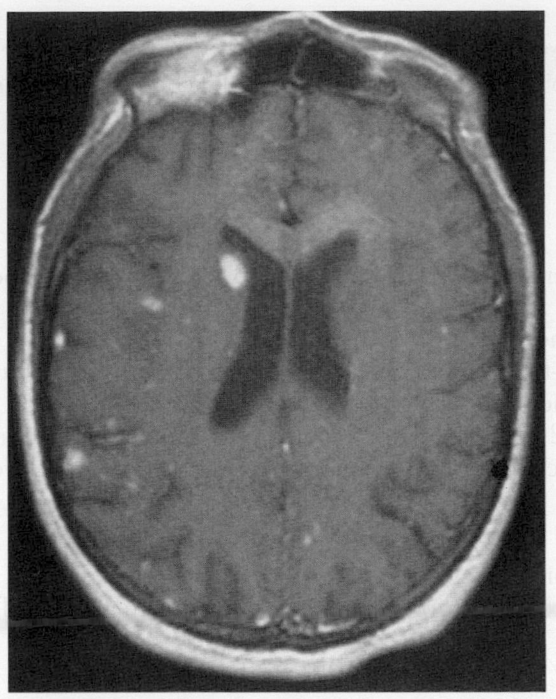

FIGURE 2.5-1. Toxoplasmosis in an AIDS patient.

Note ring-enhancing lesions. (Reproduced, with permission, from Lee SH, Rao K, Zimmerman RA [eds]. *Cranial MRI and CT.* New York: McGraw-Hill, 1999: 505.)

INFECTIOUS DISEASE

TREATMENT

- Cryptosporidia and microsporidia: Paromomycin or erythromycin.
- *Isospora*: TMP-SMZ.

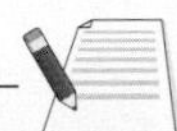

AIDS patient with diarrhea:

- Cryptosporidia (round)
- *Isospora* (oral)
- Microsporidia

A 32-year-old HIV-⊕ patient with a low CD4 count presents with 3 months of watery diarrhea. *Think: Cryptosporidiosis.* **Next step:** Check stool for ova and parasites (O&P). Effective antiretroviral treatment is best therapy + Nitazoxanide.

MYCOBACTERIUM AVIUM COMPLEX (MAC)

EPIDEMIOLOGY

- Disseminated *Mycobacterium avium* is a marker of advanced immune suppression; it typically occurs when CD4 count is < 50.
- Median survival after MAC diagnosis is 6–8 months.

SYMPTOMS

- Fever
- Cough
- Weight loss
- Night sweats
- Lymphadenopathy
- Abdominal pain
- Diarrhea

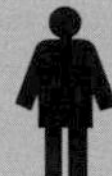

A 29-year-old HIV-⊕ patient presents with CD4 count of 100, unexplained fever, and elevated alkaline phosphatase. *Think: MAC.*

Diagnosis

- Long, slender, acid-fast bacilli (AFB) seen in biopsy specimens or sputum.
- **Other findings:**
  - Eighty-five percent of MAC patients have mycobacteremia.
  - Alkaline phosphatase level often elevated.
  - CXR: 25% have bilateral lower lobe interstitial infiltrate.
  - Blood culture confirms diagnosis (turns ⊕ within 2 weeks).

Treatment

- Clarithromycin and ethambutol.
- Prophylaxis: Azithromycin or clarithromycin when CD4 drops below 50.

Tuberculosis

See Pulmonary chapter for full discussion.

Epidemiology

- Estimated to be the cause of death in 13% of AIDS patients worldwide.
- HIV ↑ risk of developing active TB by 15–30 times.
- HIV disease progresses more rapidly in patients with active TB.

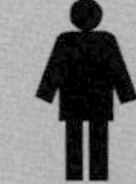

An AIDS patient being treated for TB has clinical worsening of his TB following initiation of highly active antiretroviral therapy (HAART). *Think: Immune reconstitution inflammatory syndrome (IRIS).* **Next step:** Supportive care.

Fungal Infections

- **Candidiasis:**
  - *Candida* infections are the most common fungal infections in HIV-⊕ patients, and virtually all patients experience some form of *Candida* infection during their illness.
  - Infections occur early: They are often the first sign of immunosuppression.
- **Thrush:**
  - Very early finding in immunocompromise.
  - White, cheesy exudates on posterior oropharynx.
  - Pseudohyphae detectable on wet-mount KOH preps.
- **AIDS-defining *Candida* infections:**
  - *Candida* infections of lungs, esophagus, trachea, and bronchi.
  - **Esophagitis** is most common; presents with retrosternal pain and odynophagia and diagnosed with upper GI endoscopy.

TREATMENT

- Oral and vaginal candida: Oral fluconazole; topical nystatin or clotrimazole troches are also effective.
- Severe cases including esophageal candidiasis must be treated with systemic therapy (oral itraconazole or oral/IV fluconazole).

CRYPTOCOCCOSIS

- *Cryptococcus neoformans* is the leading cause of **meningitis** in AIDS patients.
- Highest risk when CD4 count is < 50.
- Serious, life-threatening infection.

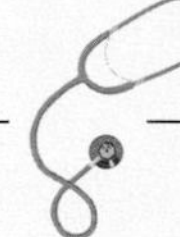

Fluconazole prophylaxis can be given to all AIDS patients once CD4 < 100/μL to prevent both cryptococcosis and candidal infections.

SIGNS AND SYMPTOMS

- **Subacute meningoencephalitis.**
- Fever (virtually all patients).
- Nausea and vomiting (40%).
- Altered mental status.
- Headache.
- Meningeal signs.

DIAGNOSIS

- Cryptococcomas.
- Variety of findings on **CT or MRI:** Can be normal or show atrophy, mass lesions, hydrocephalus, or ring-enhancing or cystic lesions.
- **Serology:** CSF or serum cryptococcal antigen or ⊕ culture from any site.
- **India ink stain of CSF** shows organism.

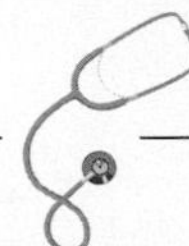

Invasive aspergillosis: Infection in immunocompromised people sometimes causing a fungus ball.

TREATMENT

- Amphotericin B for 6 weeks in combination with flucytosine for CSF disease.
- Since 50% of patients relapse after therapy is stopped, fluconazole should be given indefinitely.

ASPERGILLUS FUMIGATUS

- **Fungus ball (aspergilloma)** in preexisting lung cavity.
- Mold with septated hyphae.
- Acquired through inhalation of spores in soil and decay.
- Immunocompetent individuals can get an allergic hypersensitivity reaction; not invasive (wheezing); treat with steroids.
- **Invasive aspergillosis** is seen in immunocompromised patients and can present as rapidly progressive necrotizing pulmonary infiltrates, tracheobronchitis. Can cause **life-threatening hemoptysis.**
- Lung biopsy is needed for definitive diagnosis.
- Extrapulmonary sites: Sinusitis, CNS, skin, osteomyelitis.
- Treat with amphotericin B; some patients may benefit from surgery (removing the fungus ball). Voriconazole is usual drug of choice but interacts with antiretroviral drugs.

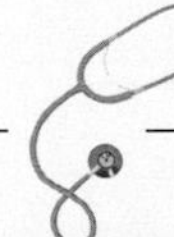

Allergic aspergillosis: A hypersensitivity reaction in immunocompetent people, causing severe obstructive lung disease, wheezing, bronchiectasis. Treat with steroids. Not an infection!

Viral Infections and AIDS/Immunocompromise

CYTOMEGALOVIRUS (CMV)

- Ninety-five percent of HIV-⊕ patients are CMV ⊕, and clinical syndromes most often represent reactivation of latent infection (see Figure 2.5-2).
- **CMV retinitis** is a dreaded HIV complications; presents with painless, progressive vision loss; may complain of "floaters."
- CMV can also cause many other systemic infections (pneumonia, hepatitis, colitis).

DIAGNOSIS

Retinitis: Fundoscopy shows perivascular hemorrhage and exudates; diagnose any systemic CMV reactivation by testing blood for CMV viral copies by PCR.

CLINICAL COURSE

Vision loss is irreversible; may be complicated by retinal detachment. Many other manifestations may reverse with therapy.

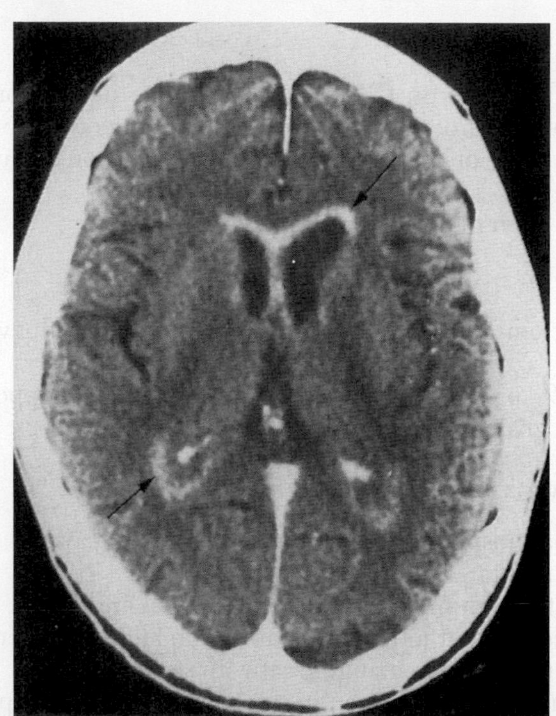

FIGURE 2.5-2. Cytomegalovirus infection in an AIDS patient.

Note diffuse periventricular enhancement. (Reproduced, with permission, from Lee SH, Rao K, Zimmerman RA [eds]. *Cranial MRI and CT.* New York: McGraw-Hill, 1999.)

TREATMENT

- Ganciclovir (ocular implants can be used) or foscarnet.
- Recurrence is common; maintenance therapy with foscarnet.
- CMV Ab–⊖ patients should receive blood products from CMV-⊖ donors if at all possible.

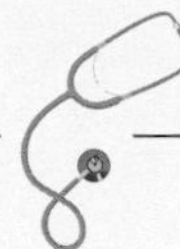

Ganciclovir causes bone marrow suppression and cannot be given with TMP-SMZ or AZT.

HERPES SIMPLEX VIRUS (HSV)

- HSV in HIV manifests as recurrent orolabial, genital, and perianal lesions.
- Can cause herpetic esophagitis (beefy red and painful esophagus).
- Can cause recurrent **herpetic whitlow** (painful nodular lesions usually found on fingers).
- Treat with acyclovir, famciclovir, or valacyclovir.

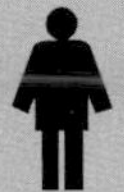

An HIV-⊕ patient presents with a painful, poorly healing, perirectal lesion. *Think: HSV.*

VARICELLA-ZOSTER VIRUS (VZV) AND HIV

- **Shingles:** The reactivation of chickenpox (or varicella-zoster) can happen in any person but is very common in AIDS patients.
  - Reactivation of latent infection.
  - Usually an early complication of HIV.
  - Painful, vesicular skin eruptions.
  - Can have extensive involvement of several dermatomes, but also may just follow one dermatome, which would classically be seen wrapping around the flank but not crossing midline.
  - Treatment with acyclovir may shorten course of disease.
- **Primary VZV infection** (chickenpox) may be *lethal* in the HIV patient. Treat aggressively with acyclovir and hyperimmune globulin.
- **Acute retinal necrosis syndrome:**
  - From zoster in the eye/orbital area (trigeminal nerve varicella-zoster or orolabial HSV).
  - Presents with pain, keratitis, and iritis.
  - Fundus exam shows widespread pale gray peripheral lesions.
  - Often complicated by retinal detachment.

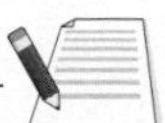

Pain from zoster may precede the rash by a couple of days. Watch for zoster in any patient presenting with pain in a dermatomal distribution!

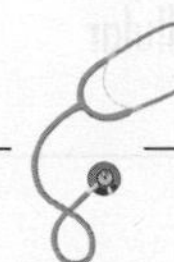

Shingles in any patient under 50 years of age mandates workup for underlying immunodeficiency.

HEPATITIS

- Ninety-five percent of HIV-⊕ patients have serologic evidence of HBV or HCV infection.
- Patients with HBV and HIV have less severe inflammatory liver disease because of immunosuppression.

Neoplastic Disease and HIV

Due to the immunosuppression, and particularly the absence of functional T cells (cellular immunity), which help find and kill abnormal cells, HIV patients are at high risk for developing neoplasms.

KAPOSI'S SARCOMA

EPIDEMIOLOGY

- Incidence has been ↓ since first recognized as an HIV-associated neoplasm.
- Mostly in homosexual men.
- Associated with human herpes virus type 8 (HHV-8).

CLINICAL FINDINGS

- Multiple vascular nodules appearing in the skin, mucous membranes, and viscera.
- Appearance is purplish macular or papular nodule on skin, or discoloration of the oral mucosa.
- Lesions often occur in sun-exposed areas.
- Pulmonary involvement can occur; presents as shortness of breath.
- May be seen with a normal CD4 count.

DIAGNOSIS

Biopsy of suspicious lesion.

TREATMENT

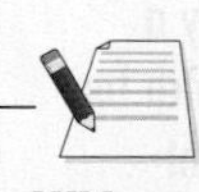

HIV-associated malignancies:

- HHV-6,8: Kaposi's sarcoma
- HPV: Cervical cancer
- HBV: Hepatocellular cancer

- Indicated when a single or multiple lesions are symptoms.
- Always give HAART.
- Can use topical all-trans retinoin or local radiation.
- Occasionally can use systemic chemotherapy.

LYMPHOMAS

EPIDEMIOLOGY

- Six percent of patients develop lymphoma at some point during their disease.
- Incidence is ↑ 120-fold in HIV compared with general population.
- **Three main types occur in HIV:**
  - Grade III or IV immunoblastic (60%).
  - Burkitt's lymphoma (20%).
  - Primary CNS lymphoma (20%).

CLINICAL PRESENTATION

- Dependent on the site of tumor.
- Persistent unexplained fever.
- Focal seizures if in CNS.
- Rapidly growing mass lesion in the oral mucosa.
- Eighty percent have extranodal disease.

TREATMENT

HAART + systemic chemotherapy.

- The following are agents with high potential for use in bioterrorism. The inhalational type is expected to be the most common form used in bioterrorism, due to ease of inoculation.
- Suspected or confirmed cases should be reported to local or state departments of health.
- Antibiotics are initially given parenterally and then switched to oral once patient improves clinically.
- In mass-casualty situations, parenteral therapy may not be possible; in this situation, oral antibiotics are administered.
- Antibiotics for treating patients infected in connection with a bioterrorist event are included in the national pharmaceutical stockpile maintained by the Centers for Disease Control and Prevention (CDC), as are ventilators and other emergency equipment.
- This information is compiled from the **CDC** Web site, where the latest surveillance information is available: *http://www.cdc.gov.*

Anthrax

INCUBATION PERIOD

Usually < 1 week.

TRANSMISSION

- **Skin:** Direct skin contact with spores; in nature, contact with infected animals or animal products (usually related to occupational exposure).
- **Respiratory tract:** Inhalation of aerosolized spores.
- **GI:** Consumption of undercooked or raw meat products or dairy products from infected animals.
- No person-to-person transmission of anthrax.

SIGNS AND SYMPTOMS OF INHALATIONAL ANTHRAX

- Initial phase consists of nonspecific symptoms such as low-grade fever, nonproductive cough, malaise, fatigue, myalgias, profound sweats, and chest discomfort.
- Upper respiratory tract symptoms are rare.
- Physical exam may reveal rhonchi, otherwise normal.
- One to five days after onset of initial symptoms, onset of high fever and severe respiratory distress (dyspnea, stridor, cyanosis) occur. Shock and death occur within 24–36 hours. An interim period of a few days of wellness can occur between the two stages, or they may occur in rapid succession.
- Hemorrhagic meningitis can also be seen.

DIAGNOSIS

- Gram-⊕ bacilli on unspun peripheral blood smear or CSF.
- **CXR** demonstrates **widened mediastinum with clear lung fields.**
- Aerobic blood culture growth of large, gram-⊕ bacilli provides preliminary identification of *Bacillus* species.

- Nasal swab for PCR available for epidemiological surveillance; not approved to make individual patient decisions.
- A blood test that detects antibodies to a component of the toxin of *Bacillus anthracis* is available, yielding results in 1 hour.

> A group of previously healthy young people develop an acute respiratory illness. CXRs demonstrate a widened mediastinum with clear lung fields. *Think: Anthrax; keep bioterrorism in mind.*

TREATMENT

- Initiate antimicrobial therapy immediately upon suspicion with ciprofloxacin, doxycycline, and amoxicillin.
- Supportive care including controlling pleural effusions.
- Contact precautions.
- Vaccine available for military personnel and lab workers who handle organism directly.

Botulism

See the Neurology chapter.

Pneumonic Plague

- There are three types of plague: pneumonic, bubonic, and septicemic.
- The most common form is bubonic, which is not transmitted person to person.

ETIOLOGY

Yersinia pestis. Indications that plague had been artificially disseminated would be the occurrence of cases in locations not known to have enzootic infection, in persons without known risk factors, and in the absence of prior rodent deaths.

INCUBATION PERIOD

Two to four days.

TRANSMISSION

Via inhalation of respiratory droplets.

SIGNS AND SYMPTOMS

- Fever, headache, weakness.
- Rapidly developing pneumonia with shortness of breath, chest pain, cough, and sometimes bloody or watery sputum.
- Pneumonia progresses for 2–4 days and causes respiratory failure and shock.

A previously healthy 29-year-old banker living in a big city contracts a severe pneumonia characterized by the rapid development of respiratory failure, shock, bleeding, and other signs of the systemic inflammatory response syndrome. Sputum reveals gram-⊖ bacilli with bipolar staining. *Think:* Yersinia pestis.

DIAGNOSIS

- Gram stain of sputum or blood may reveal gram-⊖ bacilli or coccobacilli.
- Wright, Giemsa, Wayson stain will often show bipolar staining.
- Antigen detection, IgM enzyme immunoassay, immunostaining, and PCR.

TREATMENT

- Start streptomycin within 24 hours of start of symptoms.
- Other effective agents include gentamicin, tetracycline, doxycycline, and chloramphenicol.
- Isolation of patients using respiratory droplet precautions, but then are no longer contagious after 48 hours of antibiotic treatment.

A laboratory confirmation of *Y. pestis* is made on autopsy of a healthy 40-year-old living in a big city. There was no history of handling an animal carcass or any travel to an endemic area. *Think: This could be a sentinel event for a bioterrorist attack. Be on the lookout for cases of severe acute respiratory illness in others very shortly.*

PREVENTION

- Postexposure prophylaxis for people who have had direct, close contact with infected patients (7-day course).
- A plague vaccine is not currently available for use in the United States.

Smallpox

INCUBATION PERIOD

Seven to seventeen days.

TRANSMISSION

- Face-to-face contact is required.
- Can be spread through direct contact with infected bodily fluids or contaminated objects.
- Humans are the only natural hosts of variola.

SIGNS AND SYMPTOMS

- Prodrome: 2–4 days:
  - High fever, malaise, head and body aches, and sometimes vomiting.
  - Patients are acutely ill, in contrast to varicella infection.

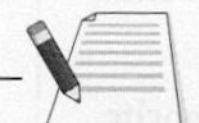

The rash of smallpox consists of lesions that are all at the ***same stage of development.*** In contrast, the lesions of varicella are at all different stages.

- Rash:
  - First, small red spots on the tongue and in the mouth that become sores that break open and spread large amounts of the virus into the mouth and throat; person becomes most contagious at that time.
  - Next, rash appears on the skin, starting on the face and spreading to the arms and legs (**centrifugal**) and then to the palms and soles. Usually, the rash spreads to all parts of the body within 24 hours. Patient may start to feel better during rash appearing.
  - On the third day, the rash becomes raised bumps.
  - By the fourth day, bumps fill with a thick fluid and often pustules (characteristic feature of smallpox). Eventually scab, which fall off and form pitted scars.

DIAGNOSIS

Made by PCR or enzyme-linked immunosorbent assay (ELISA) of throat swab, or culture of fluid from pustules or CSF.

TREATMENT

- Patients are quarantined for 17 days or until scabs fall off.
- Treatment consists of fluid replacement and antibiotics for any 2° bacterial infections.
- No treatment against the virus itself.

PREVENTION

Smallpox vaccine contains live *vaccinia* virus, a weaker relative of the *variola* virus that causes smallpox. Some military and first responders vaccinated.

Tularemia

ETIOLOGY AND TRANSMISSION

- Bacterial zoonosis caused by *Francisella tularensis* (small nonmotile, aerobic, non-spore-forming, gram-⊖ coccobacillus).
- Found in water, moist soil, hay, straw, and decaying animal carcasses.
- Very infectious.
- Mostly in south-central and western United States in summer.
- Humans infected through bite of an exposed tick, fly, or mosquito, or by direct contact with infectious animal (often carcasses) or environment (soil, water, food).
- No person-to-person transmission (no need for patient isolation).
- Rodents are reservoir.

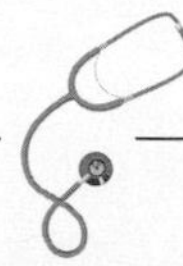

Adverse effects of tetracyclines:
- Photosensitivity
- ↑ preexisting prerenal azotemia
- Brown/yellow deposits in teeth and brittle bones (children)

INCUBATION

Symptoms usually appear at 3–5 days, but may be as long as 14 days.

SIGNS AND SYMPTOMS

- Sudden onset of high fever, chills, diarrhea, headache, myalgia, cough.
- If inhaled, hemorrhagic inflammation, pneumonia, and pneumonitis.
- Airborne *F. tularensis* can also cause ocular involvement, ulcers in broken skin, and oropharyngeal disease.

DIAGNOSIS

Gram stain, direct fluorescent antibody, or immunohistochemical stains of respiratory secretions and blood.

Treatment

- **Streptomycin** is drug of choice.
- Gentamicin, tetracyclines, and chloramphenicol are also effective.

TICK-BORNE DISEASES

Lyme Disease

Etiology

- *Borrelia burgdorferi:* Microaerophilic spirochete.
- Transmitted by *Ixodes scapularis* tick.
- Found in the northeastern United States, in wooded areas.
- **Erythema chronicum migrans** is the pathognomonic skin rash that starts at bite and progresses until there is central clearing.

Signs and Symptoms

- **Initial stage:** Fevers, headaches, arthralgias, and myalgias.
- **Second stage** (weeks to months): Recurring rash, myocarditis with first-, second-, or third-degree heart block; meningitis; cranial nerve palsy; peripheral neuropathy.
- **Third stage:** Migratory or oligoarthritis.

Diagnosis

- ELISA followed by Western blot. If clinical suspicion is high, then treat the patient before serologies come back.
- Treat with doxycycline or amoxicillin if there is no cardiac involvement.
- Treat with penicillin or cephalosporin if there is any cardiac or neurologic involvement.

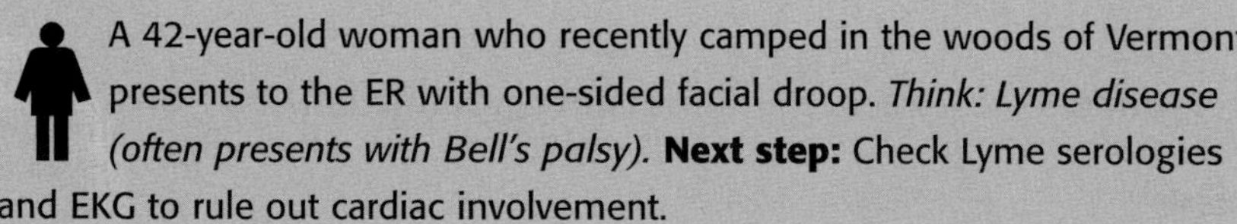

A 42-year-old woman who recently camped in the woods of Vermont presents to the ER with one-sided facial droop. *Think: Lyme disease (often presents with Bell's palsy).* **Next step:** Check Lyme serologies and EKG to rule out cardiac involvement.

Ehrlichiosis

Two types: Human monocytic ehrlichiosis (HME) and human granulocytic ehrlichiosis (HGE).

Etiology

- *Ehrlichia chaffeensis,* intracellular bacteria causing HME.
- *Ehrlichia phagocytophila,* intracellular bacteria causing HGE.

Transmission

- HME caused by the bite of the *lone star tick.*
- HGE caused by the bite of *Ixodes* tick.

SIGNS AND SYMPTOMS

Nonspecific flulike symptoms, high fever, headache, malaise, **leukopenia and thrombocytopenia** are most common presentations.

DIAGNOSIS

- Serum PCR.
- HME in southern United States and HGE in northern United States.

TREATMENT

Tetracycline or doxycycline.

Rocky Mountain Spotted Fever

ETIOLOGY

Rickettsia rickettsii, gram-⊖ coccobacillus, found in the southeastern United States.

TRANSMISSION

Bite of the wood tick *Dermacentor andersoni* or dog tick *Dermacentor variabilis*.

SIGNS AND SYMPTOMS

- Patients initially present with fever, nausea, severe headache, vomiting, and history of recent tick bite.
- After 3–4 days of symptoms, rash starts as a nonpruritic, maculopapular rash on the distal extremities starting on the wrists and ankles then involving the palms and soles, then progresses centrally to the trunk and face.
- Can be fatal if not treated aggressively.
- Disseminated intravascular coagulation (DIC) and pneumonia are serious complications of infection.

DIAGNOSIS

Indirect immunofluorescence assay or latex agglutination.

TREATMENT

Tetracyclines are the drug of choice.

Babesiosis

ETIOLOGY

Babesia microti, an intra-RBC parasite (like malaria) transmitted by the *Ixodes* tick in the Northeast and Midwest United States.

PRESENTATION

Fever, chills, myalgias, **hemolytic anemia.**

Diagnosis

Thick and thin smears of whole blood reveal ring-shaped trophozoites and the characteristic cross-shaped tetrad of merozoites known as the ***Maltese cross*** within red blood cells.

Treatment

Quinine and clindamycin.

Tularemia

Etiology

Francisella tularensis, transmitted by tick or flea bites in Arkansas and Oklahoma.

Treatment

- Gentamicin or tetracycline.
- See tularemia discussion above.

EPIDURAL ABSCESS

- **Neurosurgical emergency!**
- **If suspected, get emergent MRI.**
- Spinal abscesses are most commonly found in the immunosuppressed, IV drug users, and the elderly.
- An abscess can form anywhere along the spinal cord and as it expands, it compresses against the spinal cord and occludes the vasculature.

Etiology

- The infection is generally spread from the skin or other tissue.
- *Staphylococcus aureus*, gram-⊖ bacilli, and *Mycobacterium tuberculosis* are most common causes.

Signs and Symptoms

Presents with a triad of pain, fever, and progressive weakness of legs (focal neuromuscular weakness). Can progress over a week.

Diagnosis and Treatment

- Magnetic resonance imaging (MRI) can localize the lesion.
- Lumbar puncture (LP) is not required unless meningitis is suspected.
- Emergent surgery + antibiotics is the definitive treatment, and must be initiated early.

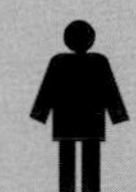

An IV drug user presents with fever of one week's duration and new-onset lower extremity weakness. *Think: Epidural abscess.* **Next step:** Order emergent MRI of spine, start empiric broad-spectrum antibiotics if ⊕.

MALARIA

PATHOPHYSIOLOGY

- **Vector:** *Anopheles* mosquito. Bites human to introduce sporozoites.
- Merozoites are then released from infected liver cells to infect RBCs.

EPIDEMIOLOGY

Three hundred million to five hundred million malaria cases, with three million deaths, occur annually worldwide.

- ***Plasmodium falciparum*** causes most deaths, endemic in Africa.
- ***Plasmodium vivax*** is endemic in India and central America.

SIGNS AND SYMPTOMS

- The organisms grow in the liver, then spread to the blood to reproduce in RBCs.
- When the RBC is full, it bursts, releasing the organism and exposing it to the host immune system; red cells burst at the same time, causing the characteristic intermittent fever.
- *P. falciparum* causes more severe disease because it infects erythrocytes of all ages. It can cause a microvascular blockade that → local anoxia affecting the brain (delirium, seizures), kidneys, lungs (pulmonary edema, acute respiratory distress syndrome [ARDS]), intestines (nausea, vomiting, diarrhea, abdominal pain), liver, and blood.
- *P. vivax* infects mostly younger erythrocytes.
- *P. vivax* and *P. ovale* cause persistent infection in the liver.
- Symptoms of fever and chills occur about 1–4 weeks after infection.
- Other symptoms include headache, ↑ sweating, back pain, myalgias, diarrhea, nausea, vomiting, and cough.
- Anemia, thrombocytopenia, and elevated liver enzymes may be present.

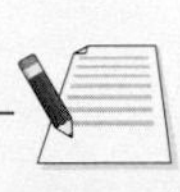

> Patients from endemic areas with **fever that follows a cyclical pattern every 48 or 72 hours** should be considered for malaria.

DIAGNOSIS

Thick and thin blood smears **show parasites in RBCs.**

TREATMENT

- Chloroquine for *P. falciparum* acquired in chloroquine-sensitive regions.
- Atovaquone when resistance is not known.
- If chloroquine resistant, use mefloquine or pyrimethamine/sulfadoxine.
- Quinidine for critically ill patients.
- Contact the CDC.

PREVENTION

- Prophylactic chloroquine or mefloquine for travelers to endemic areas.
- Check CDC recommendations.
- DEET-containing insect repellent and avoid mosquitos.

ANTIBIOTICS

(See Table 2.5-5.)

TABLE 2.5-5. Common Antibiotic Classes

ANTIMICROBIAL	MECHANISM OF ACTION	ANTIMICROBIAL SPECTRUM	SIDE EFFECTS	COMMON CLINICAL USE
Class: Beta Lactams	Inhibition of bacterial cell wall synthesis by inhibiting enzyme transpeptidases by binding to penicillin-binding proteins.			
Penicillins				
Penicillins (natural): ▪ PCN VK ▪ PCN G ▪ PCN benzathine		▪ **Gram ⊕**: *Listeria, Streptococcus* species, *Bacillus anthracis*. ▪ ***Treponema pallidum* (syphilis),** meningococci, dental infections.	Anaphylaxis, rash, pruritus, diarrhea.	**Syphilis.**
Aminopenicillins: ▪ Amoxicillin (PO) and (amoxicillin + clavulanic acid) ▪ Ampicillin (IV) and (ampicillin + sulbactam)		▪ Added gram-⊖ coverage *(H influenzae, E coli, Proteus, Salmonella)* and *Enterococcus faecalis* when compared to natural penicillins. ▪ Clavulanic acid and sulbactam add anaerobic coverage and some gram-⊖.	GI side effects.	Ampicillin is added in patients > 60 or immunocompromised in meningitis to cover *Listeria.*
Antistaphylococcal: ▪ Oxacillin (IV) ▪ Dicloxacillin (PO) ▪ Nafcillin (IV)		Added activity against beta-lactamase/ penicillinase producing *S aureus (but does not cover MRSA).*	Interstitial nephritis.	▪ Oxacillin and nafcillin are first line for non-MRSA cellulitis if IV agent is required. ▪ Dicloxacillin (or cephalexin) is first-line oral agent for cellulitis.

TABLE 2.5-5. Common Antibiotic Classes *(continued)*

Antimicrobial	Mechanism of Action	Antimicrobial Spectrum	Side Effects	Common Clinical Use
Antipseudomonal: ▪ Piperacillin (piperacillin/ tazobactam) ▪ Ticarcillin (ticarcillin / clavulanic acid)		Covers *Pseudomonas aeruginosa* and anaerobes (when in combination with beta-lactamase inhibitor like tazobactam and clavulanic acid).		Commonly used in hospital for broad pneumonia (particularly aspiration pneumonia) or gut coverage, including *Pseudomonas* and anaerobes. Also good for resistant bugs in UTIs.
Cephalosporins		Gram-⊖ coverage ↑ with increasing generations.		About 10% cross-reactivity with penicillin (less with higher generations).
First generation: ▪ Cefazolin (IV) ▪ Cephalexin, cefadroxil (PO)		MSSA and *Streptococcus,* plus some gram-⊖ (eg, *E. coli*).	▪ Rash, hypersensitivity reaction. ▪ GI upset.	Cephalexin is first-line oral agent for simple cellulitis.
Second generation: ▪ Cefuroxime, cefoxitin, cefotetan (IV) ▪ Cefaclor, cefprozil, cefuroxime axetil (PO)		▪ *E coli, Klebsiella, Proteus, Haemophilus influenzae, Moraxella catarrhalis* ▪ Cefotetan and cefoxitin cover some anaerobes also.		
Third generation: ▪ Cefotaxime, ceftriaxone, ceftazidime (IV) ▪ Ceftbuten, cefpodoxime, cefotaxime, cefdinir (PO)		▪ Second-generation coverage plus: Enterobacteriaceae, *Serratia, Neisseria gonorrhoeae.* ▪ Used for pneumonias and gonorrhea.		**Ceftriaxone:** (1) combined with azithromycin = first line for community-acquired pneumonia; (2) empiric treatment for meningitis (covers *Streptococcus pneumoniae* + *Neisseria*); (3) pyelonephritis.

TABLE 2.5-5. Common Antibiotic Classes *(continued)*

Antimicrobial	Mechanism of Action	Antimicrobial Spectrum	Side Effects	Common Clinical Use
Fourth generation: Cefepime		■ Ceftazidime, cefepime, have activity against *Pseudomonas aeruginosa.* ■ Cefepime has MSSA and streptococcal coverage.		Cefipime is first line in neutropenic fever (with or without vancomycin).
Carbepenems			Cross-reactivity in penicillin allergic patients ~ 10%.	
■ **D**oripenem ■ **I**mipenem ■ **M**eropenem ■ **E**rtapenem		■ **Very** broad coverage: gram ⊕ (but not MRSA), gram ⊖, and anaerobes (but ertapenem does not cover *Acinetobacter, Pseudomonas aeruginosa*). ■ Cilastatitin is given with imipenem as it prevents its hydrolysis in the renal tubules, and maintains the drug for longer.	Lowers seizure threshold.	■ Imipenem is used for very broad coverage for hospital infections/neutropenic fevers/immuno-compromised patients. ■ Ertapenem very good for gut coverage.
Monobactam				
■ Aztreonam	Same as other beta-lactams.	■ Covers only aerobic gram-⊖. ■ Effective in chromosomal produced beta-lactamases, but not ESBL gram ⊖.		■ Safe in penicillin-allergic patients. ■ Vancomycin + aztreonam is a common in-hospital regimen for gram-⊕ and -⊖ coverage in penicillin-allergic patients).

TABLE 2.5-5. Common Antibiotic Classes *(continued)*

Antimicrobial	Mechanism of Action	Antimicrobial Spectrum	Side Effects	Common Clinical Use
Class: Fluoroquinolones				Gram-⊕ coverage ↑ with increasing generations (whereas cephalosporin generations ↑ gram-⊖ coverage).
First generation: Nalidixic acid **Second generation:** ▪ Ofloxacin ▪ Ciprofloxacin	Inhibit bacterial DNA synthesis by inhibiting DNA gyrase/ topoisomerase IV.	▪ *E coli, Salmonella, Shigella, Enterobacter, Campylobacter,* and *Neisseria.* ▪ Intracellular organisms such as *Chlamydia, Mycoplasma, Legionella, Brucella.*	▪ Tendonitis/tendon rupture. ▪ QTc prolongation. ▪ May damage growing cartilage and cause an arthropathy; not used in children.	▪ Ciprofloxacin's excellent gram-⊖ coverage good for UTIs, gut infections, infectious diarrhea. ▪ Moxifloxacin/ levofloxacin good for pneumonias (gram ⊕ and ⊖ and atypicals).
Third generation (respiratory): ▪ Levofloxacin ▪ Trovafloxacin **Fourth generation (respiratory):** ▪ Moxifloxacin ▪ Gemfloxacin		A respiratory quinolone covers the bugs listed above, plus more gram-⊕ coverage including penicillin-resistant *S. pneumoniae* and *S aureus.*		
Class: Aminoglycosides				
▪ **Tobramycin** ▪ **Amikacin** ▪ **Gentamicin**	Prevents bacterial protein synthesis by binding to the 30S ribosomal subunit.	▪ Aerobic gram-⊖ bacteria. ▪ Synergistic activity with beta-lactams, especially for endocarditis caused by streptococci, staphylococci, and enterococci.	▪ Nephrotoxicity, ototoxicity. ▪ Avoid in patients with myasthenia gravis (causes neuromuscular blockade).	▪ Often combined with cefipime for double coverage against *Pseudomonas* in neutropenic patients. ▪ Combined with beta-lactam for synergy in endocarditis.

TABLE 2.5-5. Common Antibiotic Classes *(continued)*

Antimicrobial	Mechanism of Action	Antimicrobial Spectrum	Side Effects	Common Clinical Use
Class: Macrolides			Erythromycin and clarithromycin inhibit CYP3A4 enzymes.	
▪ Erythromycin ▪ Clarithromycin ▪ Azithromycin	Inhibits bacterial protein synthesis by binding reversibly to 50S ribosomal subunits.	▪ **Erythromycin:** Some gram ⊕ (including pneumococci, group *A streptococci,* some *Staphylococcus aureus*) and some gram ⊖ and treponemes, mycoplasmas, *Chlamydia,* and rickettsiae. ▪ **Clarithromycin:** More potent against streptococci and staphylococci + atypicals + *Helicobacter pylori.* ▪ **Azithromycin:** Good for atypical bugs (especially atypical pneumonias), plus some gram ⊕, some gram ⊖, and chlamydia and gonorrhea.	▪ **Erythromycin:** GI upset, cholestatic hepatitis. ▪ **Azithromycin:** GI upset (less common than erythromycin), LFT abnormalities. ▪ **Clarithromycin:** Metallic taste.	▪ Azithromycin is front line in uncomplicated community acquired pneumonias. ▪ For complicated pneumonias, combined with ceftriaxone.
Class: Tetracyclines ▪ Minocycline ▪ Doxycycline ▪ Tetracycline ▪ Demeclocycline	Blocks protein synthesis by binding to 30S ribosomes.	▪ More active against gram-⊕ than gram ⊖. ▪ Some microorganisms, such as *Rickettsia* and *Chlamydia.* ▪ Some atypical mycobacteria.	▪ Photosensitvity. ▪ Gray/yellow discoloration of teeth. ▪ Pseudotumor cerebri.	▪ Can be used for community-acquired MRSA infection. ▪ Treatment for chlamydia and gonorrhea and *Rickettsia* (Rocky Mountain spotted fever).

TABLE 2.5-5. Common Antibiotic Classes *(continued)*

ANTIMICROBIAL	MECHANISM OF ACTION	ANTIMICROBIAL SPECTRUM	SIDE EFFECTS	COMMON CLINICAL USE
Miscellaneous				
■ Vancomycin (a glycopeptide)	Inhibits bacterial cell wall synthesis by inhibiting elongation of peptidoglycan and cross-linking.	■ Covers only gram ⊕ including MSSA (second line), MRSA, but not some enterococci (VRE). ■ Used orally for treatment of *Clostridium difficile.*	■ **Red man syndrome:** Histamine-related reaction; avoid by giving slowly. ■ Nephrotoxicity.	MRSA.
■ Polymyxin B	Penetrates into and disrupts phospholipids in cell membranes.	Good for gram-⊖ aerobic bacilli except *Proteus, Serratia,* and *Providencia* species.	■ Nephrotoxicity, neurotoxicity. ■ Neuromuscular blockade. ■ Paresthesias around the lips, tongue, and extremities; peripheral neuropathy.	
■ Linezolid	Inhibits bacterial protein synthesis by binding to 23S ribosomal RNA of the 50S subunit.	■ Bacteriostatic against *Staphylococcus* and *Enterococcus* species. ■ Bactericidal against *Streptococcus* species.	■ Myelosuppression. ■ Linezolid is an MAOI and therefore can cause serotonin sydrome when used with SSRIs or TCAs.	■ Used primarily for VRE and MRSA infections.
■ Daptomycin	Binds to bacterial membranes resulting in depolarization, loss of membrane potential, and cell death.	Gram-⊕ coverage: *Staphylococcus, Streptococcus,* and *Enterococcus.*	■ Myopathy and rhabdomyalysis. ■ Produces false elevations in PT/INR. ■ Not for lung infections as it is denatured by pulmonary surfactant.	Covers MRSA and VRE.

ESBL: extended-spectrum beta-lactamase; INR: International Normalized Ratio; LFT: liver function test; MAOI: monoamine oxidase inhibitor; MRSA: methicillin-resistant *Staphylococcus aureus;* MSSA: methicillin-sensitive *S aureus;* PT: prothrombin time; SSRI: selective serotonin reuptake inhibitor; TCA: tricyclic antidepressant; UTI: urinary tract infection; VRE: vancomycin-resistant *Enterococcus.*

HIGH-YIELD FACTS IN

Nephrology and Acid-Base Disorders

Le Chatelier's principle is the key to understanding acid-base disorders.

General Principles

Equation

$$HCO_3^- + H^+ \rightarrow\uparrow H_2CO_3^- \rightarrow\uparrow H_2O + CO_2$$

Initial Disturbance

Understanding acid-base disorders requires only an understanding of very basic chemistry! Remember **Le Chatelier's principle:** If you change the concentration of one of the chemicals in an equilibrium, the equilibrium shifts to counteract the change.

- In a **respiratory acidosis,** hypoventilation $\rightarrow \uparrow CO_2$. This shifts the equilibrium to the left, causing a rise in H^+ (thus a fall in pH) and a rise in bicarbonate (HCO_3^-).
- In a **metabolic acidosis,** an overall gain of acid (H^+) causes the pH to fall. This shifts the equilibrium to the right causing a fall in HCO_3^-. Note that this is the case even with GI losses of bicarbonate because excess hydrochloride (HCl) in the gut $\rightarrow \uparrow$ acid reabsorption and $\uparrow$ blood acid concentration.
- In a **respiratory alkalosis,** hyperventilation $\rightarrow \downarrow CO_2$. This shifts the equilibrium to the right, causing a fall in H^+ (thus a rise in pH) and a drop in HCO_3^-.
- In a **metabolic alkalosis,** an overall loss of acid (H^+) causes the pH to rise. This shifts the equilibrium to the right, causing a rise in HCO_3^-.

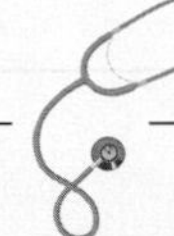

Respiratory compensation is fast and may occur in a matter of minutes. Metabolic compensation is slow and will be seen only with a chronic respiratory disturbance.

Compensation

In any acid-base disturbance, the body attempts to compensate for the disturbance (Table 2.6-1).

- In a respiratory acidosis, the kidneys attempt to generate more bicarbonate, leading to further $\uparrow$ in HCO_3^- and a compensatory $\uparrow$ in pH.
- In a metabolic acidosis, the body attempts respiratory compensation by hyperventilation. Hyperventilation $\downarrow PaCO_2$ and therefore helps shift the equilibrium to the right to $\downarrow H^+$ (and thus $\uparrow$ pH).
- In a respiratory alkalosis, the kidneys attempt to lose bicarbonate, leading to further $\downarrow$ in HCO_3^- and a compensatory $\downarrow$ in pH.
- In a metabolic alkalosis, the body attempts respiratory compensation by hypoventilation. Hypoventilation $\uparrow PaCO_2$ and therefore helps shift the equilibrium to the left to $\uparrow H^+$ and lower pH.

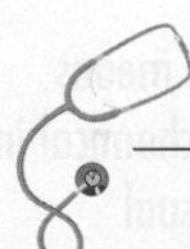

Remember, it is impossible to overcompensate for the primary disturbance. If it appears that a compensation "overcorrects" the pH, then look for a second primary acid-base disturbance.

TABLE 2.6-1. Acid-Base Disturbances

Disorder	Abnormality	Compensation	pH	$PaCO_2$	HCO_3
Metabolic acidosis	Gain H+/lose bicarb	↑ ventilation	↓	↓	↓
Respiratory acidosis	*Hypo*ventilation	Generate bicarbonate	↓	↑	↑
Metabolic alkalosis	Lose H+/gain bicarb	↓ ventilation	↑	↑	↑
Respiratory alkalosis	*Hyper*ventilation	Bicarbonate consumption	↑	↓	↓

Bold arrows indicate compensatory response

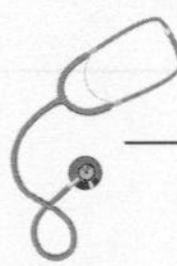

Learn this ABG sequence as these values are frequently reported in this order without labels: **Normal ABG: 7.4/40/90/24/98**

Arterial Blood Gas (ABG)

Normal Values

pH	7.4 (7.35–7.45)
$PaCO_2$	40 (35–45)
PaO_2	90 (80–100)
HCO_3	24 (21–27)
O_2 sat	98 (95–100)

- **Look for hypoxia** using PaO_2; correlate with the clinical scenario.
- **Determine the type of disturbance** using pH, $PaCO_2$, and HCO_3 (see Table 2.6-1).
- **Calculate the degree of compensation:**
  - A change in $PaCO_2$ of 10 mmHg, up or down, causes pH to ↑ or ↓ by 0.08 units (pH ↓ as $PaCO_2$ rises).
  - A pH change of 0.15 is the result of a bicarbonate change of 10 mEq/L.
- If compensation is not within the expected range, look for a second acid-base disturbance.

A high anion gap means there is another chemical in addition to the usual organic acids and albumin that is not measured by a basic metabolic panel. For example, a patient with diabetic ketoacidosis will have high ketones (acids), which will "consume" bicarbonate and generate an anion gap.

Anion Gap (Figure 2.6-1)

The concentration of serum anions not measured in routine electrolyte profiles, mostly organic acids (eg, lactic and keto acids) and albumin.

$$\text{Anion Gap} = Na - (Cl + HCO_3^-)$$

$$\text{Normal} = 8\text{–}12 \text{ mEq/L}$$

Though chiefly used to determine the etiology of a metabolic acidosis, it should be calculated on every patient with an acid-base disturbance to evaluate for an underlying anion gap metabolic acidosis.

Use Winter's formula to determine if compensation is appropriate in the setting of metabolic acidosis: **$1.5 \times (HCO_3^-) + 8 \pm 2 = pCO_2$**

Metabolic Acidosis

- ↓ in pH with ↓ in HCO_3.
- Etiology depends on presence or absence of an anion gap.

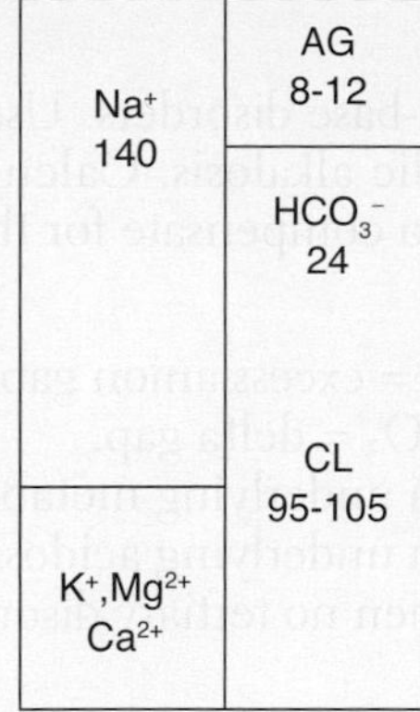

FIGURE 2.6-1. Anion Gap

The sum of the positive and negative charges within the box (including AG) must be neutral. If negative, the there are unmeasured anions resulting in an anion gap metabolic acidosis.

Normal Anion Gap Metabolic Acidosis

Etiology

- Renal losses:
  - Renal tubular acidosis (RTA).
  - Medications (acetazolamide, spironolactone, beta blockers).
- GI losses:
  - Diarrhea
  - Ileostomy

Always check the anion gap. It is the easiest way to pick up a secondary metabolic acidosis.

Anion Gap Metabolic Acidosis

See Table. 2.6-2.

TABLE 2.6-2. Causes of Anion Gap Metabolic Acidosis: MUDPILES

Cause	Findings/Diagnostic Tool
Methanol	Tox screen, vision changes, ↑ osmolal gap
Uremia	History of renal failure, ↑ creatinine
Diabetic ketoacidosis	Diabetes, ↑ serum glucose
Paraldehyde	Tox screen
Isoniazid, **I**ron	Medication history
Lactic acidosis	Serum lactate
Ethanol, **E**thylene glycol	Tox screen, history of alcohol abuse
Salicylates	Respiratory alkalosis and metabolic acidosis, tox screen

Delta Gap or Delta-Delta

Used to calculate tertiary acid-base disorders. Use only to diagnose anion gap metabolic acidosis or metabolic alkalosis. Calculates whether the body is excreting bicarbonate properly to compensate for the presence of unmeasurable anions.

- Anion gap – 12 (nl gap) = excess anion gap.
- Excess anion gap + HCO_3 = delta gap.
- If delta gap is > 30, then underlying metabolic alkalosis is present.
- If delta gap is < 23, then underlying acidosis is present.
- If between 23 and 30, then no tertiary disorder is present.

Treatment

- Correct underlying cause.
- Often, HCO_3^- is given in IV solution (bicarb drip) when pH < 7.0, but this practice has **not** been proven to improve mortality.

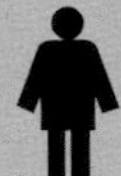

A 34-year-old diabetic man with renal insufficiency has normal anion gap. K is high; bicarbonate level is low. *Think: Type IV RTA (hyporeninemic hypoaldosteronism).*

Respiratory Acidosis

- Hypoventilation from any cause ↑ the $PaCO_2$ and ↓ the serum pH.
- There is a compensatory ↑ in bicarbonate. Remember the equation.
- With an ↑ in CO_2, the equation shifts to the left, creating more H^+ and HCO_3^-.
- More H^+ means the pH ↓.

Etiology

- Pulmonary (chronic obstructive pulmonary disease [COPD], severe alveolar infiltrates, pulmonary edema, interstitial restrictive lung disease).
- Airway obstruction (foreign body, severe bronchospasm, laryngospasm).
- Thoracic disorders (pneumothorax, flail chest).
- Alveolar hypoventilation (myasthenia gravis, severe hypokalemia causing weak muscles of respiration, muscular dystrophy).
- Peripheral nervous system disorders (Guillain-Barré syndrome, botulism, tetanus, organophosphate poisoning).
- Depression of central respiratory drive (narcotic overdose, general anesthesia, ↑ intracranial pressure [ICP]).

Signs and Symptoms

Confusion, encephalopathy, coma.

Treatment

- Treat underlying cause.
- Mechanical hyperventilation will ↓ the amount of CO_2 retention in severely hypoxic patients.

Respiratory Alkalosis

- Elevated arterial pH and hyperventilation, resulting in ↓ PCO_2 and compensatory ↓ in serum bicarbonate. Remember the equation.
- With a ↓ in CO_2, the equation shifts to the right, H^+ ↓, so the pH ↓ and the HCO_3^- ↓ (though often the bicarb change is minimal).

Etiology

- Most commonly caused by anxiety, which provokes hyperventilation.
- Other causes include shock, sepsis, pulmonary disease, cerebrovascular accident (CVA), normal pregnancy, liver disease, hyperthyroidism, salicylates.

Signs and Symptoms

- Rapid, deep breathing.
- Chest tightness, chest pain, and anxiety.
- Circumoral paresthesias, tetany in severe cases.

Treatment

- Reassurance, if anxiety.
- If patient can be calmed enough, have him or her breathe into a paper bag. This ↑ PCO_2 and helps restore pH.
- ↓ the minute volume in the mechanically ventilated patient.

Metabolic Alkalosis

- Elevated pH, ↑ plasma bicarbonate, and a compensatory ↑ in $PaCO_2$.
- Usually seen in cases of volume contraction.
- Remember, an ↑ in HCO_3^- pushes the equation to the right and uses up H^+, therefore ↑ pH and ↑ CO_2.
- Also, in metabolic alkalosis, the respiratory compensation is hypoventilation, → a further ↑ in PCO_2.

Etiology

Divided into chloride-responsive and chloride-resistant forms:

- **Chloride-responsive:** Urine chloride < 20 mEq/L:
  - Vomiting or prolonged NG tube drainage.
  - Pyloric stenosis.
  - Laxative abuse.
  - Diuretics (urine chloride is high during active diuretic use and low after discontinuation of diuretic therapy).
  - Post-hypercapnic states.
- **Chloride-resistant:** Urine chloride > 20 mEq/L:
  - Severe Mg or K deficiency.
  - Diuretics (thiazides or loops).
  - ↑ mineralocorticoids (Cushing's syndrome, primary aldosteronism, renal artery stenosis).
  - Licorice, chewing tobacco.
  - Inherited disorders (Bartter's syndrome, Gitelman's syndrome, and Liddle's syndrome).

Signs and Symptoms

- Irritability and neuromuscular hyperexcitability.
- Concomitant signs of hypokalemia (muscular weakness, cramping, ileus).
- Suspect metabolic alkalosis when the physical exam suggests hypovolemia and chronic GI volume loss.

Treatment

- Mild metabolic alkalosis requires no specific treatment.
- Hydration if cause is volume contraction.
- In severe hypokalemia and hypermineralocorticoid states the alkalosis is chloride resistant and cannot be corrected until potassium is replaced. Specific therapy must address hypermineralocorticoid state.

COMPENSATION FORMULAS

You will not need to calculate the appropriateness of the compensation for an exam, but it may help you during your rotation when trying to decide if there is more than one acid-base disturbance. If you find that the measured change differs significantly from the expected, look for a second acid-base disturbance.

Important Rules

1. There can be only three acid-base disorders at the same time.
2. The body can **never** overcompensate for the primary acid-base disorder.

Respiratory Acidosis

- **Acute:** $\uparrow$ in HCO_3 by 1 for every 10 $\uparrow$ in CO_2.
- **Chronic:** $\uparrow$ in HCO_3 by 3 for every 10 $\uparrow$ in CO_2.

pH $\downarrow$ by 0.08 for every $\uparrow$ in CO_2 by 10 in acute, and pH $\downarrow$ by 0.04 for every $\uparrow$ CO_2 by 10 in chronic.

Respiratory Alkalosis

- **Acute:** $\downarrow$ in HCO_3 by 2 for every $\downarrow$ in CO_2 by 10.
- **Chronic:** $\downarrow$ in HCO_3 by 4 for every $\downarrow$ in CO_2 by 10.

Metabolic Acidosis

Calculate Winter's formula to determine what the CO_2 should be in a primary metabolic acidosis.

$$1.5 \times (HCO_3^-) + 8 \pm 2 = pCO_2$$

A quick way to estimate the expected CO_2 should be is to look at the last two digits of the pH (ie, if the pH is 7.28, the CO_2 in a metabolic acidosis should be 28).

Metabolic Alkalosis

CO_2 $\uparrow$ by .06 for every $\uparrow$ in HCO_3 by 1.

Putting It All Together

The primary distubance is always the factor that changes in the same directions as the pH. For example, in acidosis, the primary disturbance will be identified by either a low HCO_3 or a low CO_2.

1. Look at pH: If < 7.40, acidosis is present; if > 7.40, alkalosis is present.
2. Next, look at the CO_2. If acidosis is present and the CO_2 is < 40, the primary disorder is metabolic acidosis; if the CO_2 is > 40, the primary disorder is respiratory acidosis. If alkalosis is present and the CO_2 is < 40, the primary disorder is respiratory alkalosis. If the CO_2 is > 40, the primary disorder is metabolic alkalosis.
3. Calculate compensation for the primary disorder using the calculations above to diagnose secondary acid-base disorder.
4. Calculate the anion gap if an acidosis is present.
5. Calculate delta gap to diagnose tertiary acid-base disorder.

ELECTROLYTE DISORDERS

Body Fluids

- Total body water (TBW) is approximately 60% of lean body mass.
- Intracellular fluid (ICF) is two-thirds of TBW:
  - The major cations in ICF are K^+ and Mg^{2+}.
  - The major ICF anions are proteins and organic phosphates (adenosine triphosphate [ATP], adenosine diphosphate [ADP], adenosine monophosphate [AMP]).
- Extracellular fluid (ECF) is one-third of TBW:
  - Consists of interstitial fluid (third space) and plasma.
  - The major ECF cation is Na^+.
  - The major ECF anions are Cl^- and HCO_3^-.
  - Plasma comprises one-fourth of the ECF (one-twelfth of TBW). The major plasma proteins are albumin and globulins.
  - Interstitial fluid is three-fourths of the ECF (one-fourth of TBW). The electrolyte composition of interstitial fluid is the same as plasma. However, interstitial fluid contains little protein (ultrafiltrate).

Fluid Shifts Between Compartments

- Water shifts between ECF and ICF so the osmolarities of the two compartments remain equal.
- Solutes that do not cross the cell membranes freely contribute to ECF osmolarity (glucose, sodium, mannitol, IV contrast materials).
- **Serum osmolarity:**
  - Normal range: 280–300 mOsm/kg.
  - Serum osmolarity can be estimated with the following formula:

    Serum Osmolarity = 2(Na + K) + Glucose/18 + BUN/2.8

  - Elevated in dehydration, hypernatremia, diabetes insipidus, uremia, hyperglycemia, mannitol therapy, toxin ingestion, hypercalcemia, diuretic therapy.
  - ↓ in syndrome of inappropriate antidiuretic hormone (SIADH), hyponatremia, overhydration with 5% dextrose solution, Addison's disease, hypothyroidism.
  - Major toxins that ↑ the serum osmolarity: EtOH, methanol, ethylene glycol.

Hyponatremia

Plasma sodium < 134 mEq/L.

Etiology and Classification

Calculate serum osmolarity and determine fluid status of a patient to determine classification of hyponatremia. Hyponatremia is subdivided into three categories based on the serum osmolarity and fluid status (Table 2.6-3):

- **Hypotonic hyponatremia** is further subdivided into three categories:
  1. *Hypervolemic:* CHF (↑ free H_2O), nephrotic syndrome (↓ albumin), cirrhosis (↓ albumin).
  2. *Isovolemic:* Renal failure, SIADH, glucocorticoid deficiency (hypopituitarism or Addison's disease), hypothyroidism with myxedema, primary polydypsia, and medications.
  3. *Hypovolemic:*
     - Loss of both sodium and water.
     - Renal losses (diuretics, partial urinary tract obstruction, salt-wasting nephropathies).
     - Extrarenal losses (vomiting, diarrhea, extensive burns, third-spacing (pancreatitis, peritonitis).
- **Isotonic hyponatremia** (normal serum osmolarity):
  - SIADH.
  - Isotonic infusions (glucose, mannitol).
- **Hypertonic hyponatremia** (↑ serum osmolarity):
  - *Hyperglycemia:* Each 100 mg/dL ↑ in serum glucose above normal (100 mg/dL) ↓ plasma sodium concentration by 1.6 mEq/L. To avoid missing a potentially severe *hypernatremia,* you must calculate the corrected serum sodium: Corrected Na = [(serum glucose –100)/100] × 1.6.
  - *Hypertonic infusions:* Mannitol, glucose.

Signs and Symptoms

- Moderate hyponatremia or gradual onset: Confusion, muscle cramps, lethargy, anorexia, nausea.
- Severe hyponatremia or rapid onset: Seizures or coma (no exact number, but $Na^+ < 115$ is always severe).

TABLE 2.6-3. Causes of Hyponatremia

		Urine Osm	Urine Sodium
Hypovolemic	Extrarenal: GI losses, skin losses, lung losses, third-spacing (fistula, burns, vomiting, diarrhea, GI suction, edema, pancreatitis).	↑	↓ < 10 mEq/L
	Renal: Diuretics, intrinsic renal damage (including acute tubular necrosis), partial urinary tract obstruction, salt-wasting nephropathies.	↑	↑ > 20 mEq/ L
	Adrenal insufficiency (Addison's).	↑	↑
Isovolemic	Water intoxication.	↓	↓
	SIADH.	↑	↑
Hypervolemic	CHF, liver cirrhosis, and the nephrotic syndrome.	↑	↓

CHF, congestive heart failure; SIADH, syndrome of inappropriate antidiuretic hormone.

Diagnosis

- **Normal osmolarity:** Consider pseudohyponatremia and overinfusion of non-sodium-containing isotonic solutions such as glucose and mannitol.
- **Low osmolarity:** Clinically assess the extracellular fluid volume. Look for tachycardia, hypotension, poor skin turgor (indicative of **hypovolemia**). Also look for peripheral edema (indicative of **hypervolemia**). Normal vital signs and no edema usually indicate **isovolemia.**
- **High osmolarity:** Measure serum glucose concentration to consider hyperglycemia. Also consider overinfusion of hypertonic, non-sodium-containing solutions (mannitol, glucose, glycine).

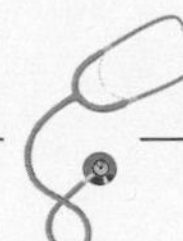

If kidneys are still functional in a hypovolvemic patient, urine Na^+ should be < 10 mEq/L as the kidneys will be trying to conserve Na^+ to maintain intravascular volume.

Pseudohyponatremia

- Simply an error in measurement of sodium due to an ↑ in other plasma components.
- Since plasma is 93% water and 7% plasma protein and lipid, and sodium ions are only dissolved in the plasma water, increasing the nonaqueous phase artificially lowers the Na^+ concentration.
- This occurs in multiple myeloma (due to ↑ plasma protein) or hyperlipidemia.

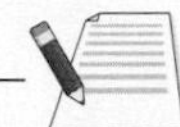

Urine Na^+ can distinguish between renal and extrarenal causes of hypovolemic hyponatremia. Renal cause: UNa^+ > 20 µEq/L since kidneys cannot conserve Na^+ or H_2O. Nonrenal cause: UNa < 10 µEq/L.

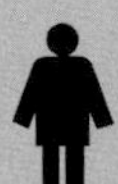

A patient presents with multiple myeloma and hyponatremia, but calculated serum tonicity is normal. *Think: Pseudohyponatremia/ paraproteinemia.*

Treatment

General Rules

- Treatment approach is twofold: Correction of the serum sodium and treatment of the underlying disorder.
- Serum sodium should be corrected only halfway to the lower range of normal within the first 24 hours.
- Unless patient has acute hyponatremia with seizure, do not correct sodium faster than 1 mEq/L/hr with a maximum correction of 10 mEq/L/24 hrs. Central pontine myelinolysis (CPM), seizures, coma, and death can result.

Type-Specific Treatment

- **Hypovolemic hyponatremia:** 0.9% NaCl (**normal saline**) infusion to correct volume deficit. Monitor the serum sodium to prevent complications of rapid correction. Hypertonic saline is rarely indicated.
- **Hypervolemic hyponatremia:** Sodium and **water restriction.** In congestive heart failure (CHF), the combination of captopril and furosemide is effective.

Pseudohyponatremia is suspected if the measured and calculated serum osmolarities are different.

Complications

Central pontine myelinolysis (CPM):

- Sometimes termed osmotic demyelination syndrome, occurs as a treatment complication of severe or chronic hyponatremia (< 110 mEq/L).

- A symmetric zone of demyelination occurs in the basis pontis (and extrapontine areas), leading to stupor, lethargy, quiet and confused delirium, and quadriparesis.
- CPM can be avoided by increasing the serum sodium no faster than 1 mEq/L/hr. Some patients treated symptomatically will recover in 3–4 weeks; however, in some, the damage is irreversible.

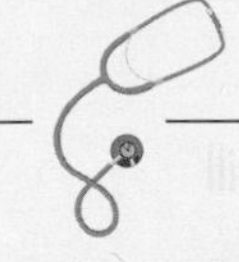

Formula: Water deficit (WD) in hypernatremic patients:
WD (in liters) = 0.6 × body weight (kg) × (Measured Na/Normal Na) – 1)

Hypernatremia

Serum Na > 145 mEq/L.

Etiology and Classification

See Table 2.6-4.

- **Hypovolemic** (most common):
  - Loss of water and sodium (water loss >> than sodium loss).
  - Renal losses (diuretics, glycosuria); GI, respiratory, or skin losses; adrenal deficiencies.
- **Isovolemic:**
  - ↓ TBW, normal total body sodium, and ↓ ECF.
  - Diabetes insipidus (neurogenic and nephrogenic), skin losses (hyperthermia), iatrogenic causes, reset osmostat.
- **Hypervolemic:**
  - ↑ TBW, markedly ↑ total body sodium, and ↑ ECF.
  - Iatrogenic (hypertonic fluid administration).
  - Mineralocorticoid excess (Conn's tumor, Cushing's syndrome).
  - Excess salt ingestion.

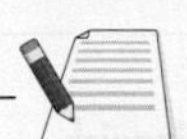

Giving DDAVP (desmopressin) to a patient with hypernatremia will result in increased urine osmolarity and improvement in hypermatremia in central diabetes insipidus.

Signs and Symptoms

- Fatigue
- Confusion (can progress to coma and seizures)
- Lethargy
- Edema

NEPHROLOGY AND ACID-BASE DISORDERS

TABLE 2.6-4. Causes of Hypernatremia

		Urine Osm	Urine Sodium
Hypovolemic	Renal loss: Osmotic diuresis (glycosuria, urea), acute/chronic renal failure, partial obstruction.	N/↓	↑
	Extrarenal loss: Hyperpnea, excessive sweating.	↑	↑
	Extrarenal loss: Diarrhea, burns, moderate sweating.	↑	↓
	Iatrogenic (bicarbonate, dialysis, salt tablets).	↑	↑
Isovolemic	Diabetes insipidus (from any cause).	↓	↓
Hypervolemic	Mineralocorticoid excess (eg, Conn's syndrome).	N/↓	N/↓

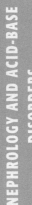

TREATMENT

- **Hypovolemic hypernatremia:** Fluid replacement with normal saline. Correct plasma sodium no faster than 0.5mEq/L/hr.
- **Isovolemic hypernatremia:**
  - Fluid replacement with half normal (0.45%) saline. Correct only half of the estimated water deficit in the first 24 hours.
  - The correction rate should not exceed 1 mEq/L/hr in acute hypernatremia and 0.5 mEq/L/hr in chronic hypernatremia.
  - Vasopressin for central diabetes insipidus.
- **Hypervolemic hypernatremia:**
  - Fluid replacement with half normal (0.45%) saline (to correct hypertonicity).
  - Loop diuretic therapy (eg, furosemide) to ↑ sodium excretion.

In hypovolemic hypernatremia, always correct fluid deficit with normal saline before anything else.

Hypokalemia

Plasma potassium < 3.3 mEq/L.

ETIOLOGY AND CLASSIFICATION

- Extra- to intracellular potassium shifting (redistribution) and undetermined mechanisms:
  - Alkalosis (each 0.1 ↑ in pH ↓ serum K^+ by 0.4–0.6 mEq/L).
  - Insulin (drives K^+ into cells).
  - Vitamin B_{12}.
  - Beta-adrenergics.
  - Correction of digoxin toxicity with digitalis antibody fragments (Digibind).
- **↑ renal potassium excretion:**
  - Medications (diuretics, amphotericin B, cisplatin, aminoglycosides, corticosteroids).
  - Renal tubular acidosis type I (distal) or type II (proximal).
  - Hypomagnesemia.
  - Osmotic diuresis (mannitol).
  - Bartter's syndrome: JG-cell hyperplasia causing ↑ renin/aldosterone, metabolic alkalosis, hypokalemia, hypercalciuria, muscle weakness, and tetany (seen in young adults).
  - Gitelman's syndrome: Defective distal tubule thiazide-sensitive Na^+ Cl^- transporter → metabolic alkalosis, hypokalemia, hypomagnesemia, and hypocalciuria. Presents similar to Bartter's syndrome, but less severe in presentation.
  - ↑ mineralocorticoid activity (primary hyperaldosteronism [tumor] or secondary hyperaldosteronism [CHF, cirrhosis, dehydration]), Cushing's syndrome.
- **GI losses:**
  - Vomiting, nasogastric suctioning.
  - Diarrhea, laxative abuse.
  - Inadequate dietary intake (anorexia nervosa).
  - Cutaneous losses from excessive sweating.

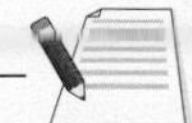

Patients taking digitalis must have their potassium checked regularly because hypokalemia ↑ the risk and severity of digitalis toxicity.

SIGNS AND SYMPTOMS

- Impaired gastric motility, nausea, and vomiting.
- Mild muscle weakness to overt paralysis depending on severity.
- Rhabdomyolysis.
- Atrial and ventricular dysrhythmias.

TREATMENT

Replace potassium (PO or IV, depending on severity). IV infusion of K^+ should not exceed 20 mEq/L/hr, but may be combined with simultaneous oral administration.

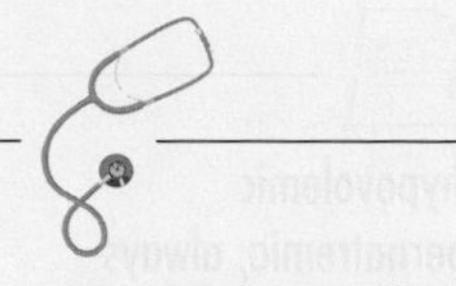

A 10-mEq infusion will raise the serum K by 1.0 mEq/L.

Hyperkalemia

Serum K > 5.5 mEq/L.

ETIOLOGY

Chronic, slowly developing hyperkalemia is better tolerated than acute changes (ie, less likely to have cardiac changes).

- Always consider pseudohyperkalemia (falsely elevated measurement due to hemolysis of specimen and leakage of potassium from lysed cells in the tube). This is the most common cause of elevated potassium based on lab results. Repeat test.
- **Intra- to extracellular potassium shifting** occurs in acidosis, heavy exercise, insulin deficiency, and digitalis toxicity.
- ↑ **potassium load** occurs with IV potassium supplementation, potassium-containing medications, and ↑ cellular breakdown.
- ↓ **potassium excretion** occurs with oliguric renal failure, potassium sparing diuretics, beta blockers, angiotensin-converting enzyme (ACE) inhibitors, aldosterone deficiency, and obstructive uropathies.

Perform a STAT ECG on patients with moderate to severe hyperkalemia.

SIGNS AND SYMPTOMS

- GI: Nausea, vomiting, diarrhea.
- Neuro: Muscle cramps, weakness, paresthesias, paralysis, areflexia, tetany, focal neurologic deficits, confusion.
- Respiratory insufficiency.
- Cardiac: Arrhythmias, arrest.

DIAGNOSIS

Electrocardiogram (ECG) changes:

- 6.5–7.5 mEq/L: **Tall peaked T-waves in ALL ECG leads** (see Figure 2.6-2), short QT interval, prolonged PR.
- 7.5–8.0 mEq/L: QRS widening, flattened P-wave.
- 10–12 mEq/L: QRS may degrade into a "sine-wave" pattern.
- V-fib, complete heart block, or asystole may occur.

Treatments for hyperkalemia—

Controlling K Immediately Diverts Bad Arrhythmias

Calcium
Kayexalate, Diuretics
Insulin and glucose
Dialysis
Bicarbonate
Albuterol

TREATMENT

- **Immediate:** The following therapies are only **temporizing measures** of lowering potassium until definitive therapy is initiated. *Remember:* Your job is not done until definitive potassium lowering therapy is given.
  - IV calcium gluconate: **Goal is immediate cardiac membrane stabilization;** acts in minutes.
  - Insulin has the most potent effect on driving potassium into cells. Also can use albuterol (beta-adrenergic agonist), and lastly bicarbonate. Goal is shifting K^+ from ECF to ICF; acts in minutes.
  - If giving insulin, must make sure to give the patient glucose, usually in the form of D50 IV push, to prevent hypoglycemia.
- **Definitive therapy:** The following therapies provide removal of total body potassium.
  - Cation exchange resin such as Kayexalate, diuretics, and hemodialysis are used with goal removal of potassium from the body; takes hours to work.

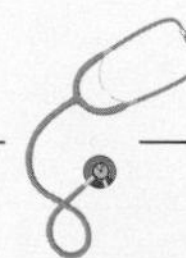

Kayexalate and diuretics are the only treatments of hyperkalemia (other than dialysis) that remove potassium from the body.

NEPHROLOGY AND ACID-BASE DISORDERS

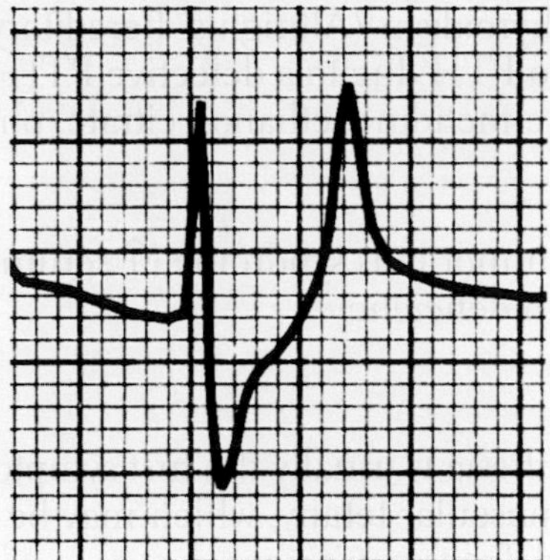

FIGURE 2.6-2. Peaked T-wave due to hyperkalemia.

- Diuretics (eg, furosemide) ↑ K^+ excretion and may be given with IV fluids if patient is euvolemic.
- Refractory hyperkalemia, or hyperkalemia with life-threatening arrhythmias, requires hemodialysis as the most effective therapy to lower total body potassium.

Hypocalcemia

- Serum Ca < 8.5 mg/dL.
- Calcium can be found bound to plasma proteins, complexed with anions (eg, phospate), or free (ionized). The free (ionized) fraction is biologically active.

Etiology

- Always consider hypoalbuminemia. Since a large amount of calcium is bound to albumin, patients with hypoalbuminemia (eg, liver failure, nephrotic syndrome) have low total calcium levels but normal ionized calcium levels.
- You can calculate a corrected calcium as follows for an estimate of effective calcium level, or you can check an ionized calcium level to be sure:

$$\text{Corrected Calcium} = \text{Measured Calcium} + [(4 - \text{Measured Albumin})] \times 0.8$$

- Parathyroid hormone (PTH) insufficiency. PTH secretion is stimulated by low free calcium and inhibited by increasing free calcium. Three major actions:
  1. In bone, PTH causes resorption of both calcium and phosphate.
  2. In the kidney, PTH facilitates resorption of calcium and excretion of phosphate.
  3. Also in the kidney, PTH stimulates conversion of 25-OH vitamin D to 1,25 dihydroxyvitamin D_3 (active vitamin D). Renal failure results in vitamin D deficiency → low Ca^+ → ↑ PTH. Vitamin D causes retention of both calcium and phosphate.

  Therefore, the net effect of PTH is to ↑ serum calcium and ↓ serum phosphate.
- Vitamin D deficiency (intestinal malabsorption, cholestyramine, primidone, renal disease).

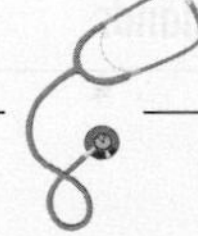

Correcting for hypoalbuminemia: The measured Ca should be adjusted upward by 0.8 mg/dL for each 1.0 g/dL of albumin below normal.

- Pseudohypoparathyroidism (Albrights' hereditary osteodystropy) = end-organ resistance to PTH due to a defective PTH receptor.
- Toxins: Fluoride, cimetidine, ethanol, citrate, phenytoin.
- Sepsis.
- Pancreatitis.
- Rhabdomyolysis, tumor lysis syndrome (↑ serum phosphate).
- Severe magnesium deficiency.

SIGNS AND SYMPTOMS

- Circumoral paresthesia is usually the first symptom.
- The next sign is muscular tetany, which may be observed by examining for Chvostek's and Trousseau's signs.
  - **Chvostek's sign:** Facial muscle spasm with tapping of the facial nerve.
  - **Trousseau's sign:** Carpal spasm after occluding blood flow in forearm with blood pressure cuff.
- Acute severe hypocalcemia may cause laryngospasm, seizures, confusion, or cardiovascular collapse with bradycardia and decompensated heart failure.

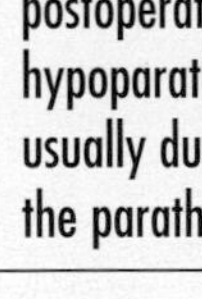

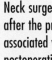

Neck surgery, even long after the procedure, can be associated with postoperative hypoparathyroidism, usually due to ischemia of the parathyroid glands.

DIAGNOSIS

- Clues to diagnosis can be provided by careful bedside evaluation, looking for evidence of prior neck surgery, a thorough evaluation of medications, as well as detailed family history looking for cases of hypocalcemia, hypoparathyroidism, or pseudohypoparathyroidism.
- ECG findings: Prolonged QT and ST intervals (peaked T-waves are also possible, as in hyperkalemia).

TREATMENT

- For PTH deficiency: Replacement therapy with vitamin D or calcitriol combined with high oral calcium intake. Thiazide diuretics are used to lower urinary calcium and prevent calcium urolithiasis.
- Repletion of magnesium for hypomagnesemia.
- Oral calcium supplementation, dietary phosphate restriction, and calcitriol for chronic renal failure.
- Vitamin D and calcium supplementation for pseudohypoparathyroidism.
- IV calcium for severe, life-threatening hypocalcemia.

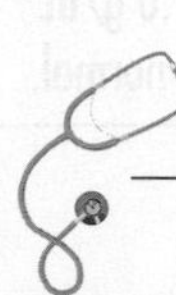

Primary hyperparathyroidism is the most common cause of hypercalcemia in the outpatient. Malignancy is the most common cause in the inpatient.

Hypercalcemia

Serum Ca > 10.2 mg/dL.

ETIOLOGY

- **Drugs:**
  - Calcium supplementation (IV).
  - Excess vitamin D ↑ intestinal calcium absorption.
  - Antacid abuse.
  - Thiazides (inhibit renal calcium excretion).
  - Lithium.

- **Malignancies:**
  - Colon, lung, breast, prostate (all cause metastasis to bone).
  - Multiple myeloma.
  - Zollinger-Ellison syndrome (as part of multiple endocrine neoplasia type I (MEN I).
- **Endocrinopathies:**
  - Hyperparathyroidism
  - Hyperthyroidism
  - Acromegaly
  - Addison's disease
  - Paget's disease (of bone)
- **Other:**
  - Immobility (→ ↑ bone turnover with ↑ bone resorption).
  - Granulomatous diseases such as sarcoidosis, tuberculosis (1,25-[OH]$_2$-vitamin D_3 production by macrophages within granulomatous tissue).

Causes of hypercalcemia—CHIMPANZEES

Calcium supplementation
Hyperparathyroidism/**H**yperthyroidism
Immobility/**I**atrogenic
Metastasis/**M**ilk alkali syndrome
Paget's disease
Addison's disease/**A**cromegaly
Neoplasm
Zollinger-Ellison syndrome
Excessive vitamin A
Excessive vitamin D
Sarcoidosis

Signs and Symptoms

- Malaise, fatigue, headaches, diffuse aches and pains.
- Patients are often dehydrated and a vicious cycle ensues. Dehydration ↓ renal calcium excretion, while at the same time patients are losing fluids from vomiting and nausea induced by the hypercalcemia.
- Lethargy and psychosis occur when hypercalcemia is severe.
- Metastatic calcifications may occur in skin, cornea, conjunctiva, and kidneys.
- Severe hypercalcemia may cause QT interval shortening and variable degrees of AV block.

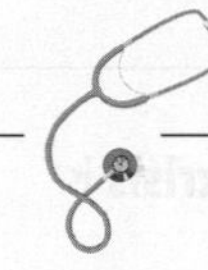

Acute pancreatitis can be precipitated by hypercalcemia.

Treatment

- IV fluids +/– Lasix.
- Calcitonin.
- Bisphosphonate derivatives (↓ osteoclastic activity).
- Dialysis for severe or symptomatic hypercalcemia.
- Parathyroidectomy if hyperparathyroid is cause.

Malignancy and Hypercalcemia

- **Humoral hypercalcemia of malignancy**: Tumor production of PTH-related peptide (PTH-rp). Stimulates bone resorption and renal calcium reabsorption. PTH-related peptide is not detected by the usual PTH immunoassay. Specific immunoassay exists for PTH-related peptide.
- **Local osteolytic hypercalcemia:** Malignant cells in multiple myeloma or solid tumors with bone metastases may cause osteoclast stimulation. Osteoclast-activating factors (OAFs) are interleukins, transforming growth factors, and other cytokines.

Management of Severe Hypercalcemia

- Rehydration with normal saline to initiate calciuresis.
- IV infusion of **pamidronate** (bisphosphonate) should be initiated simultaneously.
- May also use calcitonin.
- May also use furosemide to ↑ diuresis once patient is hydrated.
- Dialysis if severe or refractory to medical treatment.

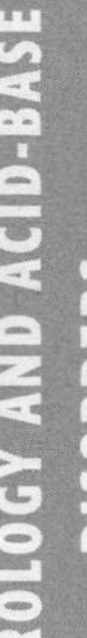

Transient hypoparathyroidism can occur after removal of a parathyroid adenoma because the remaining glands take a few days to begin secreting PTH again.

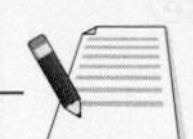

Hypercalcemia: "Stones, bones, groans, and psychiatric overtones."

Hypercalcemic crisis is an uncommon manifestation of primary hyperparathyroidism. It presents with severe hypercalcemia, volume depletion, and altered mental status.

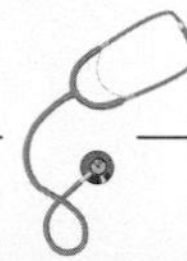

Hungry bone syndrome is the rapid transfer of calcium and phosphate into bones following removal of a hyperactive parathyroid nodule.

Hyperparathyroidism

PRIMARY

- Elevated parathyroid hormone and elevated serum calcium.
- May occur in conjunction with MEN I or MEN IIa (all glands are hyperplastic).
- Usually, only one parathyroid gland is enlarged, and hypercalcemia suppresses the function of the remaining glands.

EPIDEMIOLOGY

More common in middle-aged to elderly women.

SIGNS AND SYMPTOMS

- Usual presentation is asymptomatic hypercalcemia noted on routine laboratory examination.
- Patients may also have nonspecific complaints like fatigue, weight loss, depression, abdominal pain, or arthralgias.
- Hypercalciuria from the kidneys' inability to reabsorb the large calcium load may → nephrocalcinosis or renal calculi.
- Elevated PTH levels → bone remodeling and ↓ bone mass.

DIAGNOSIS

- Hypercalcemia.
- PTH level in the high-normal range.
- Hypophosphatemia.
- Hypercalciuria.

SECONDARY/RENAL OSTEODYSTROPHY

PATHOPHYSIOLOGY

- In chronic kidney disease, (CKD), nephron loss reduces phosphate excretion, causing hyperphosphatemia.
- This lowers serum calcium (thereby increasing PTH secretion) and impairs calcitriol formation.
- ↓ calcitriol formation (also due to nephron loss) reduces intestinal calcium absorption.
- This provides further stimulation for PTH secretion.
- The ↑ PTH → excessive bone resorption/turnover.

ETIOLOGY AND CLASSIFICATION

Three types of bone lesions are associated with secondary hyperparathyroidism:

1. **Osteitis fibrosa cystica:** Normal bone is replaced by fibrous tissue, primitive woven bone, and cysts due to high bone turnover.
2. **Osteomalacia:** Associated with vitamin D deficiency, characterized by defective osteoid mineralization.
3. **Adynamic bone disease:** Cause is unknown, but the disease is due to excessively low bone turnover.

SIGNS AND SYMPTOMS

- Bone pain.
- Proximal muscle weakness.
- Pruritus.
- Soft-tissue ulcerations.
- Diffuse soft-tissue calcifications.

TREATMENT

Goal is to normalize the calcium–phosphate balance:

- Dietary phosphate restriction.
- Reduce intestinal absorption of phosphate with aluminum-containing antacids and/or phosphate binders (PhosLo, Renagel, etc.).
- Vitamin D with calcitriol to ↑ serum calcium and reverse some of the bone changes.
- Cinacalcet (Sensipar), which mimics the action of calcium on the parathyroid gland reducing PTH levels.
- Subtotal parathyroidectomy may benefit patients who do not respond to medical therapy.
- Frequent dialysis.
- Renal transplant in selected patients.

Hypophosphatemia

- Serum phosphate < 2.5 mg/dL.
- Usually, alcoholism or malnutrition is the cause. Also seen with diabetic ketoacidosis (DKA) and hyperparathyroidism.
- Symptoms are neuro (mental status change, agitation) and muscle weakness.
- Severe hypophosphatemia (< 1 mg/dL) can result in rhabdomyolysis or seizures.
- Treat with phosphate supplementation orally, or if phosphate < 1 mg/dL intravenously.

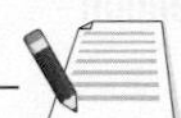

Phosphate is especially important for weaning patients off ventilators since the diaphragm requires a lot of ATP (adenosine tri*PHOSPHATE*) for energy.

Hyperphosphatemia

Plasma phosphate > 5 mg/dL.

ETIOLOGY

Renal failure, tumor lysis syndrome (rapid necrosis of tumor after chemotherapy), iatrogenic (excessive amounts given IV or PO).

TREATMENT

Oral calcium carbonate (binds phosphate in gut and ↓ absorption), low-phosphate diet, aluminum-containing antacids, phosphate binders (PhosLo, Renagel, etc.) depending on the level and cause of hyperphosphatemia.

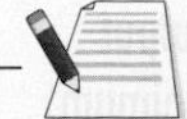

A common cause of high phosphate serum values is *in vitro* hemolysis. Most labs will report that the specimen was hemolyzed, however.

Hypomagnesemia

Serum magnesium < 1.8 mg/dL.

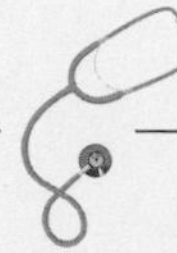

When supplementing calcium or potassium, always check for hypomagnesemia. The calcium and potassium levels will not elevate if magnesium is low.

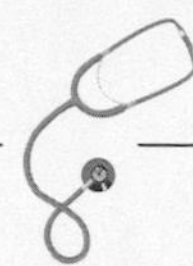

IV magnesium infusion requires:

- Cardiac monitor
- Vitals q 10 min
- Monitor deep tendon reflexes
- Monitor urine output

ARF with oliguria has a worse prognosis. In addition, interventions to change renal failure from oliguric to nonoliguric (using high-dose diuretics) do not change the prognosis.

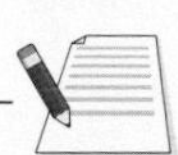

Oliguria: Urine output < 400 mL/day. Minimum volume needed to excrete daily production of metabolites and waste products.

ETIOLOGY

- Drugs (loop diuretics, amphotericin, gentamicin), insulin, hungry bone syndrome.
- Low magnesium causes hypokalemia and hypocalcemia *refractory* to replacement.
- **You will be unable to correct the potassium or calcium deficit until magnesium is corrected.**
- ECG changes similar to hypokalemia.
- Treat with oral or IV supplementation.

Hypermagnesemia

Serum magnesium > 2.3 mg/dL.

ETIOLOGY

Iatrogenic (during treatment of eclampsia/preeclampsia), magnesium-containing drugs (some laxatives, antacids) if given to a patient with renal failure.

TREATMENT

IV fluids, calcium if there are ECG changes; dialysis if refractory.

General Principles of Electrolyte Disorder Management

- Always check the other electrolytes—isolated electrolyte abnormalities are uncommon.
- Abnormal calcium level is meaningless without an albumin level in an asymptomatic patient.
- Redraw labs if *in vitro* hemolysis is a possibility.
- If severe, place patient on continuous ECG monitoring.
- Neurological exam soon after treatment begun—focus on level of consciousness, presence of confusion, and deep tendon reflexes. Serial neuro exams during treatment can guide therapy while labs are pending.

ACUTE RENAL FAILURE (ARF)

- Also called **acute kidney injury (AKI).**
- Clear-cut definition does not exist.
- Usually rapid onset of increasing blood urea nitrogen (BUN) and creatinine.
- Often occurs in the hospitalized patient.
- May be heralded by ↓ urine production (oliguria).

CLASSIFICATION

Prerenal, postrenal, or intrinsic renal failure.

GENERAL APPROACH

- **Prerenal** (due to ↓ kidney perfusion):
  - BUN rising out of proportion to creatinine (> 20:1).
  - Volume depletion from hemorrhage, dehydration, surgery.
  - CHF causing ↓ cardiac output and secondary renal hypoperfusion.

- Third-spacing from cirrhosis, nephrotic syndrome, sepsis, burns.
  - Most common cause of inpatient renal insufficiency is due to ↓ renal perfusion.
  - Exacerbated by nonsteroidal anti-inflammatory drugs (NSAIDs), angiotensin-converting enzyme (ACE) inhibitors, and diuretics.
- **Postrenal** (due to obstruction of urinary excretion):
  - Bilateral ureteral obstruction: Urothelial tumor, benign prostatic hypertrophy (BPH), cervical cancer.
  - Unilateral ureteral obstruction from renal stones, stricture, or tumor may cause significant ↓ in glomerular filtration rate (GFR) and unilateral kidney failure.
  - Urethral obstruction: Bladder cancer.
  - Retroperitoneal fibrosis.
  - Renal sonogram: May show bilateral hydronephrosis; retrograde ureterogram is more sensitive for obstruction.
  - Reversible if obstruction removed in time.
  - If lower obstruction cannot be removed, nephrostomy tubes relieve the obstruction and prevent further kidney injury.
  - Postobstructive diuresis: Frequent temporary sequela of obstruction removal. Presents with overdiuresis by kidneys, resulting in dehydration and electrolyte disturbance. If present, hydrate and follow electrolytes.
- **Intrinsic:**
  - Acute tubular necrosis (ATN) due to ischemia (after prerenal insult/hypoperfusion), toxins such as medications (aminoglycosides, cisplatin, pentamidine, lithium, amphotericin), myoglobin from rhabdomyolysis, IV contrast.
  - Acute allergic interstitial nephritis (AIN).
  - Vascular disorders and atheromatous emboli.
  - Glomerular disorders (nephrotic and nephritic syndromes).
- **Urinary sodium:**
  - Prerenal failure has low urine sodium (< 15 mEq/L) and high urine osmolarity (> 500 mOsm/L). The urine specific gravity is usually around 1.020. This is a result of the kidney's trying to concentrate the urine and conserve volume when perfusion is ↓.
  - Intrinsic renal failure has high urine sodium (> 15 mEq/L) and low urine osmolarity (< 400 mOsm/L) because the kidneys are unable to concentrate the urine.
- **Urinary sediment:** Intrinsic renal disease shows large amounts of protein and an "active" sediment (blood, protein, and red and white cell casts) that often will point toward the underlying cause of the renal disease:
  - **Acute glomerulonephritis:** Red blood cell (RBC) casts with hematuria and proteinuria and low urine specific gravity.
  - **ATN:** Many renal epithelial cells and muddy brown granular casts.

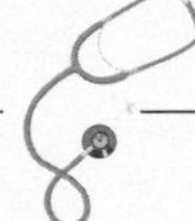

The fractional sodium excretion (FeNa+) is the best discriminator between prerenal and intrinsic renal failure:

FeNa <1% is pre-renal, FeNa >2% is intrinsic renal failure. A value between 1% – 2% is indeterminant.

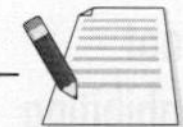

Dopamine, diuretics, mannitol, and saline confound use of fractional sodium excretion in finding etiology of renal failure.

NEPHROLOGY AND ACID-BASE DISORDERS

Tubulointerstitial Diseases

- Most common cause of intrinsic ARF.
- Includes ATN and interstitial nephritis.
- Tubulointerstitial causes of renal failure are the most common etiologies of ARF in hospitalized patients, and are associated with the best outcomes if recognized early.

Acute Tubular Necrosis (ATN)

Acute necrosis of renal tubules due to ischemic or toxic insult.

Etiology

- **Ischemic:** Shock, trauma, sepsis, hypoxia.
- **Toxic:** IV contrast media, aminoglycosides, rhabdomyolysis (heme pigments), and tumor lysis.

Course

- Patients present with dramatic renal failure.
- Most survive and recover normal renal function.
- Severity correlates with survival.
- Failure lasts 1–2 weeks, during which intensive care and sometimes hemodialysis are required while kidneys recover.
- Approximately 50% have normal urine output (less severe).

Diagnosis

- Muddy brown granular casts.
- High urine sodium.
- Rising creatinine.
- FeNa is > 1%.

The fractional sodium excretion (FeNa) is the best discriminator between prerenal and intrinsic renal failure. **FeNa <1% is pre-renal, FeNa >2% is intrinsic renal failure. A value between 1% – 2% is indeterminant.**

Prevention

- Monitor creatinine in patients receiving nephrotoxic substances.
- Maintain adequate intravascular volume for patients pre and post surgical procedures.
- Provide hydration to patients that will receive iodinated contrast media as tolerated (typically use normal saline IV).
- Maintain good cardiac output.

Treatment

- Normal saline for volume replacement.
- Match fluid and salt intake to daily urine output.
- Discontinue precipitating cause/offending or exacerbating agents (eg, medications).
- Manage electrolyte disturbances.

NSAIDs usually do not cause AIN, but by inhibiting prostaglandin synthesis they ↓ the GFR, which can precipitate renal failure in a patient with underlying renal problems.

Acute Interstitial Nephritis (AIN)

Inflammation of the renal parenchyma.

Etiology

- **Systemic diseases:** Sarcoidosis, Sjögren's syndrome, lymphoma.
- **Systemic infections:** Syphilis, toxoplasmosis, cytomegalovirus, Epstein-Barr virus, HIV.
- **Medications:** Beta-lactam antibiotics, diuretics, and NSAIDs, proton pump inhibitors, allopurinol.

TABLE 2.6-5. ATN vs. AIN

	ATN	AIN
Classic clinical setting (but not limited to)	Hypotension/post-hypotension (shock)	■ Drugs (beta-lactam antibiotics) ■ Infections (*Legionella, Streptococcus*)
Findings	Muddy brown granular and epithelial casts	■ Rash, fever ■ Eosinophilia ■ Eosinophils in urine ■ White and red cell casts
Treatment	Fluids and treat hypotension	■ Stop drug ■ Give steroids (if severe)

A patient was treated with penicillin for streptococcal pharyngitis. Now he has a diffuse rash and renal failure. Urinalysis shows white and red cell casts. Complete blood count shows elevated eosinophils.
Think: Acute interstitial nephritis. **Next step:** Stop antibiotic, give steroid.

CLINICAL AND LAB FINDINGS

- Clinical and lab findings similar to ATN (see Table 2.6-5).
- Drug-induced interstitial nephritis is associated with eosinophilia and eosinophiluria and may be accompanied by other signs of systemic hypersensitivity reaction (eg, rash).

TREATMENT

- Address underlying cause/discontinue offending agent.
- Manage renal failure as for ATN.
- Renal function recovers in most cases following discontinuation of offending agent.
- High-dose prednisone may improve recovery if infection is not a concern.

GLOMERULAR DISORDERS

Nephrotic Syndrome

- Glomerular lesion causing proteinuria > 3 g/day.
- Indicates a defect in the glomerular filtration barrier.
- Defined by the triad of proteinuria, hyperlipidemia, and peripheral edema.

PATHOPHYSIOLOGY

- Onset of glomerular permeability to plasma proteins, resulting in proteinuria and loss of albumin (hypoalbuminemia).
- Hypoalbuminemia → a ↓ in oncotic pressure, resulting in edema and serosal effusions.
- Hyperlipidemia, particularly hypercholesterolemia, is also common.
- Hypercoagulability due to loss of proteins C and S and antithrombin III.

> ***Rule of Thirds* for membranous nephropathy:**
> One-third progress to CRF; one-third have spontaneous remission; one-third remain nephrotic but do not progress.

COMMON CAUSES

- **Minimal change disease** (nil disease, lipoid nephrosis):
  - Usually idiopathic, usually found in children.
  - Electron microscopy shows podocyte (epithelial) foot process fusion, but light microscopy shows no change.
  - Usually responds to steroid therapy, though sometimes cytotoxic therapy is required, especially in recurrent cases.
  - Recurs frequently.
  - Rarely progresses to chronic renal failure (unlike the other causes of nephrotic syndrome).
- **Focal segmental glomerulosclerosis (FSGS):**
  - Glomerular scarring involving limited number of glomeruli (segmental involvement).
  - May be primary (idiopathic) or secondary to a known disease.
  - Causes of secondary FSGS include HIV, hepatitis B virus (HBV), heroin abuse, vesicoureteric reflux, morbid obesity causing glomerular hyperfiltration.
  - Immunoglobulin and complement deposition may be detected by immunofluorescence.
  - → hypertension and chronic renal failure.
  - Treatment may include corticosteroids or cytotoxic therapy, as well as ACE inhibitors or angiotensin receptor blockers (ARBs) if nonnephrotic. If secondary FSGS, treatment must also be directed against the primary disease.
- **Membranous nephropathy:**
  - Common cause of adult nephrotic syndrome.
  - Caused by subepithelial immune complex deposition.
  - Idiopathic, or associated with systemic lupus erythematosus (SLE), HBV, or solid tumors.
  - Treat with steroids and cytotoxic agents (chlorambucil or cyclophosphamide).
  - Rule of thirds.
- **Systemic causes:**
  - Sickle cell anemia (papillary damage due to sickling in hyperosmotic medullary interstitium).
  - Diabetic glomerulopathies (diffuse glomerulosclerosis, nodular glomerulosclerosis). Most common secondary cause of nephrotic syndrome.
  - Multiple myeloma (Bence Jones proteinuria from immunoglobulin light chains or their breakdown products).

Nephritic Syndrome (Glomerulonephritis)

- Indicates inflammation and glomerular damage.
- Involves abrupt-onset hematuria with RBC casts, mild proteinuria; often includes hypertension, edema, and azotemia.
- Acute glomerulonephritis (AGN): Nephritic syndrome (synonym).

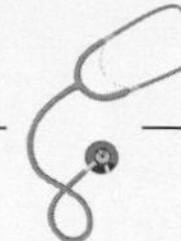

RBC casts are pathognomonic of any glomerulonephritis.

Poststreptococcal Glomerulonephritis (PSGN)

- Also called **postinfectious glomerulonephritis.**
- Associated with group A, beta-hemolytic *Streptococcus* (usually associated with preceding pharyngitis or impetigo).
- On immunofluorescence, immune complex deposition with complement (IgG, C3) in a "lumpy-bumpy" pattern between the glomerular epithelial cell and the GBM → glomerular damage.
- Presents ~ 2 weeks after infection with dark urine and edema (periorbital or generalized).
- Usually reversible but occasionally progresses (children often have complete recovery).

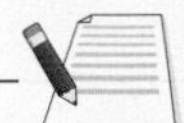

If a patient presents with hematuria immediately after an infection, think *IgA nephropathy.* If a patient presents 2 weeks after infection, think *postinfectious glomerulonephritis.*

Labs

Nephritic sediment (RBC casts), low complement, antistreptolysin O (ASO) antibody titers are helpful in diagnosis.

Treatment

- Treat underlying infection.
- Immunosuppressive drugs are ineffective.

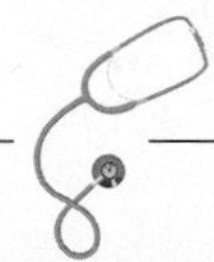

Antimicrobial therapy of the initial streptococcal infection does **not** prevent the onset of PSGN (as opposed to rheumatic fever).

IgA Nephropathy (Berger's Disease)

- Most common glomerulonephritis.
- Presents as hematuria during a viral infection or after exercise.
- On immunofluorescence, immune complex deposition of IgA and C3 in mesangial matrix ("mesangial hypercellularity"). Mesangial proliferation on light microscopy.
- Conservative management with ACE inhibitors or ARBs in patients with normal renal function and minimal proteinuria.
- Pulse corticosteroids in severe cases may be beneficial.

Membranoproliferative Glomerulonephritis (MPGN)

- Idiopathic, associated with hepatitis C and cryoglobulinemia, bacterial endocarditis, and autoimmune diseases such as lupus and Sjögren's syndrome.
- On immunofluorescence, subendothelial immune deposits are seen. Basement membrane proliferation causes basement membrane to look double layered ("tram-track"); also mesangial proliferation.
- **Labs:** Nephritic sediment and low complement levels (C3 and C4).
- Frequently progresses to renal failure.
- **Treatment:** Depends on underlying disease, for example, successful treatment of hepatitis C, or plasmapheresis for patients with cryoglobulinemia.

RAPIDLY PROGRESSIVE GLOMERULONEPHRITIS (RPGN)

- Any glomerulonephritis that progresses can subsequently become RPGN.
- Also called *crescentic* GN because biopsy shows epithelial cell proliferation (crescents) in glomeruli.
- Characterized by fulminant renal failure with proteinuria, hematuria, and RBC casts.
- Uncommon.

Anti–glomerular basement membrane Ab disease:
In 60–90% of patients, the anti-GBM Ab cross-react with pulmonary alveolar basement membranes—you get both lung and renal manifestations.

CLASSIFICATION

Three categories:

1. **Pauci-immune RPGN** (antineutrophil cytoplasmic antibody [ANCA]-associated vasculitis):
   - 50% of RPGN.
   - No immune complex or complement deposition.
   - ANCA is serologic marker for pauci-immune RPGN associated with systemic vasculitis.
   - **Examples:** Churg-Strauss, Wegener's (c-ANCA ⊕), polyarteritis nodosa (p-ANCA ⊕), microscopic polyangiitis (c- or p-ANCA ⊕).
2. **Immune complex RPGN** (granular immunoflourescence):
   - 40% of RPGN.
   - Can be associated with certain medications, syphilis, some malignancies.
   - **Examples:** Postinfectious glomerulonephritis, lupus nephritis, IgA nephropathy, membranoproliferative glomerulonephritis, idiopathic RPGN.
3. **Anti–glomerular basement membrane Ab disease** (linear immunofluorescence):
   - 10% of RPGN.
   - Anti-GBM Ab present in blood—can be seen on GBM with immunofluorescent microscopy.
   - Cytotoxic T-cells contribute to the pathogenesis.
   - **Example: Goodpasture's syndrome.**

PROGNOSIS AND TREATMENT

- Eighty percent of untreated patients progress to end-stage renal disease in 6 months.
- Treat with steroids and cyclophosphamide.

OTHER DISEASES ASSOCIATED WITH ACUTE NEPHRITIC SYNDROME

Secondary (multisystem-associated) glomerular diseases:

- **Collagen vascular disorders:**
  - Polyarteritis nodosa
  - SLE
  - Wegener's granulomatosis
  - Henoch-Schönlein purpura (HSP)
- **Hematologic disorders:**
  - Thrombotic thrombocytopenic purpura (TTP)
  - Hemolytic-uremic syndrome
  - Serum sickness

- **Glomerular basement membrane diseases:**
  - Alport's syndrome
  - Goodpasture's syndrome
  - Thin basement membrane disease

CHRONIC KIDNEY DISEASE (CKD)

↓ renal function (GFR < 60 mL/min per 1.73m^2) or evidence of kidney injury for > 3 months.

Etiology

- **Diabetes mellitus:** Diffuse glomerulosclerosis, nodular glomerulosclerosis (Kimmelstiel-Wilson lesions).
- **Hypertension:** Nephrosclerosis.
- Idiopathic failure.
- **Chronic glomerulonephritis:** RBC casts.
- **Chronic tubulointerstitial diseases:** Sodium wasting, no proteinuria, prolonged obstructive uropathies.
- **Polycystic kidney disease.**

Pathophysiology

- Nephrons are lost and remaining healthy nephrons compensate by increasing their GFR. This process damages the healthy nephrons causing disease progression.
- Loss of renal endocrine function: ↓ synthesis of activated vitamin D, ammonia, and erythropoietin.

Renal Function in CKD

- Usually asymptomatic until GFR < 30 mL/min per 1.73m^2.
- **Water and sodium balance:**
  - Initially: ↓ urine concentrating ability, easy dehydration, sodium wasting.
  - Later: Volume overload once the kidneys are no longer able to excrete dietary sodium.
- **Potassium:** Once GFR becomes markedly diminished, the ability to excrete dietary potassium is lost. The distal tubule compensates for the loss of excretory function until there is oliguria.
- **Acid-base balance:** With decreasing GFR, the tubular excretion of H^+ is impaired secondary to the impaired renal production of ammonia, resulting in anion gap metabolic acidosis.
- **Calcium and phosphate:**
  - Hypocalcemia, hyperphosphatemia.
  - ↓ activation of vitamin D due to loss of 1-hydroxylase activity.
  - Secondary hyperparathyroidism.
  - Renal osteodystrophy: Severe bone resorption.
  - Ectopic calcifications.
- Serum **creatinine** ↑ (creatinine clearance ↓ with ↓ GFR).
- **BUN** ↑, but to a lesser extent than the creatinine.

Renal biopsy should be performed **prior** (ie, don't wait) to development of end-stage renal disease (ESRD) to provide any hope of identifying the etiology and providing treatment. Once ESRD is established, biopsy will likely only show chronic scarring.

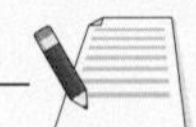

Anemia is common in CKD and is associated with ↑ cardiovascular disease risk as well as accelerated CKD progression. It is due, primarily, to erythropoietin deficiency and is treated to a target hemoglobin of 11 g/dL with erythropoiesis-stimulating agents.

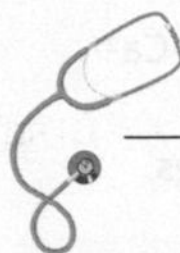

Why creatinine is a measure of kidney function:
Creatinine is neither secreted nor reabsorbed by the nephron, it is only filtered. Therefore, the creatinine clearance is directly proportional to the GFR.

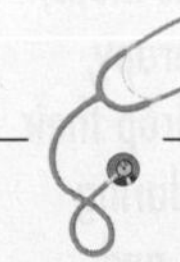

GFR and creatinine clearance:
For each doubling of the serum creatinine, the GFR has ↓ by 50%.

Large kidneys can be seen on sonogram in diabetes, amyloidosis, polycystic kidney disease, and HIV nephropathy, though in diabetes and HIV, they can ultimately become atrophic and small.

Indications for Emergent Hemodialysis

A E I O U

Acidosis
Electrolytes (K^+, Ca^{2+}, PO_4^-)
Ingestions (drugs, toxins)
Overload (volume)
Uremia

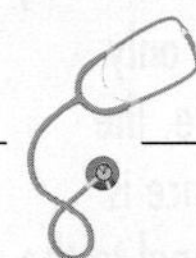

Patients on chronic medications (cardiac meds, warfarin, chemotherapy, etc.) dramatically drop their serum drug levels during dialysis. The timing and dosing of medication must be decided with the dialysis schedule in mind.

Signs and Symptoms

- Uremic syndrome, nephrotic syndrome.
- Ultrasound often reveals shrunken kidneys with cortical thinning.
- Rule out urinary tract infection (UTI) with urine culture.

Treatment

- ACE inhibitors may slow progression.
- Treat reversible causes.
- Diet: Modest protein restriction with near normal caloric intake ↓ nitrogen intake and avoids catabolism.
- Dialysis (see below).

Dialysis

- Chronic hemodialysis (HD) is the mainstay of therapy for chronic renal failure, but chronic ambulatory peritoneal dialysis (CAPD) is also an alternative.
- There is no absolute lab value that requires dialysis.
- **The decision is clinical** and based on a constellation of factors.

Absolute Indications for Dialysis

- Uremic pericarditis with or without cardiac tamponade.
- Progressive motor neuropathy.
- Intractable volume overload.
- Life-threatening and intractable hyperkalemia or acidosis.
- Toxins (eg, ethylene glycol).

Clinical Findings Responding to Dialysis (Relative Indications)

- Fluid and electrolyte imbalances.
- Volume-dependent hypertension.
- Central nervous system (CNS) abnormalities.
- Anemia and bleeding diatheses.
- Anorexia, nausea, and vomiting.
- Weight loss.
- Pruritus and ecchymoses.

Hemodialysis

- The two most commonly used vascular access sites are arteriovenous fistulae (AVF), (usually in the forearm) and artificial grafts inserted between an artery and a vein. Dialysis needles are placed directly into the graft.
- A tunneled dialysis catheter (TDC) is usually placed in the right internal jugular vein and serves as a bridge that allows hemodialysis to take place until AVF or graft is placed.
- Dialysis patients are frequently instrumented, and combined with the dialysis patient's impaired immunity, infection is common. Infective endocarditis may occur if the infections are not recognized early and treated correctly.
- Viral hepatitis is also a risk of hemodialysis, possibly from other patients using the same dialysis machine. For that reason, patients with hepatitis are dialyzed with separate machines.

Chronic Ambulatory Peritoneal Dialysis

- A permanent catheter is inserted into the peritoneum, allowing dialysis to be provided to the patient outside the hospital.
- Approximately 2 L of dialysis fluid is infused rapidly and allowed to remain in the peritoneal cavity for 4–6 hours. The fluid is then drained, and new fluid is immediately infused.
- Peritoneum acts as a dialysis membrane.
- Infusion of hypertonic glucose solution allows for concurrent volume reduction.
- Spontaneous bacterial peritonitis (SBP) is a common problem.
- Hypoalbuminemia, hypertriglyceridemia, hypokalemia, and anemia are common.

Uremic Syndrome

Uremia is a syndrome associated with chronic renal failure that affects multiple organ systems.

Signs and Symptoms

- Appearance: Pale complexion, wasting, purpura, excoriation.
- Complaints: Pruritus, polydipsia, nausea, anorexia, vomiting.
- Urinalysis: Isosthenuria, proteinuria, abnormal sediment with tubular casts.

Isosthenuria: Inability of kidney to concentrate urine; fixes specific gravity at 1.010.

Systemic Effects

- **CNS:** Foot drop, carpal tunnel syndrome, clonus, asterixis, seizures.
- **Cardiac and pulmonary:**
  - Hypertension → left ventricular hypertrophy (LVH) and diastolic dysfunction.
  - Accelerated atherosclerosis, development of ischemic heart disease.
  - Pleuropericardial inflammation (pericarditis with effusion and tamponade).
  - Calcification of mitral and aortic valves.
  - Pulmonary edema and pleural effusions.
- **Hematologic:**
  - Normochromic, normocytic anemia due to ↓ erythropoietin synthesis, among other reasons.
  - Defective platelet function—prolonged bleeding time.
  - White cell function and absolute counts are reduced, resulting in ↑ likelihood of infection.
- **GI:** Mild GI bleeding, nausea/vomiting, anorexia.
- **Metabolic:** Elevated triglycerides, ↓ insulin clearance may → hypoglycemia and perceived improvement in diabetes mellitus.

Polycystic Kidney Disease

- Autosomal dominant.
- Kidneys are enlarged and have multiple cysts.
- Patients typically present in their 30s or 40s with flank pain or hematuria.
- Approximately 50% of patients will develop end-stage renal disease by the age of 60.
- Associated extrarenal manifestations are berry aneurysms (subarachnoid hemorrhage), hepatic cysts, pancreatic cysts. and diverticula.

- Complications of polycystic kidneys are hypertension, recurrent UTIs, and kidney stones (calcium oxalate and uric acid stones).
- Diagnose via ultrasound or computed tomography (CT) scan.

Renal Tubular Acidosis

Defect in renal tubular ability to excrete daily acid load created by the metabolism of protein or to reabsorb filtered bicarbonate, which results in a metabolic acidosis with a normal anion gap.

Etiology

- There are three types (see Table 2.6-6): 1, 2, and 4 (there is no type 3).
- May be inherited or acquired via medications or disease states.
- Types 1 and 4 occur in the distal tubules.
- Type 2 occurs in the proximal tubule.

Pathophysiology

- **Type 1** is caused by a distal tubule defect in hydrogen secretion causing acidosis and hypokalemia.
  - Can be caused by autoimmune diseases (SLE, rheumatoid arthritis, Sjögren's syndrome), medication (lithium, amphotericin B).
  - Patients may also get renal stones due to hypercalcemia.
- **Type 2** is caused by a defect in proximal bicarbonate reabsorption (bicarbonate wasting), usually in the setting of Fanconi's syndrome (generalized proximal tubule dysfunction).
  - The bicarbonate loss is self-limiting as the distal tubules can absorb some bicarbonate and bicarbonate levels reach a new, lower set point.
  - Can be caused by multiple myeloma, heavy metals, carbonic anyhydrase inhibitors (acetazolamide).
  - Potassium can be low to normal.
- **Type 4 = hypoaldosteronism** and is caused by a defect in aldosterone secretion or aldosterone sensitivity by the renal tubules and ammonium excretion. The effect is similar to that of a potassium-sparing diuretic.
  - Patients usually have low renin and aldosterone levels.
  - The hallmark of type 4 RTA is **hyperkalemia,** and patients are usually managed with potassium-wasting diuretics or fludrocortisone.
  - May be a primary defect or caused by diabetic nephropathy, obstructive uropathy, or other kidney diseases.

Urolithiasis

Calculi in the urogenital system.

TABLE 2.6-6. RTA Types

	Defect	Plasma Bicarbonate Level	Urine pH	Plasma K^+
Type 1 RTA	Impaired acidification of urine	Low	> 5.3	Low
Type 2 RTA	↓ bicarbonate resorption	12–20	< 5.3	Low to normal
Type 4 RTA	↓ aldosterone	Typically > 17	< 5.3	**High**

EPIDEMIOLOGY

- One of the most common diseases of the urinary tract.
- Two to five percent of the population will form a urinary stone at some point in their lives.
- Majority of stones form between the ages of 20 and 50.
- Male-to-female ratio of 3:1.
- Familial tendency in stone formation.
- Tendency for recurrence—36% of patients with a first stone will have another stone within 1 year.

TYPES OF STONES

- **Calcium oxalate stones** (75%):
  - Strongly radiopaque.
  - Treat with thiazides to ↓ calciuria.
  - ↑ incidence in inflammatory bowel disease (↑ oxalate), hypercalcemia (hyperparathyroidism), ↓ citrate (forms stable soluble complex with calcium), uricosuria (small urate crystals serve as nidus for larger calcium stones).
- **Struvite (Mg NH4 PO4) stones** (15%):
  - Moderately radiopaque.
  - Common in *Proteus* UTIs due to high urinary pH (*Proteus* makes urease, which cleaves urinary urea, yielding two molecules of ammonia—the conjugate base of ammonium ion).
  - Treat by lowering urine pH.
- **Uric acid stones** (< 1%):
  - Radiolucent.
  - ↑ incidence in myeloproliferative diseases and gout (due to ↑ purine turnover).
  - Treat by raising urine pH.
- **Cystine stones** (< 1%):
  - Moderately radiopaque.
  - Seen in congenital cystinuria (*not* homocystinuria).
  - Hexagonal crystals, positively birefringent.
  - Treat by raising urine pH.

PREDISPOSING FACTORS

- Dietary history—large calcium and alkali intake.
- Prolonged immobilization.
- Residence in hot climate.
- History of UTIs.
- History of calculus in the past and in family members.
- Drug ingestion (analgesics, alkalis, uricosuric agents, protease inhibitors).
- Prior history of gout.
- Underlying gastrointestinal disease (Crohn's, ulcerative colitis, peptic ulcer disease).

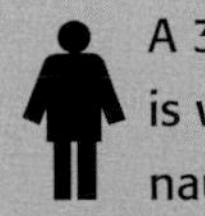

A 39-year-old man presents with severe back pain and hematuria. He is writhing in the bed, unable to find a comfortable position, and is nauseous. *Think: Renal colic due to urolithiasis.* **Next step:** Order noncontrast CT abdomen and pelvis to determine size and location of stone.

TABLE 2.6-7. Interpretation of the Urinalysis

Finding	Significance
Color	▪ Red or brown indicates presence of hemoglobin, myoglobin (as with rhabdomyolysis), or red food (beets).
Clarity	▪ Normal urine should be clear. ▪ Turbidity or cloudiness can be caused by excessive cellular material (often as WBCs in pyuria or casts), protein, or precipitation of salts.
pH	Normal pH ranges from 4.5 to 7.5. ▪ Alkaline urine indicates type 1 RTA or UTI with *Proteus* or *Ureaplasma.* ▪ Acidic urine can be seen with aspirin overdose or type 2 RTA.
Specific gravity	▪ Normal specific gravity is 1.002–1.035. ▪ High (> 1.010) indicates dehydration. ▪ Inability to concentrate urine in the setting of dehydration indicates renal disease.
Protein	▪ Proteinuria indicates glomerular dysfunction. ▪ Microalbuminuria is a marker for early diabetic nephropathy. ▪ Protein loss in urine of > 3 g/day is nephritic syndrome.
Glucose	▪ Glucose in urine can indicate hyperglycemia.
Ketones	Seen in diabetic ketoacidosis, isopropyl alcohol intoxication, and starvation ketosis.
Nitrite	▪ Normal is ⊖. ▪ ⊕ nitrite indicates bacteria present in the urine, usually gram-⊖ rods.
Leukocyte esterase	▪ ⊕ findings indicate the presence of white cells and infection.
RBCs	Present in glomerulonephritis, tumor, trauma, renal stones, renal infarct, malignant hypertension (also often erroneously ⊕ in menstruating females).
WBCs	▪ Also called pyuria; seen in UTIs, prostatitis, vaginitis.
Eosinophils	▪ Seen in acute interstitial nephritis (AIN).
Squamous epithelial cells	▪ From the skin surface or outer urethra; a measure of contamination.
Casts	▪ Urinary casts are formed in the distal convoluted tubule and the collecting duct. ▪ RBC casts: Glomerulonephritis. ▪ WBC casts: Pyelonephritis or glomerulonephritis. ▪ Muddy brown granular casts: ATN. ▪ Hyaline casts: Prerenal azotemia.
Crystals	▪ Renal stones, ethylene glycol intoxication.
Bilirubin	▪ Extravascular hemolysis.
Hemoglobin	▪ Intravascular hemolysis.

SIGNS AND SYMPTOMS

- Severe, abrupt onset of colicky pain that begins in the flank and may radiate toward the groin. In males, the pain may radiate toward the testicle. In females, it may radiate toward the labia majoris.
- Nausea and vomiting are almost universal with acute renal colic.
- Abdominal distention from secondary ileus.
- Gross hematuria.

DIAGNOSIS

- **Urinalysis** (Table 2.6-7).
  - Vast majority of patients (about 85%) will have RBCs in the urine. However, a lack of RBCs on urinalysis does not rule out renal stones.
  - Urinary pH can aid in differentiating the type of stone present. Normal urinary pH is about 5.85. If the pH is > 6, one should suspect the presence of urea-splitting organisms (*Proteus*). A low urine pH (≤ 5) suggests uric acid stones.
  - WBCs or bacteria may suggest underlying urinary tract infection and should be aggressively treated.
- **Radiographic studies:**
  - See Infectious Disease chapter for table on common genitourinary procedures.
  - Plain abdominal film (KUB) will reveal only radiopaque stones (60–70%).
  - Renal ultrasound is useful to detect hydronephrosis and is easy, cheap, and doesn't require subjecting the patient to IV contrast. It misses small stones.
  - Noncontrast renal CT is most useful to diagnose small stones. It can accurately locate stones in the renal collecting system and detect the presence of hydronephrosis. Overall sensitivity is about 95%.
  - Intravenous pyelogram (IVP) has been the gold standard for the diagnosis of renal and ureteral calculi. It can clearly outline the entire urinary system making it easy to see hydronephrosis and the presence of any type of stones. In addition, an IVP can demonstrate renal function and allow for verification that the opposite kidney is functioning properly.

TREATMENT

- Analgesia.
- Hydration.
- **Passage of stones:**
  - Ninety percent of stones < 5 mm will pass spontaneously.
  - Fifteen percent of stones 5–8 mm will pass.
  - Five percent of stones > 8 mm will pass.
- **For stones unlikely to pass spontaneously:**
  - Extracorporeal shock wave lithotripsy (ESWL) has been effective for stones located in the kidney with 85% success rate.
  - Percutaneous nephrolithotomy, which establishes a tract from the skin to the collecting system, is used when stones are too large or too hard for lithotripsy.
  - New laser techniques are becoming mainstays of therapy for extracting large stones.

HIGH-YIELD FACTS IN

Pulmonology

HYPOXIA

↓ delivery/utilization of oxygen at tissue level. A variety of cardiorespiratory diseases can cause hypoxia by some basic mechanisms:

A married couple comes to the hospital complaining of "flulike" symptoms, including headache, nausea, vomiting, and disorientation. The wife thinks they caught the virus from a neighbor when they borrowed his home generator. *Think: Carbon monoxide poisoning.* **Next step:** Check carboxyhemoglobin levels.

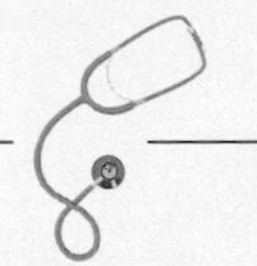

The most important determinant of the amount of oxygen delivery to tissues is *hemoglobin.*

- **V/Q mismatch:** When perfusion and ventilation to different areas of lungs are not proportionately matched, causing some of the ventilation or perfusion to go to waste. *Responds to supplemental oxygen.*
  - **Examples:** Chronic obstructive pulmonary disease (COPD), congestive heart failure (CHF), pulmonary fibrosis, and asthma.
  - **Dead space ventilation:** When a part of the lungs receives ventilation, but the blood supply is interrupted as in pulmonary embolism (PE).
- **Right-to-left shunt:** Intrapulmonary shunting of blood, due to perfusion of the nonventilated lung (as in lung consolidation), or extrapulmonary, such as congenital heart disease.
- **Diffusion defect:** Gas exchange compromised due to a defect in the alveolar interface, as seen in interstitial lung disease.
- In the *absence* of cardiorespiratory disease, hypoxia may be the result of:
  - **Anemia:** ↓ hemoglobin ↓ oxygen carrying capacity, has a normal PaO_2, ↓ PvO_2 (due to ↑ extraction from the tissues).

    Arterial oxygen content = $PaO_2 \times 0.0031 + 1.36 \times Hb \times SaO_2$

  - **Improper utilization of delivered oxygen in the tissues:** Cytochrome impairment due to cyanide poisoning, diphtheria toxin, etc.
  - **Low inspired oxygen:** At high altitude or other low-oxygen environment.
  - **Carbon monoxide (CO) poisoning:** CO has much higher affinity for hemoglogin than oxygen; carboxyhemoglobin is unavailable for oxygen transport; O_2 unloaded at much lower oxygen tensions, resulting in impaired delivery to tissues. CO poisoning does not cause cyanosis. At highly toxic levels, it can cause a "cherry red" discoloration of lips and nails.
  - **Hypoventilation:** Occurs with obesity-hypoventilation syndrome, neuromuscular disorders (Guillain-Barré, myasthenia gravis, amyotrophic lateral sclerosis [ALS]).

LUNG PHYSICAL EXAM

- **Inspection:** Best done with the patient standing.
  - Look for evidence of respiratory distress such as nasal flaring, accessory muscle use, pursed-lip breathing (common in COPD), and intercostal retractions.

- Also look for chest wall deformities such as kyphoscoliosis or pectus excavatum.
- Look for evidence of recent trauma such as bruising, bleeding, or "flail chest."
- **Auscultation:** See Table 2.7-1.
- **Breath sounds:**
  - **Normal** (vesicular): Breath sounds are low pitched and are heard throughout inspiration and most of early expiration.
  - **Bronchial:** Breath sounds are high pitched and heard equally well during both inspiration and expiration.
  - **Crackles (rales):** Short, discontinuous nonmusical sounds heard mostly during inspiration ("crunchy").
  - **Wheezes/rhonchi:** Continuous, musical, high-pitched sounds heard mostly during expiration. Both terms are usually used interchangeably.
  - **Pleural rub:** Grating sound produced by motion of pleura, heard best at end of inspiration/beginning of expiration.
  - **Stridor:** Discontinuous sound usually best heard during inspiration. Signifies upper airway narrowing or obstruction by foreign body, tumor, or laryngospasm.
  - **Egophony:** Spoken words by the patient are ↑ in intensity and take on different quality during auscultation. Patient says "eeee" and will be heard as "aaaa." Signifies "solid" lung tissue in communication with a patent bronchus, as in areas of consolidation and in areas of compressed lung above the upper level of a pleural effusion.
- **Palpation:**
  - **Tactile fremitus:** Performed by placing ulnar side of hand or palm against the patient's chest wall and having the patient say "ninety-nine." Vibrations are felt through the chest wall and can be compared from one side to the other. A local or unilateral difference in tactile fremitus is of clinical importance.
    - ↑ tactile fremitus = ↑ density of the lung parenchyma (consolidation).
    - ↓ tactile fremitus = excess subcutaneous tissue on the chest, air or fluid in pleural cavity (pneumothorax, pleural effusion) or overexpansion of lung.

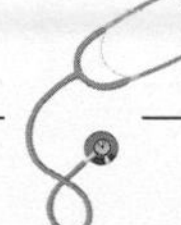

Clinical Pearl: Sound travels better through *solid* (lung consolidation) than *liquid* (pleural effusion). For example, if you put your ear to the ground, you can hear the train coming, but if you are under water, you won't be able to hear your friend shout your name.

TABLE 2.7-1. Lung Auscultation

Term	Mechanism	Causes
Crackle (rale)	Excessive airway secretions.	Bronchitis, pneumonia, pulmonary edema, atelectasis, fibrosis.
Wheeze	Rapid airflow through obstructed airway.	Asthma, pulmonary edema, bronchitis.
Rhonchus	Transient airway plugging.	Bronchitis.
Pleural rub	Inflammation of the pleura.	Pneumonia, pulmonary infarction.

- **Percussion:** Tapping the chest wall to evaluate underlying structures. The sound produced depends on the air-tissue ratio of the structure involved.
    - **Dull:** Dullness over the chest implies ↑ density, as when the air in the lungs is replaced by fluid or solid tissue. Examples include consolidation, a lung mass, or fluid surrounding the lung as in pleural effusion. (Percussion over the liver will reveal *dull* sounds.)
    - **Flat:** Large muscle mass (thigh).
    - **Tympanic:** Hollow, air-containing structure (percussion over the stomach will yield *tympanic* sounds).
    - **Resonant:** Structure composed of air within tissue (normal lung).
    - **Hyperresonant:** Structure with ↓ density and ↑ amount of air, such as in emphysema, or a large pneumothorax.

PLEURAL EFFUSION

Abnormal accumulation of fluid within the space between the parietal and visceral pleural membranes of the lungs. Pleural effusion is classified as a transudative or exudative.

- **Transudative** pleural effusions are due to:
    - ↑ hydrostatic pressure as in heart failure.
    - ↓ oncotic pressure, as in nephrotic syndrome.
- **Exudative** pleural effusions are due to ↑ capillary permeability, usually secondary to an inflammatory process.

DIAGNOSIS

- Any pleural effusion of unclear etiology should be tapped for diagnostic pleural fluid analysis.
- Any pleural fluid should be analyzed for total and differential cell count, protein, glucose, lactate dehydrogenase (LDH), and pH (if there is suspicion of empyema).
- **Light's criteria** *(learn this for exam):* The effusion is an **exudate** if **one** or more of the following is present:
    - Ratio of pleural to serum protein > 0.5.
    - Ratio of pleural to serum lactic dehydrogenase (LDH) > 0.6.
    - Pleural fluid LDH > ⅔ upper normal limit of serum LDH.
- An effusion is a **transudate** if **none** of the above criteria is fulfilled.

Transudates
- **CHF**
- Cirrhosis
- Nephrosis

Exudates
- **Infection**
- Tumor
- Trauma

COMMON ASSOCIATIONS

- **Parapneumonic effusion:** As the name suggests, it should be suspected if an effusion develops in the setting of a pneumonia. Any parapneumonic effusion is an exudate, with a high neutrophil count.
    - A "simple" parapneumonic effusion can become "complex" and "complicated" if any of the following is present:
        - pH < 7.2
        - Glucose < 40 mg/dL
        - LDH > 1000
        - ⊕ Gram stain or culture

- When frank pus can be aspirated, the term *empyema* is used. Complicated parapneumonic effusions and empyemas can also become loculated.
- **Gross blood:**
  - Tumor (breast cancer, lung cancer, lymphoma).
  - Pulmonary infarction.
  - Hemothorax: Defined as pleural fluid hematocrit > 50% of serum hematocrit; this is a **surgical emergency!** Causes include trauma and aortic dissection.
- **Low glucose:**
  - Complicated parapneumonic effusion and empyema.
  - Rheumatoid arthritis (glucose extremely low, usually < 15 mg/dL).
  - Tumor: Indicator of poor prognosis.
  - Tuberculosis.
- **High amylase:**
  - Pancreatitis.
  - Renal failure.
  - Tumor.
  - Esophageal rupture: High *salivary* amylase is useful in diagnosis. **Surgical emergency** with high mortality if not treated immediately!

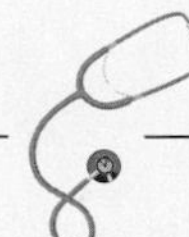

Empyema (pus in pleural space), ⊕ cultures, or loculated effusions always require chest tube.

PULMONARY FUNCTION TESTS (PFTs)

- **Spirometry:** Measures the rate at which the lung volume *changes* during forced breathing.
- **Forced vital capacity (FVC):** Patient inhales maximally, then exhales as rapidly and completely as possible for > 6 sec. The exhalation and subsequent inhalation are recorded as a flow volume curve.
- **FEV_1:** The volume of air exhaled in the first second of the FVC maneuver.
- FEV_1, FVC, and the ratio between them (FEV_1/FVC) are important parameters to determine the nature of lung disease and severity (see Table 2.7-2). The values obtained in a patient are compared with the expected normal values for that age, sex, height, and ethnic background.
  - Normal FEV_1 = > 80% of predicted.
  - Normal FVC = > 80% of predicted.
  - Normal FEV_1/FVC ratio = > 0.7.
- **Obstructive lung disease:** FEV_1 is disproportionately reduced compared to FVC; therefore FEV_1/FVC ratio is low. FEV_1/FVC ratio of < 70% is a key parameter to diagnose obstruction. Seen with airway diseases like chronic bronchitis, emphysema, and asthma.

TABLE 2.7-2. Pulmonary Function Tests

Normal Spirometry	Obstructive Lung Disease	Restrictive Lung Disease
▪ FVC normal ▪ FEV_1 normal ▪ FEV_1/FVC > 0.7	▪ FVC normal or ↓ ▪ FEV_1 ↓ ▪ FEV_1/FVC < 0.7 ▪ Lung volume normal or ↑	▪ FVC ↓ ▪ FEV_1 normal or ↓ ▪ FEV_1/FVC > 0.7 ▪ Lung volume *always* ↓

- **Restrictive lung disease:** Seen with interstitial lung diseases, neuromuscular diseases (ALS, myasthenia gravis, Guillain–Barré), chest wall disorders (obesity, kyphoscoliosis). Both FEV_1 and FVC are low, but their ratio is usually normal or elevated.
- **Lung volume measurements:** Lung volumes such as total lung capacity (TLC), functional residual capacity (FRC), and residual volume (RV) can be measured by using body plethysmography or helium dilution techniques.
- **Diffusion capacity of carbon monoxide (DL_{CO}):** Using trace amounts of CO in the inhaled gas mixture, diffusion of alveolar air across pulmonary capillaries can be assessed. DL_{CO} is a very useful test for diagnosis and follow up for patients with interstitial lung diseases, in which this value is usually ↓.

LUNG INFECTIONS

Pneumonia

Infection of the lung parenchyma by any microorganism.

- **Community-acquired pneumonia (CAP):** Pneumonia diagnosed in patients within 48 hours of hospital admission who do not meet criteria for health care–associated pneumonia.
- **Health care–associated pneumonia (HCAP):** Pneumonia diagnosed within 48 hours of hospital admission in patients who have ≥ 1 of the following risk factors for being infected with organisms resistant to multiple antibiotics:
  - Hospitalization for ≥ 2 days in an acute-care facility within previous 90 days (most common and also most likely to cause infection with resistant organisms).
  - Residence in a nursing home or long-term care facility.
  - Antibiotic therapy, chemotherapy, or wound care within 30 days of current infection (lower risk).
  - Hemodialysis treatment at a hospital or clinic (lower risk).
  - Home infusion therapy or home wound care (low risk).
- **Hospital acquired pneumonia (HAP):** Pneumonia developing at least 48 hours after hospital admission. HAP may be due to multidrug-resistant (MDR) organisms if any of the following are present:
  - Antibiotic therapy within 90 days of infection.
  - Current hospitalization of > 5 days.
  - High frequency of antibiotic resistance in the specific hospital unit.
  - Immunosuppressive disease or therapy.
  - Presence of HCAP risk factors for MDR.

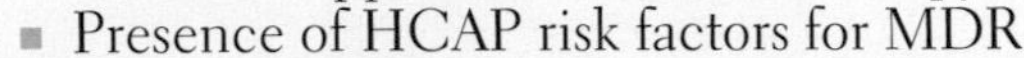

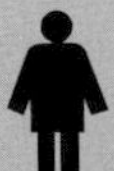

A 27-year-old patient has pneumonia, bullous myringitis, and a chest film that looks worse than expected. *Think:* Mycoplasma pneumoniae.

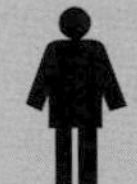

A patient with HIV who has a CD4 count of 52 does not take antiretroviral medications or trimethoprim-sulfamethoxazole, is hypoxic on room air, and has a diffuse bilateral infiltrates on chest film. *Think:* Pneumocystis jiroveci *pneumonia (PCP).*

An elderly man presents with pneumonia, GI symptoms, bradycardia, and hyponatremia. *Think: Legionella.*

ETIOLOGY

See Table 2.7-3 for organisms affecting immunocompetent host and Table 2.7-4 for those affecting immunocompromised hosts.

PATHOPHYSIOLOGY

Pathogenic bacteria reach alveoli in one of the following ways:

- **Inhalation:** Aspiration of (colonized) nasopharyngeal, oral, or gastric contents.
- **Hematogenous spread:** Direct inoculation (stab wounds, endotracheal tube).

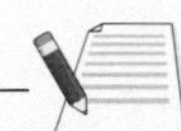

Pneumonias causing relative bradycardia (slower-than-expected heart rate for temperature or disease, but above 60 bpm):
- *Legionella*
- *Salmonella*
- *Chlamydia psittaci*

SIGNS AND SYMPTOMS

Patients with pneumonia may have few signs or symptoms, or may be extremely ill.

- **Typical symptoms:**
  - Fever
  - Cough with sputum production
  - Pleuritic chest pain

TABLE 2.7-3. Likely Organisms Causing Pneumonia in Immunocompetent Host

Community acquired, typical
1. *Streptococcus pneumoniae*
2. *Haemophilus influenzae*
Community acquired, atypical
1. *Chlamydia pneumoniae*
2. *Legionella pneumophila*
3. *Mycoplasma pneumoniae*
Hospital acquired
1. *Pseudomonas aeruginosa*
2. *Staphylococcus aureus*
3. Enteric organisms

TABLE 2.7-4. Causes of Pneumonia in Immunocompromised Host

HIV Infection	CD4 Count/dL
Mycobacterium tuberculosis	< 500
Pneumocystis jiroveci (PCP)	< 200
Histoplasma capsulatum	< 200
Cryptococcus neoformans	< 200
Mycobacterium avium-intracellulare	< 50
Cytomegalovirus	< 50
Neutropenia: 1. *Pseudomonas aeruginosa* 2. Enterobacteriaceae 3. *Staphylococcus aureus* 4. *Aspergillus*	
Splenectomy, sickle cell anemia: Encapsulated organisms **Chronic steroid use:** 1. *M tuberculosis* 2. *Nocardia*	
Alcoholics: 1. *Streptococcus pneumoniae* 2. *Haemophilus influenzae* 3. *Klebsiella pneumoniae* 4. *M tuberculosis*	

- Atypical symptoms:
  - Dry cough
  - Headache
  - Malaise
  - Gastrointestinal (GI) symptoms

Physical Exam

- Dullness to percussion.
- Rales.
- Tactile fremitus in consolidated lobe or segment.
- Egophony (E to A changes) with stethoscope.
- Respiratory distress depending on severity.

Diagnosis

- **Chest x-ray (CXR):** Most patients with pneumonia will have an infiltrate on x-ray corresponding to a lobe or segment. Sometimes they can have bilateral infiltrates. In some cases, the localization and/or nature of infiltrates can give clues to the etiologic agents:
  - Upper lobe (*Mycobacterium tuberculosis, Klebsiella*).
  - Small cavities without air-fluid levels (*M tuberculosis*).
  - Large cavities with air-fluid levels (*Staphylococcus* spp, anaerobes, gram-$\ominus$, coccidiomycosis, nocardiosis).
  - Diffuse bilateral infiltrate (PCP, *Mycoplasma*).
- **Gram stain:** An adequate sputum sample should contain:
  - < 10 epithelial cells per low-power field (the fewer the better).
  - > 25 leukocytes per low-power field.
- **Culture:** Once an organism is identified on sputum culture, antibiotics should be tailored to cover this organism if possible.

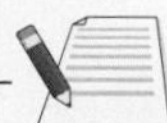

If a patient develops a postinfluenza pneumonia, think *Pneumococcus.*

If there are no bacteria on Gram stain, consider *Legionella* and *Mycoplasma.*

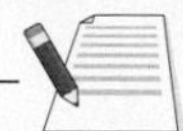

If you see **currant jelly sputum,** think *Klebsiella.*

Severity Assessment

- Mainly used for CAP to determine need for admission and strategy for management.
- There are many scoring systems available. One of the simpler ways to assess severity of pneumonia is the **CURB-65 score** (see Table 2.7-5):
  - **0–1 point:** Low risk. Consider outpatient treatment.
  - **2 points:** Higher severity. Consider short hospitalization or closely observed outpatient therapy.
  - **3–5 points:** Severe pneumonia. Hospitalization strongly recommended, consider ICU care if higher score.
- Remember, there are many scoring systems out there, but they serve only as *guides.* The most important tool you have is your clinical judgment. If you feel a patient is very ill and requires more aggressive care, you should always provide it.

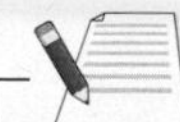

If you see **rusty sputum,** think *Pneumococcus.*

Loeffler's pneumonia is idiopathic eosinophilic pneumonia.

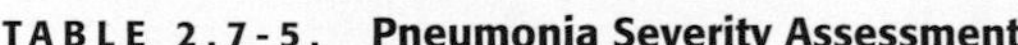

TABLE 2.7-5. Pneumonia Severity Assessment

CURB-65	**Points**
Confusion	1
Blood **U**rea nitrogen > 19 mg per dL	1
Respiratory rate $\geq$ 30 breaths per minute	1
Systolic **B**lood pressure < 90 mmHg or Diastolic blood pressure $\leq$ 60 mmHg	1
Age $\geq$ **65** years	1
Total points:	

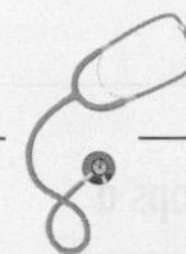

Steroid administration in PCP prevents respiratory failure and improves survival. Give for:

- A-a gradient > 35
- $PaO_2 < 75$

TREATMENT

The best choices for empiric coverage until cultures are completed depend on the type of pneumonia as defined above.

- **Community-acquired** (cover for both typicals and atypicals):
  - No risk factors: Macrolide (azithromycin).
  - Risk factors present (CHF, diabetes, etc.): Macrolide and second-/third-generation cephalosporin.
  - Alternatively, respiratory flouroquinolone such as moxifloxacin or levofloxacin.
- **Hospital-acquired:** Need *Pseudomonas* coverage with imipenem or piperacillin-tazobactam), if severe add coverage for methicillin-resistant *Staphylococcus aureus* (MRSA) with vancomycin.
- **Immunocompromised:** Add PCP coverage (trimethoprim-sulfamethoxazole ([TMP-SMZ]).

Tuberculosis

Tuberculosis (TB) is a leading cause of death worldwide. In the United States, the incidence of TB ↓ every year until 1984, with a resurgence during the HIV epidemic.

PATHOPHYSIOLOGY

Transmission occurs by inhalation of droplet nuclei produced by the cough or sneeze of a patient with pulmonary TB disease. Particles may remain suspended in air for several hours:

- Five percent of those infected will develop TB disease in 2 years.
- Five percent more will develop TB disease in their lifetime.
- Ninety percent will remain infected but disease free.

Sites of TB disease:

- Lungs (85% of all cases)
- Central nervous system (TB meningitis)
- Lymphatics
- Genitourinary system
- Bones (Pott's disease)
- Disseminated TB (miliary)

EPIDEMIOLOGY

- **High-prevalence groups:**
  - HIV-infected persons.
  - Close contacts of persons with TB disease.
  - IV drug users.
  - Immunocompromised persons (non-HIV).
  - Foreign-born persons.
  - Residents of medically underserved communities.
  - Prisoners.
  - Homeless.
- **High risk for active tuberculosis once infected:**
  - HIV-infected persons.
  - IV drug users.
  - Immunocompromised persons (non-HIV).
  - Abnormal CXR.

SYMPTOMS

- Productive cough
- **Night sweats**
- **Hemoptysis**
- Anorexia
- Weight loss
- Fever, chills, fatigue
- Chest pain

DIAGNOSIS

- **Findings:**
  - ⊕ purified protein derivative (PPD): Indicative of infection, *not* active disease.
  - Infiltrate or granuloma in upper lobes of lungs.
  - Acid-fast bacilli (AFB) on sputum microscopy.
- **How to use the TB skin test:**
  1. Screen patients in high-prevalence groups.
  2. Gives a ⊕ reaction 2–10 weeks after infection.
  3. Plant 0.1 mL of PPD intradermally on volar aspect of the forearm.
  4. Read 48–72 hours after placement.
  5. Measure induration, not erythema (see Table 2.7-6).
- **False ⊕:**
  - *Bacillus Calmette–Guérin (BCG)* vaccination will result in false ⊕ for a period of 10–15 years. Immigrants receiving BCG vaccine as children should not be ⊕ as adults over 25–30 years old.
  - Nontuberculous mycobacterial infection.
- **False ⊖:**
  - Ten to twenty-five percent of patients with TB infection have ⊖ skin tests.
  - The two-step TB skin test is used in high-prevalence patients who have a ⊖ first test: The first test boosts the immune response to a second skin test, which will turn ⊕ in infected patients.

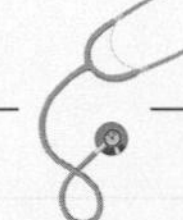

Anergy (does not mount response) can be screened for, by planting the common antigens *mumps* and *Candida* intradermally. If no response, PPD testing is useless.

TREATMENT

- **Latent TB:**
  - Isoniazid (INH) daily for 9 months (may be given twice weekly if directly observed therapy [DOT] is used).
  - Rifampin daily for 4 months if in contact with people with INH-resistant TB.
  - Close contacts of active tuberculosis patients with ⊖ PPD should be retested in 10 weeks.
  - Pregnant women should wait until after delivery for treatment unless high risk (eg, HIV).

TABLE 2.7-6. Interpretation of PPD Skin Test

Measured Induration		
≥ 15 mm	**≥ 10 mm**	**≥ 5 mm**
All patients are considered infected	Considered infected if: ▪ IV drug user ▪ Foreign born ▪ Medically underserved ▪ Nursing home resident ▪ Prisoner ▪ Child under age 4 ▪ Health care worker (you) ▪ Other medical problems	Considered infected if: ▪ HIV ▪ Close contact ▪ Abnormal CXR ▪ Immunocompromised

- **Active TB:**
  - Standard regimen for pulmonary TB: 2 months of INH, rifampin, pyrazinamide, and ethambutol followed by 4 months of INH/rifampin.
  - Pregnant with TB: 2 months of INH, rifampin, and ethambutol followed by INH and rifampin (no ethambutol) for 7 more months.
  - Meningeal, skeletal, and sometimes lymph node TB are treated with longer duration of antituberculous antibiotics.
- **Infectivity:** People are considered no longer infectious when they are undergoing appropriate therapy, improving clinically, and have had three consecutive sputum smears on different days ⊖ for TB.

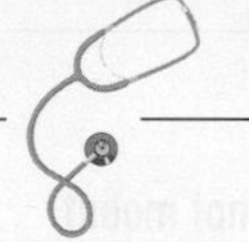
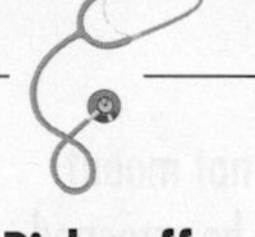

Pink puffers (emphysema):

- Barrel-shaped chest
- Thin and emaciated
- High PCO_2, normal to low PO_2

TOXICITY OF TB MEDICATION

- **INH:**
  - Peripheral neuropathy (can be prevented with administration of pyridoxine).
  - Seizures in overdose: These can be very difficult to break with standard measures—remember to give pyridoxine!
  - Hepatitis (check liver function tests each month).
- **Rifampin:**
  - Induces hepatic microsomal enzymes; also hepatotoxic.
  - Is excreted as a **red-orange compound in urine,** stool, sweat, and tears; will discolor contact lenses.
- **Ethambutol:** Optic neuritis and impaired color vision are related to cumulative dose.

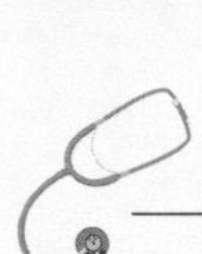
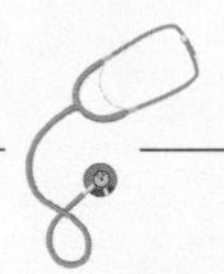

Blue bloaters (chronic bronchitis):

- Right heart failure
- Polycythemia
- High PCO_2, low PO_2

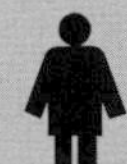

A patient is brought in by ambulance in status epilepticus. The patient's family member says he has no medical history except TB. *Think: INH toxicity.* **Next step:** Treat with pyridoxine.

OBSTRUCTIVE AIRWAY DISORDERS

Chronic Obstructive Pulmonary Disease (COPD)

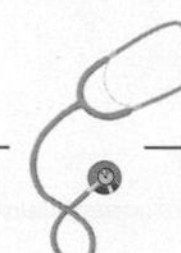

Patients with severe emphysema will lose weight for a variety of reasons. For example, the work of breathing is highly taxing metabolically; in addition, stopping to chew food and swallow prevents adequate oxygenation, so patients avoid eating in severe cases.

Chronic bronchitis and emphysema are forms of chronic obstructive pulmonary disease. COPD is defined by a chronic obstruction to expiratory airflow, largely irreversible, as evidenced by a ↓ in FEV_1. The term *COPD* is preferred to describe both chronic bronchitis and emphysema, as many patients have elements of each disease.

- **Chronic bronchitis:** Defined as chronic productive cough on most days for ≥ 3 months in each of 2 successive years; may or may not be accompanied by chronic expiratory airflow obstruction.
- **Emphysema:** Permanent enlargement of the air space distal to the terminal bronchioles due to destruction of alveolar septa. A pathological entity whose clinical correlate is chronic expiratory airflow obstruction with evidence of hyperinflation.

PATHOPHYSIOLOGY OF EMPHYSEMA

- **Centrilobular** emphysema affects the respiratory bronchioles and surrounding alveoli. Usually in smokers, predominantly in the *upper lobes.*
- **Panlobular or panacinar emphysema** occurs in patients with α_1-antitrypsin deficiency. α_1-antitrypsin protects against the degradation of lung elastin. The whole of pulmonary lobules are destroyed. Seen predominantly in *lower lobes.*

EPIDEMIOLOGY

- Higher prevalence in men.
- Mortality rates are higher in whites.
- Only 15% of smokers develop COPD.

RISK FACTORS

- Smoking.
- α_1-antitrypsin deficiency (autosomal recessive inheritance, more common in Mediterraneans).

DIAGNOSIS/FINDINGS

- **Clinical presentation:** Usually with slowly progressive shortness of breath on exertion.
- **Physical exam:** Barrel chest, ↓ air entry with prolonged expiration, wheezes.
- **CXR:** Hyperinflated lungs, low and flattened diaphragm.
- **PFTs:** Irreversible obstructive pattern (low FEV_1, low FEV_1/FVC. The severity of COPD is defined by the extent of loss of FEV_1.
- **Electrocardiogram (ECG):** May show right-sided strain pattern. Also, multifocal atrial tachycardia is a common supraventricular tachycardia seen in these patients.
- **Computed tomography (CT):** Shows loss of alveolar walls in emphysema.

TREATMENT

Supplemental oxygen is the only therapy for COPD proven to extend life.

- **Smoking cessation:** The only intervention proven to slow down the loss of pulmonary function.
- **Oxygen:** Has also been shown to **improve** COPD patients' IQ, exercise tolerance, and **mortality**! Oxygen should be given to:
  - Patients with a resting PaO_2 of < 55 mmHg.
  - Patients with PaO_2 of 55–59 who have cor pulmonale, erythrocytosis, or who desaturate during exercise.
- Maintain vaccination against influenza and *Streptococcus pneumoniae.*
- Beta agonists and anticholinergics (ipratropium bromide, tiotropium) improve FEV_1 modestly.
- Inhaled corticosteroids (eg, fluticasone, budesonide) are helpful in patients with severe COPD (FEV_1 < 50% predicted and frequent infective exacerbations).
- Antibiotics for acute infective exacerbations of COPD reduce the duration of COPD exacerbation symptoms by 20% and ↓ hospital admissions by 50%. A course of steroids can also help in resolution of COPD exacerbations.

NSAIDs can precipitate an asthma attack. Watch for this in a patient with a history of asthma who takes ibuprofen for a headache.

Asthma

A chronic condition characterized by airway inflammation, bronchoconstriction, and hypersecretion. It is reversible (typically with bronchodilators).

Pathophysiology

- Airway inflammation occurs in response to allergen exposure. The early phase of asthma is immunoglobulin E (IgE) mediated, associated with histamine release from mast cells.
- The late phase is associated with cytokine release and eosinophil infiltration, and is improved by steroids.

Triggers

- Exposure to various allergens from pets, dust, pollen, etc., → inflammation and airway hyperreactivity.
- Once airway hyperreactivity is established, an asthma attack may be induced by nonspecific triggers like exercise, cold air, strong smells, etc.

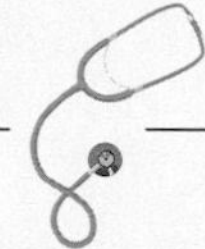

Cough-variant asthma: Cough is the patient's only symptom. The diagnosis of asthma is demonstrated by response to asthma-specific treatment.

Signs and Symptoms

The hallmark of airflow obstruction associated with asthma is its variability from day to day, at different times of the day and from season to season. Predominant symptoms include:

- Chest tightness
- Wheezing
- Shortness of breath
- Cough, usually dry (especially at night)

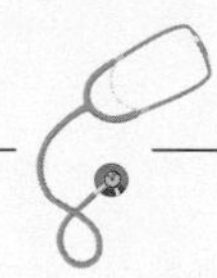

MDIs deliver smaller particles than nebulizers and therefore reach the smallest airways better. Nebulizers are favored for hospital treatment because of ease of use.

Physical Exam

- Wheezing on exhalation.
- ↓ air entry, ↑ expiratory phase.
- ↓ peak flow and FEV_1.
- **Clinical features of acute severe asthma:**
  - Patient too breathless to complete a full sentence.
  - Respiratory rate > 30/min.
  - Use of accessory muscles.
  - ↓ air entry on auscultation.
  - Heart rate > 120/min, and presence of pulsus paradoxus > 20 mmHg.
  - Patient is drowsy or tells you that they're "tiring out."
  - Arterial blood gas analysis showing normal or ↑ CO_2 level (see below).

Treatment (Table 2.7-7)

- **Short-acting β_2 agonists** (eg, albuterol, terbutaline) (rapid onset):
  - Delivered by metered-dose inhaler (MDI) or nebulizer.
  - Promote bronchodilation.
- **Ipratropium bromide** (rapid onset):
  - Delivered by nebulizer or MDI.
  - Dries up bronchial secretions.
  - Effects of beta agonists and ipratropium bromide are additive.

TABLE 2.7-7. Asthma Classification and Treatment

CLASSIFICATION	FREQUENCY OF SYMPTOMS	TREATMENT
Mild intermittent	1–2 episodes per month	**PRN:** Short-acting β_2 agonists as needed.
Mild persistent	> 2 per week but < 1 per day	**PRN:** Short-acting β_2 agonists as needed. **Maintenance:** May add oral or inhaled steroids or cromolyn or leukotriene modifier.
Moderate persistent	Daily	**Maintenance:** Oral or inhaled steroids and long-acting β_2 agonist; may also use cromolyn or leukotriene modifier. **PRN:** Short-acting β_2 agonist as needed.
Severe persistent	Continuous	**Maintenance:** Oral or inhaled steroid + long-acting β_2 agonist. **PRN:** Short-acting β_2 agonist.

- **Steroids** (take 6 hours to work):
  - Reduce inflammation.
  - Inhaled corticosteroids, often used in combination with long acting β_2 agonists (eg, salmeterol, fomoterol) are the cornerstone of preventive and maintenance therapy for bronchial asthma.
  - Oral or IV use for acute exacerbations.
- Other preventative medications:
  - Leukotriene modifiers such as montelukast.
  - Mast cell stabilizers such as cromolyn.
- **Methylxanthines** such as theophylline are no longer regularly used for asthma due to the narrow therapeutic window and the frequency of adverse effects, including nausea, vomiting, headache, and, in severe toxicity, seizures and arrhythmias.
- **Allergen removal:** Common environmental triggers should be addressed, including smoking, dust, pets, carpets, cockroaches, and seasonal allergens.

INTERPRETATION OF ARTERIAL BLOOD GASES IN ASTHMA

The notation for arterial blood gases is: pH/P_{CO_2}/PO_2/calculated HCO_3/calculated SaO_2.

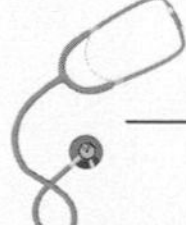

If an asthmatic in respiratory distress has a normal pH and normal P_{CO_2}, beware of *impending respiratory failure:* intubate (he is tiring out).

Sample ABGs

- **Normal:** 7.4/40/98.
- Mild asthma: 7.48/30/60 (acute respiratory alkalosis).
- Severe asthma: 7.40/40/55 (the "normalization" of the pH and P_{CO_2} in the presence of continued symptoms and hypoxia indicate that the patient is getting fatigued and is no longer able to maintain CO_2 balance).

Obstructive Sleep Apnea (OSA)

Brief periods of breathing cessation (apnea) or marked reduction in tidal volume (hypopnea) occurring during sleep due to occlusion of upper airways.

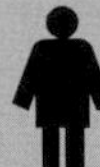

Why does an obese patient known to snore have daytime sleepiness?
Obstructive sleep apnea/obesity hypoventilation syndrome.

Signs and Symptoms

- Snoring.
- Persistent daytime sleepiness.
- Morning headache.
- Obesity.
- Hypertension.
- Large neck circumference.
- OSA ↑ the risk of morbidity and mortality from hypertension and other cardiovascular disorders.

Differential Diagnosis

- Simple snoring.
- Central sleep apnea.
- Other disorders causing daytime sleepiness (insufficient sleep, circadian rhythm disturbances, narcolepsy, periodic limb movement disorder).

Diagnosis

- Made with polysomnography (sleep study).
- OSA is defined by ≥ 5 episodes of apnea and hypopnea per hour of sleep (apnea-hypopnea index).

Treatment

- Lateral sleeping position, avoidance of alcohol or sedative medications, weight loss.
- Continuous positive airway pressure (CPAP) during sleep: Very effective, if consistently used by the patient.
- Surgery (tonsillectomy, uvulopalatopharyngoplasty, tracheostomy).

UPPER RESPIRATORY TRACT DISEASES

Acute Cough

- Cough is a common presenting complaint of patients.
- Acute cough, or cough of < 3 weeks' duration, is most commonly caused by the postnasal drip associated with the common cold.
- See Table 2.7-8 for causes of acute cough.

Chronic Cough

Cough of > 3 weeks' duration.

Etiology

- Postnasal drip.
- Asthma.
- Gastroesophageal reflux disease (GERD).
- See Table 2.7-9 for a complete list of causes.

TABLE 2.7-8. Causes of Acute Cough

PREVALENCE	CAUSE
Very common	Postnasal drip (due to common cold, acute bacterial sinusitis, allergic rhinitis, environmental irritant rhinitis)
Common	Pertussis COPD exacerbation
Less common	Asthma Congestive heart failure Pneumonia Aspiration syndromes Pulmonary embolism

Postnasal Drip Syndrome (PNDS)

PNDS is thought to be the single most common cause of both acute and chronic cough. It is now called upper airway cough syndrome.

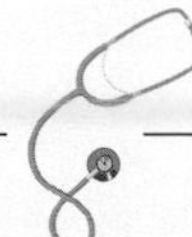

PNDS, asthma, and GERD account for nearly 100% of causes of chronic cough in nonsmokers with normal CXR, who are not on angiotensin-converting enzyme (ACE) inhibitors.

Etiology

All causes of rhinosinusitis can cause postnasal drip and cough.

Pathophysiology

PNDS may be caused by a mucus hypersecretory phenotype that develops following chronic exposure of the respiratory tract to particulate matter, allergens, irritants, and pathogens. The mechanical action of secretions dripping into the hypopharynx triggers the cough reflex.

TABLE 2.7-9. Causes of Chronic Cough

PREVALENCE	CAUSES
Common	PNDS Asthma GERD
Less common	Chronic bronchitis Bronchiectasis Postinfectious cough (pertussis)
Uncommon	Bronchogenic carcinoma ACE inhibitors
Rare in adults	Psychogenic cough

ACE, angiotensin-converting enzyme; GERD, gastroesophageal reflux disease; PNDS, postnasal drip syndrome.

Signs and Symptoms

- Cough, more on lying down and more at night when the patient sleeps.
- Nasal discharge or nasal obstruction.
- Dripping sensation or tickle in the throat; drainage may be present on the posterior pharyngeal wall.

Treatment

- PNDS is treated with a first-generation antihistamine and a decongestant. Nonsedating antihistamines have been shown to be less effective in this case.
- Intranasal corticosteroids are used in cases where PNDS is secondary to allergic rhinitis or symptoms are more persistent.
- Treatment of PNDS due to sinusitis is addressed below.

Sinusitis

- Sinusitis is a common cause of PNDS and cough.
- Acute sinusitis is a bacterial infection that usually involves an obstructed maxillary sinus.
- Chronic sinusitis is the persistence of sinus inflammation for ≥ 3 months.
- Also associated with allergic rhinitis, dental infections, foreign body or tumor, cystic fibrosis, and asthma.

Signs and Symptoms

- Purulent nasal discharge.
- Sinus pain worse on bending forward.
- Fever.
- Tenderness to percussion over sinuses.

Diagnosis

- Transillumination findings are inconsistent.
- CT scan is extremely sensitive but is not specific to sinusitis, and many false ⊕ occur. CT scan should be reserved for hospitalized patients, or for the diagnosis of chronic sinusitis.

Treatment

- **Acute sinusitis:** Routine treatment with antibiotics is *not* indicated. If initial symptomatic treatment with antihistamines and anti-inflammatory medications is not effective, nasal corticosteroids are to be tried.
- If severe symptoms persist or there are indications of spreading infections, antibiotics are started and should be directed against the most likely bacterial organisms: *S. pneumoniae*, *Haemophilus influenzae*, and *Moraxella catarrhalis*. Amoxicillin or TMP-SMZ or amoxicillin–clavulanic acid for 1–2 weeks.
- **Persistent chronic sinusitis:** May require subspecialist involvement.

Complications of Untreated Severe Acute/Chronic Sinusitis

- Preseptal or periorbital cellulitis.
- Orbital cellulitis.
- Epidural, subdural, or cerebral abscess.
- Meningitis.
- Dural sinus venous thrombosis.

Pertussis (Whooping Cough)

Caused by *Bordetella pertussis,* a gram-⊖ coccobacillus.

EPIDEMIOLOGY

- Thought to be a common cause of cough in adults.
- The classic "whoop" caused by rapid air inspiration against a closed glottis is rarely seen in adults.

IMMUNIZATION

- Before routine immunization, whooping cough was a common cause of infant death.
- DTP (killed whole-cell) or DTaP (acellular) at 2, 4, 6, 18 months, and 4–6 years.

SIGNS AND SYMPTOMS

- **Catarrhal stage:**
  - Lasts 1–2 weeks.
  - Characterized by mild upper respiratory infection (URI) symptoms.
- **Paroxysmal stage:**
  - Lasts 2–4 weeks.
  - Characterized by prolonged paroxysmal cough.
  - Often worse at night.
- **Convalescent stage:** Characterized by gradual improvement of symptoms.

DIAGNOSIS

Nasopharyngeal swab and culture.

TREATMENT

- Macrolide antibiotics, such as erythromycin, will reduce the severity of the disease if started within 8 days.
- Identification and treatment of adult patients is important to help prevent transmission to unimmunized or incompletely immunized children.

MISCELLANEOUS LUNG DISORDERS

Acute Respiratory Distress Syndrome (ARDS)

- A condition that results from ↑ permeability of alveolar capillaries causing fluid to fill alveoli.
- Also known as noncardiogenic pulmonary edema.

ETIOLOGY

- Shock
- Septicemia
- Aspiration
- Severe pancreatitis
- Blood transfusion

DIAGNOSIS

- Ratio of $PaO_2/FiO_2 \le 200$.
- Bilateral fluffy infiltrates.
- Pulmonary artery capillary pressure, which reflects pressures in the left side of the heart, < 18 mmHg (thereby ruling out cardiogenic pulmonary edema).

Clinical Pearl: ARDS is a diagnosis of exclusion. You must be certain that there is no other explanation for the acute onset of bilateral "fluffy" infiltrates.

TREATMENT

- O_2 treatment does not improve hypoxia in ARDS. Fluid-filled, consolidated, or collapsed alveoli lead to effective arteriovenous shunting.
- Treatment usually involves hemodynamic support and treatment of the underlying disease.

A 54-year-old male with pancreatitis goes into respiratory failure. CXR shows bilateral infiltrates. Diagnosis? ARDS (sepsis is the most common cause of ARDS).

Bronchiectasis

- A chronic condition characterized by pathological dilatation of the medium-sized airways.
- Usually caused by an abnormal inflammatory response to an initial infectious or toxic insult.

ETIOLOGY

- **Localized:** Usually the result of previous pneumonia.
- If **severe or bilateral,** the following causes should be considered:
  - Cystic fibrosis.
  - Immotile cilia syndromes (Kartagener's).
  - Immunodeficiency: Hypogammaglobulinemia, HIV.

A patient with cystic fibrosis has chronic hypoxia that causes pulmonary hypertension and then cor pulmonale and right heart failure.

PATHOPHYSIOLOGY

- The resulting airway damage allows bacterial colonization, buildup of secretions, and continued bronchial destruction.
- Bronchiectasis is the cause of chronic cough in about 4% of cases.

SIGNS AND SYMPTOMS

- Chronic cough often with large amount of expectoration.
- Hemoptysis is often the major or only presenting symptom.
- Wheezing.
- Failure to thrive.

Most common organisms to colonize bronchiectatic lung:

- *H influenzae*
- *S aureus*
- *Pseudomonas aeruginosa*

DIAGNOSIS

- High-resolution CT scan will detect bronchial dilatation and destruction in 60–100% of cases.
- Patients with cystic fibrosis will have abnormal pancreatic function and an abnormal sweat test.

TREATMENT

- Chest physiotherapy and postural drainage.
- Antibiotics.
- Bronchodilators, mucolytics.

Hemoptysis

- Coughing up of blood due to bleeding from the lower respiratory tract.
- See Table 2.7-10 for a list of causes.
- **Massive hemoptysis** is defined as bleeding > 600 mL in 48 hours (200–600 mL/24 hr), or any amount of bleeding causing clinical impairment of respiratory function.

> A patient presents with hemoptysis, sinusitis, and glomerulonephritis. On physical exam, you notice a "saddle-nose" deformity. *Think: Wegener's granulomatosis.* **Next step:** Send for circulating antineutrophil cytoplasmic antibody (c-ANCA).

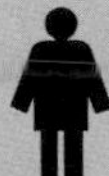

> A patient presents with dyspnea, hemoptysis, and acute renal failure. *Think: Goodpasture's syndrome.* **Next step:** Send for anti–glomerular basement membrane antibodies.

Diagnosis

CXR, high-resolution CT, bronchoscopy.

TABLE 2.7-10. Causes of Hemoptysis

Incidence	Cause
Common	Bronchitis TB Pneumonia Lung cancer Bronchiectasis Unknown
Uncommon	Coagulopathy Congestive heart failure Pulmonary embolism Wegener's granulomatosis Goodpasture's syndrome
Rare	Pulmonary hypertension Trauma Vasculitis Foreign body Collagen vascular disease Pulmonary arteriovenous malformation

Treatment

- Supplemental oxygen.
- Position patient with bleeding side down.
- Suppress cough reflex (ie, codeine).
- Patients with massive hemoptysis usually require surgical involvement. Initial therapy includes:
  - Protection of the good lung often by intubation with a double-lumen tube (selective intubation).
  - Endobronchial cold saline or epinephrine.
  - Bronchial artery embolization.

Pulmonary Embolism (PE)

- Usually results from the dislodging and migration of a deep venous thrombus, causing blockage of pulmonary blood flow beyond the embolus.
- Very large PEs that impede blood flow in both the right and left pulmonary arteries are called **saddle emboli.**

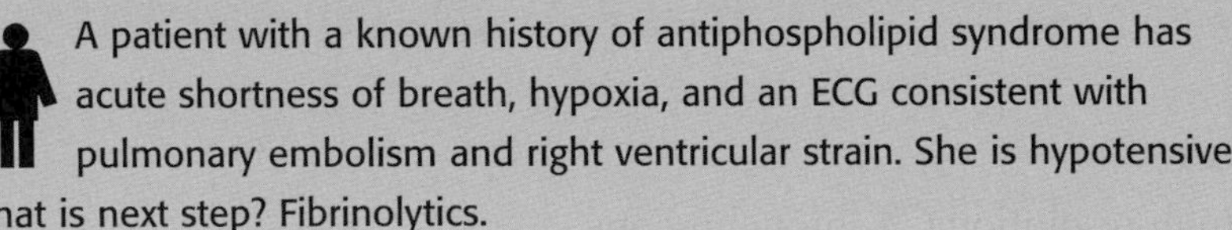

A patient with a known history of antiphospholipid syndrome has acute shortness of breath, hypoxia, and an ECG consistent with pulmonary embolism and right ventricular strain. She is hypotensive. What is next step? Fibrinolytics.

Risk Factors for Venous Thromboembolism (VTE)

- Immobilization.
- Leg fracture or leg surgery.
- Hypercoagulable state (active malignancy, pregnancy, genetic).
- Medications: Oral contraceptives, tamoxifen.

Signs and Symptoms

No sign or symptom is specific for PE.

- Sinus tachycardia (most common rhythm disturbance).
- Dyspnea.
- Cough.
- Tachypnea.
- Pleuritic chest pain.
- Hemoptysis.
- Hypoxia, often in presence of a clear CXR.

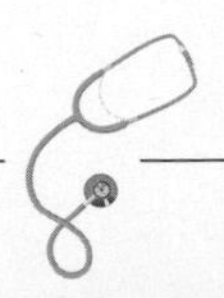

Westermark's sign: Oligemia seen on the CXR distal to the PE. (Rare finding in the times of CT angiograms; however, a favorite topic on rounds with attendings).

Diagnosis

Any of the following three is reasonable:

- **Helical (spiral) CT:** Also called CTPA (CT of pulmonary arteries); to look for embolus in the pulmonary vasculature. Most common. Fast and convenient, fairly sensitive. Downside: IV contrast can damage kidneys.
- **Pulmonary angiogram:** The gold standard for detection of PE. Very sensitive. Downside: Invasive test.

- **Ventilation-perfusion scan (V/Q scan):** To look for perfusion defects at site of PE. Does not affect kidneys. Okay for pregnant patients. Downside: long test and not useful in patients with underlying lung disease.
- Other findings:
  - **ECG:** Often normal! Sinus tachycardia is the most common finding. S in lead I, Q and inverted T waves in lead III, when found is characteristic. ECG may show diffuse ST changes and tachycardia (see Figure 2.7-1) (S1Q3T3 is the mnemonic).

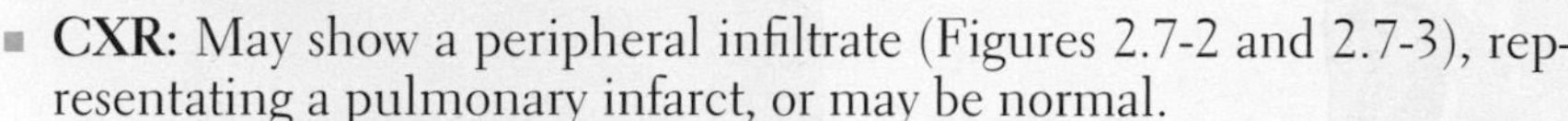

  - **CXR:** May show a peripheral infiltrate (Figures 2.7-2 and 2.7-3), representating a pulmonary infarct, or may be normal.
  - **ABGs:** Usually reveal hypoxemia, hypocapnia, and respiratory alkalosis (if big PE).
  - **D-dimer:** Measures products of fibrin degradation (will be elevated).
  - A low D-dimer with low clinical suspicion essentially rules out PE as cause of symptoms.
  - **Leg ultrasonography (venous duplex):** To detect DVT—⊕ will make one more suspicious of PE if symptoms.

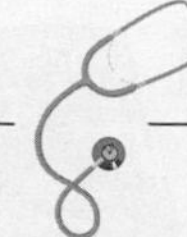

Hampton's hump: Wedge-shaped infiltrate seen on CXR.

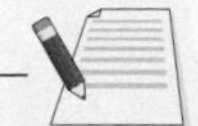

Angiography is the gold standard in the diagnosis of:

- Deep venous thrombosis
- Dissecting aortic aneurysm
- Ischemic bowel syndrome
- Pulmonary embolism

Treatment

- Acute:
  - Anticoagulation with heparin or low-molecular-weight heparin. Usually the only therapy in stable patients.

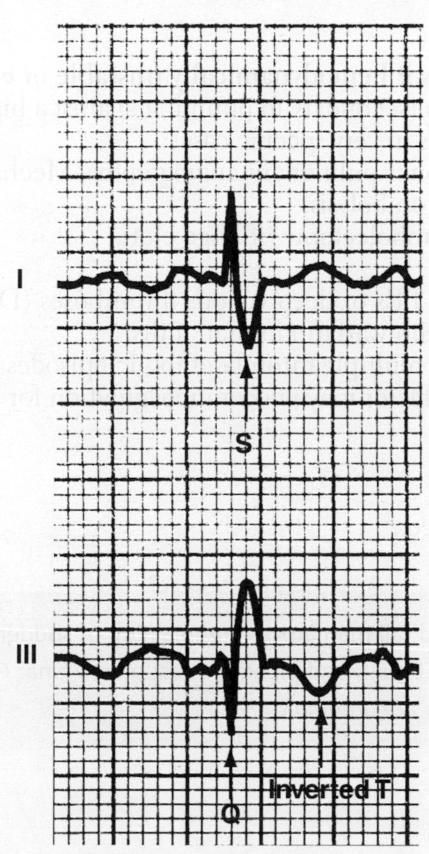

FIGURE 2.7-1. Pulmonary embolism. S_1-Q_3-T_3 pattern.

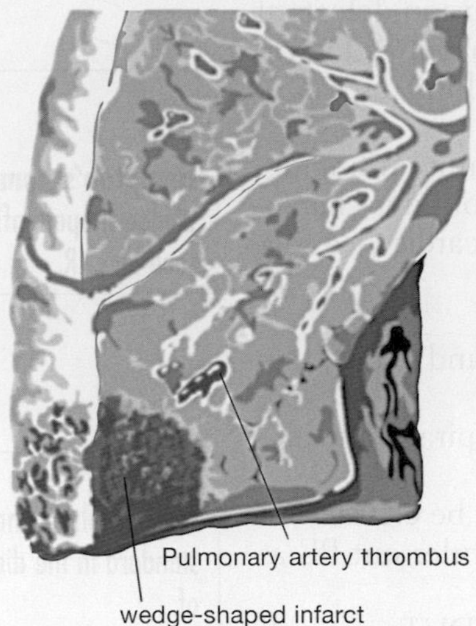

FIGURE 2.7-2. Drawing depicting Hampton's hump.

(Reproduced, with permission, from Schwartz DT. *Emergency Radiology: Case Studies.* New York: McGraw-Hill, 2008: 38.)

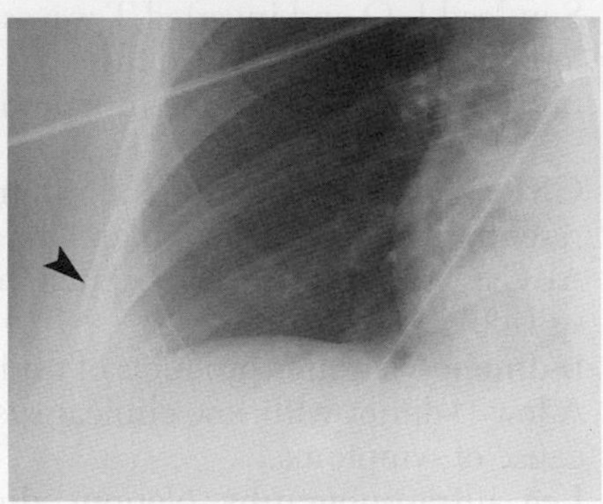

FIGURE 2.7-3. Hampton's hump.

Note the wedge-shaped infiltrate. Can be mistaken for pneumonia, so a careful history is very important if this finding is seen. (Reproduced, with permission, from Schwartz DT. *Emergency Radiology: Case Studies.* New York: McGraw-Hill, 2008: 38.)

- Thrombolysis **if hemodynamically unstable** or echo shows right ventricular strain (secondary to pumping against a big clotted artery).
- Other options in very specific cases:
  - Interventional pulmonary angiography: Mechanical disintegration or local thrombolysis.
  - Surgery: Embolectomy (if huge clot).
- **Prolonged:**
  - Patients with PEs or deep venous thromboses (DVTs) are orally anticoagulated with warfarin for 6 months.
  - Patients with multiple thromboembolic episodes and patients with an ongoing risk factor may need anticoagulation for indefinite period.

Pneumothorax

Air in the pleural space.

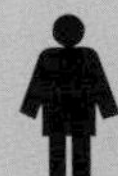

A 20-year-old tall man arrives complaining of sudden onset of severe shortness of breath and pleuritic chest pain. *Think: Primary spontaneous pneumothorax.*

EPIDEMIOLOGY

- Spontaneous pneumothorax affects approximately 20,000 persons annually, usually from rupture of a subpleural bleb or pleural necrosis due to lung disease.
- Primary spontaneous pneumothorax occurs in an otherwise healthy person, while secondary spontaneous pneumothorax occurs in patients who have underlying lung disease.

ETIOLOGY

- **Primary spontaneous pneumothorax:**
  - Male smokers
  - Patients tall for weight
- **Secondary spontaneous pneumothorax:**
  - COPD
  - Cystic fibrosis
  - Pneumonia
  - Cancer

SIGNS AND SYMPTOMS

- Chest pain.
- Dyspnea.
- Hyperresonance on affected side.
- ↓ breath sounds on affected side.
- Tracheal deviation *away* from affected side (in tension pneumothorax).

DIAGNOSIS

Upright CXR is ~ 83% sensitive; demonstrates an absence of lung markings where the lung has collapsed.

TREATMENT

- 100% oxygen.
- For pneumothoraces > 20% of lung volume or with hemodynamic compromise, perform tube thoracostomy to remove air.
- Pleurodesis to adhere the visceral and parietal pleura, in cases of recurrent pneumothorax.

Mediastinum

MASSES

- **Anterior (4 Ts):**
  - Thymoma
  - Teratoma
  - Thyroid
  - Terrible lymphoma
- **Middle:**
  - Vascular lesions
  - Lymph nodes
- **Posterior:** Neurogenic tumor

Mediastinitis

Causes

- Esophageal perforation.
- Postmedian sternotomy.
- Inhalation anthrax (hemorrhagic mediastinitis).
- TB, histoplasmosis (chronic).

Symptoms

- Initial symptoms similar to viral syndrome.
- After 1–3 days, fever, and dyspnea develop. Patients die from airway obstruction and hypoxia.

Treatment

High-dose penicillin, ciprofloxacin, or doxycycline is recommended.

Pneumomediastinum

Causes

- Esophageal rupture is the first possibility to be considered (often associated with left hydropneumothorax).
- **Boerhaave's syndrome:** Ruptured esophagus from violent retching. Associated with very high mortality if not identified and managed surgically.
- Rupture of alveolus, bronchus, or trachea.

> **Physical finding in pneumomediastinum: Hamman's sign:** A crunching sound occurring with the heartbeat.

Treatment

Treat underlying cause.

INTERSTITIAL LUNG DISEASE

- A group of diverse disorders involving the parenchyma of the lung that cause alveolitis, interstitial inflammation, and fibrosis or a granulomatous response.
- There are known and idiopathic etiologies (Table 2.7-11).

Symptoms

- Dyspnea (chronic, progressive)
- Exercise intolerance
- Nonproductive cough
- Tachypnea

Exam Findings

- End-inspiratory crackles
- Clubbing of digits
- Pulmonary hypertension

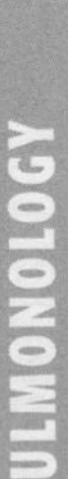

TABLE 2.7-11. Interstitial Lung Disease Causes

Known Causes	Idiopathic
Environmental/occupational (dusts, fumes)	Sarcoidosis
Drugs (amiodarone, gold)	Idiopathic pulmonary fibrosis
Radiation	Collagen vascular disease
Infections	Goodpasture's syndrome
Hypersensitivity pneumonitis	Alveolar proteinosis
Pulmonary edema	Amyloidosis
Neoplasms (lymphatic carcinoma, lymphoma)	Bronchiolitis obliterans with organizing pneumonia now known as "Crypotogenic Organizing Pneumonia or COP"
	Neurofibromatosis, tuberous sclerosis
	Lymphangioleiomyomatosis
	Eosinophilic pneumonias
	Lymphocytic interstitial pneumonia

Diagnosis

- Usually requires biopsy.
- High-resolution CT, can be used as diagnostic modality for idiopathic pulmonary fibrosis (IPF).
- CXR (may show diffuse bilateral reticular infiltrates).
- PFTs (mostly demonstrate restrictive abnormalities and reduced gas transfer).

Treatment

- Removal/cessation of exposure to known environmental causes. Often, there is no effective treatment.
- Supplemental oxygen as needed.
- Steroids (possibly in combination with cyclophosphamide or azathioprine).
- Lung transplant.

Examples of Environmental Lung Disease

- **Asbestosis:** A diffuse interstitial lung disease caused by dust of mineral silicates. Asbestos exposure is associated with an ↑ risk of **mesotheliomas** (also lung cancers). Smokers with asbestos exposure are particularly at a high risk for developing lung cancer.
- **Silicosis:** Nodular fibrosis of the lung caused by exposure to silica flour, sand blasting, or the manufacture of abrasive soaps. These patients are at a greater risk of developing pulmonary TB disease.
- **Coal workers' pneumoconiosis:** An occupational hazard of ~ 50% of all coal miners; they develop progressive massive fibrosis, usually involving upper lung fields.
- **Byssinosis (cotton dust exposure):** Patients experience "chest tightness" with an associated ↓ in FEV_1 with exposure to cotton dust. Clinically behaves like COPD. Treatment is to wear protective equipment and to use bronchodilators.
- **Farmer's lung:** A *hypersensitivity pneumonitis* caused by exposure to spores of thermophilic actinomycetes. Thought to be associated with a suppressor T-cell defect, is IgG mediated. Symptoms include fever, chills, cough, and dyspnea, and episodes occur more frequently during

wet weather. Treat with steroids, and avoid exposure. Long-term complications include pulmonary fibrosis and weight loss.

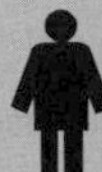

A farmer presents with fever, cough, and difficulty breathing after several days of filling his silo with grain. *Think: Hypersensitivity pneumonitis.*

CAUSES OF LUNG FIBROSIS

- *Upper* lung zone fibrosis: Remember the mnemonic **CHARTS:**
  - Coal workers' pneumoconiosis
  - Histiocytosis, Langerhans' cell; Hypersensitivity pneumonitis (chronic)
  - Ankylosing spondylitis
  - Radiation (usually unilateral, radiation for breast cancer)
  - Tuberculosis
  - Silicosis, Sarcoidosis (chronic)
- *Lower* lung zone fibrosis: Remember the mnemonic **I SOAR:**
  - Idiopathic pulmonary fibrosis (IPF)
  - Systemic sclerosis
  - Others (eg, drug induced)
  - Asbestosis
  - Rheumatoid arthritis

LUNG CANCER

Two types of cancer share a **"s"**entral location:

- **Small cell**
- **Squamous cell**

TYPES

- **Small cell lung cancer:**
  - Central location.
  - Sensitive to chemotherapy.
  - Surgery is *not* indicated.
  - Poor prognosis with high recurrence after initial response to chemotherapy.
- **Non–small cell lung cancer:**
  - Includes squamous cell, large cell, and adenocarcinoma.
  - Poor response to chemotherapy.
  - Treated with surgery if early stage.
  - Prognosis varies with stage.

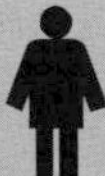

A 61-year-old heavy smoker presents with shoulder pain, ptosis, and anhydrosis. What does he have? Pancoast tumor (metastasis to supraclavicular lymph node in lung cancer).

EPIDEMIOLOGY

- Leading cause of cancer death in both men and women in the United States.
- Cases have been decreasing in men, but increasing in women.
- Smoking is by far the most important causative factor in the development of lung cancer.

Bronchoalveolar cancer, a type of adenocarcinoma, is not linked to smoking and is more common in women.

ETIOLOGY

- Smoking
- Passive smoke exposure
- Radon gas exposure
- Asbestos
- Arsenic
- Nickel

SIGNS AND SYMPTOMS

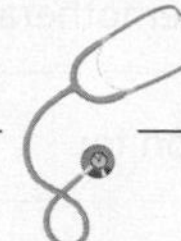

Chronic cough is the most common symptom of lung cancer.

- Cough.
- Hemoptysis: Common with central tumors.
- Dyspnea: Results from significant endobronchial obstruction with collapse of distal lung, pleural effusion, lymphangitic spread of tumor within the lung.
- Symptoms from mediastinal involvement either from spread of the tumor or large mediastinal lymphadenopathy:
  - Hoarseness (recurrent laryngeal nerve paralysis).
  - Dysphagia.
  - Superior vena cava syndrome.
  - Associated (paraneoplastic) syndromes (see Table 2.7-12)

TABLE 2.7-12. Syndromes Associated with Lung Cancer

Horner's syndrome	Sympathetic nerve paralysis produces enophthalmos, ptosis, miosis, amd ipsilateral anhidrosis.
Pancoast's syndrome	Superior sulcus tumor injuring the eighth cervical nerve and the first and second thoracic nerves and ribs, causing shoulder pain radiating to arm.
Superior vena cava syndrome	Tumor causing obstruction of the superior vena cava and subsequent venous return, producing facial swelling and plethora, cough, headaches, epistaxis, syncope. Symptoms worsened with bending forward and on awakening in the morning.
Syndrome of inappropriate antidiuretic hormone (SIADH)	Ectopic antidiuretic hormone release in the setting of plasma hyposmolarity, producing hyponatremia without edema. Seen in small cell lung cancer.
Eaton-Lambert syndrome	Presynaptic nerve terminals attacked by antibodies, decreasing acetylcholine release. Treated by plasmapheresis and immunosuppression, 40% associated with small cell lung cancer, 20% have other cancer, 40% have no cancer.
Trousseau's syndrome	Venous thrombosis associated with metastatic cancer.
PTH-like hormone	Results in high calcium, low phosphate; seen in squamous cell lung cancer.

TABLE 2.7-13. Distinction Between Small and Non–Small Cell Lung Cancer

CHARACTERISTIC	SMALL CELL LUNG CANCER	NON–SMALL CELL LUNG CANCER
Histology	Small, dark nuclei; scant cytoplasm.	Copious cytoplasm, pleomorphic nuclei.
Ectopic peptide production (causing paraneoplastic syndromes)	▪ ACTH—causes a Cushing syndrome ▪ ADH—causes SIADH (low Na^+) ▪ Eaton-Lambert syndrome ▪ Gastrin—can cause stomach ulcer ▪ Calcitonin—can cause low Ca^+ ▪ ANF	▪ PTHrP (PTH related peptide). Presents with hypercalcemia. Classically in squamous subtype.
Response to radiotherapy	80–90% will shrink	30–50% will shrink
Response to chemotherapy	Very responsive to chemo	Somewhat responsive to chemo
Surgical resection for	Not indicated	Stages I, II, IIIA
Included subtypes	Small cell only	Adenocarcinoma, sqamous cell, large cell, bronchoalveolar
5-year survival rate all stages	5%	10% in later stages; up to 90% in early stages

ACTH, adrenocorticotropic hormone; ADH, antidiuretic hormone (also known as arginine vasopressin [AVP]); ANF, atrial natriuretic factor; PTH, parathyroid hormone.

TREATMENT

The two main types of lung cancer, small cell and non–small cell cancer, have different responses to radiotherapy, chemotherapy, and surgery (see Table 2.7-13). Generally, small cell—always chemo, never surgery; non–small cell—surgery if cancer is local, chemo only if there is metastatic disease.

HOW TO PRESENT A CHEST RADIOGRAPH (CXR)

- First, confirm that the CXR belongs to your patient.
- If possible, compare to a previous film.
- Then, present in a systematic manner:
  1. *Technique:* Rotation, anteroposterior (AP) or posteroanterior (PA), penetration, inspiratory effort.
  2. *Bony structures:* Look for rib, clavicle, scapula, and sternum fractures.
  3. *Airway:* Look for tracheal deviation, pneumothorax, pneumomediastinum.
  4. *Pleural space:* Look for fluid collections, which can represent hemothorax, chylothorax, pleural effusion.

5. *Lung parenchyma:* Look for infiltrates and consolidations: These can represent pneumonia, pulmonary contusions, hematoma, or aspiration. The location of an infiltrate can provide a clue to the location of a pneumonia:
   - Obscured right (R) costophrenic angle = Right lower lobe.
   - Obscured left (L) costophrenic angle = Left lower lobe.
   - Obscured R heart border = Right middle lobe.
   - Obscured L heart border = Left upper lobe.
6. *Mediastinum:* Look at size of mediastinum—a widened one (> 8 cm) goes with aortic dissection. Look for enlarged cardiac silhouette (more than one-half thoracic width at base of heart), which may represent congestive heart failure (CHF), cardiomyopathy, or pericardial effusion.
7. *Diaphragm:* Look for free air under the right hemidiaphragm (suggests bowel perforation). Look for stomach, bowel, or nasogastric tube (NGT) above diaphragm (suggests diaphragmatic rupture).
8. *Tubes and lines:*
   - Identify all tubes and lines.
   - An endotracheal tube should be 2 cm above the carina. A common mistake is right mainstem bronchus intubation.
   - A chest tube (including the most proximal hole) should be in the pleural space (not in the lung parenchyma).
   - An NGT should be in the stomach and uncoiled.
   - The tip of a central venous catheter (central line) should be in the superior vena cava (not in the right atrium).
   - The tip of a Swan-Ganz catheter should be in the pulmonary artery.
   - The tip of a transvenous pacemaker should be in the right ventricle.

A sample CXR presentation may sound like:

> This is the CXR of Mr. Jones. The film is an AP view with good inspiratory effort. There is an isolated fracture of the eighth rib on the right. There is no tracheal deviation or mediastinal shift. There is no pneumo- or hemothorax. The cardiac silhouette appears to be of normal size. The diaphragm and heart borders on both sides are clear; no infiltrates are noted. There is a central venous catheter present, the tip of which is in the superior vena cava.

HIGH-YIELD FACTS IN

Rheumatology

Rheumatology is a broad discipline covering diseases of the joints, connective tissue, and certain immunological disorders. Also covered in this chapter are conditions that are not typically classified as rheumatologic, but nonetheless affect the musculoskeletal system. Table 2.8-1 discusses laboratory data commonly used in rheumatology.

LOWER BACK PAIN

Leading causes of back pain: **ACTIONS.**

- Arthritis (rheumatoid, osteoarthritis, ankylosing spondylitis).
- Congenital anomalies (spina bifida, spondolysis [not covered here]).
- Trauma (strains, sprains, fractures, and lumbar disk herniation).
- Infection (abscess).
- Osteoporosis (secondary fracture, compression).
- Neoplasms (primary or metastatic).
- Spinal stenosis.

TABLE 2.8-1. Laboratory Data Commonly Used in Rheumatology

Finding	Significance
ESR	Determined by filling a tube with whole blood and measuring the rate of sedimentation of red cells—changes in the rate are seen with ↑ plasma proteins. Certain proteins called *acute-phase reactants* (negatively charged proteins) are produced at an ↑ rate during an inflammatory response. These proteins cause RBCs to adhere to one another like stacks of coins called **rouleaux,** which fall through the plasma faster than free RBCs. This is a very nonspecific test. An ↑ ESR is seen in infections, tissue infarctions, malignancies, collagen vascular diseases, and states of ↑ physiologic stress (pregnancy, extreme exercise).
ANA	Found in many rheumatologic disorders, such as: ▪ SLE ▪ Rheumatoid arthritis ▪ Scleroderma ▪ Polymyositis and dermatomyositis
RF	This is an IgM antibody directed against the Fc portion of IgG. Found mainly in rheumatoid arthritis but also in **vasculitides.**
Complement levels	Complement levels drop when there is ↓ production in the liver or ↑ loss—either through the formation of immune complexes or from glomerular disease. Complement levels can be low with: ▪ Liver disease (viral hepatitis) ▪ SLE nephritis ▪ Glomerulonephritis (C3 is the most reduced) ▪ Bacterial endocarditis ▪ Serum sickness ▪ Rheumatoid arthritis with vasculitis

ANA, antinuclear antibody; ESR, erythrocyte sedimentation rate; IgG, immunoglobulin G; IgM, immunoglobulin M; RBC, red blood cell; RF, rheumatoid factor; SLE, systemic lupus erythematosus.

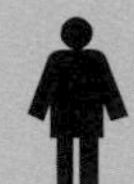

An athlete presents with nonspecific lower back pain of 2 months' duration. On examination he does not have any restriction of movement, no neurological signs, and ⊖ straight leg-raising test. *Think: Acute low back pain.* **Next step:** Education, conservative management.

Lumbar Disk Herniation

- Disk herniation is a common cause of chronic lower back pain.
- L4–L5 and L5–S1 are the most common sites affected.
- Herniation occurs when the nucleus pulposus prolapses through the annulus fibrosis.
- More common in men and overweight individuals.

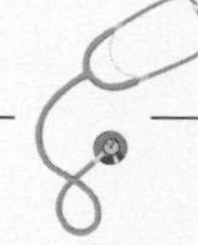

The nucleus pulposus is a thick gel. Herniation of the nucleus pulposus is like toothpaste being squeezed out of the tube.

Signs and Symptoms

- Occurs due to activities that involve sudden movement or heavy lifting.
- Pain is worse with coughing, sneezing, Valsalva, and spinal flexion.
- Pain (sciatica) and paresthesia with a dermatomal distribution.
- Specific signs depend on nerve root involved:

	Sensory Loss/ Pain Distribution	Motor Deficit	Reflex
L4	Anterior thigh	Impaired dorsiflexion and inversion at the ankle (anterior tibialis)	Knee jerk
L5	Lateral calf and first web space	Extends big toe (extensor hallucis longus)	—
S1	Lateral and plantar aspect of foot	Foot plantar flexion and eversion (peroneus longus and brevis)	Ankle jerk

Treatment

- Nonsteroidal anti-inflammatory drugs (NSAIDs) and epidural injection for symptomatic relief.
- Surgical treatment is indicated only for refractory pain and/or neurological deficits.

Vertebral Compression Fracture

- The most common manifestation of osteoporosis.
- Also seen in patients on long-term steroids and in patients with lytic bony metastases.
- Thoracic spine is the most common site affected (see Figure 2.8-1).

Signs and Symptoms

- Height loss.
- Sudden back pain after mild trauma.
- Local radiation of pain—the extremities are rarely affected (unlike a herniated disk).

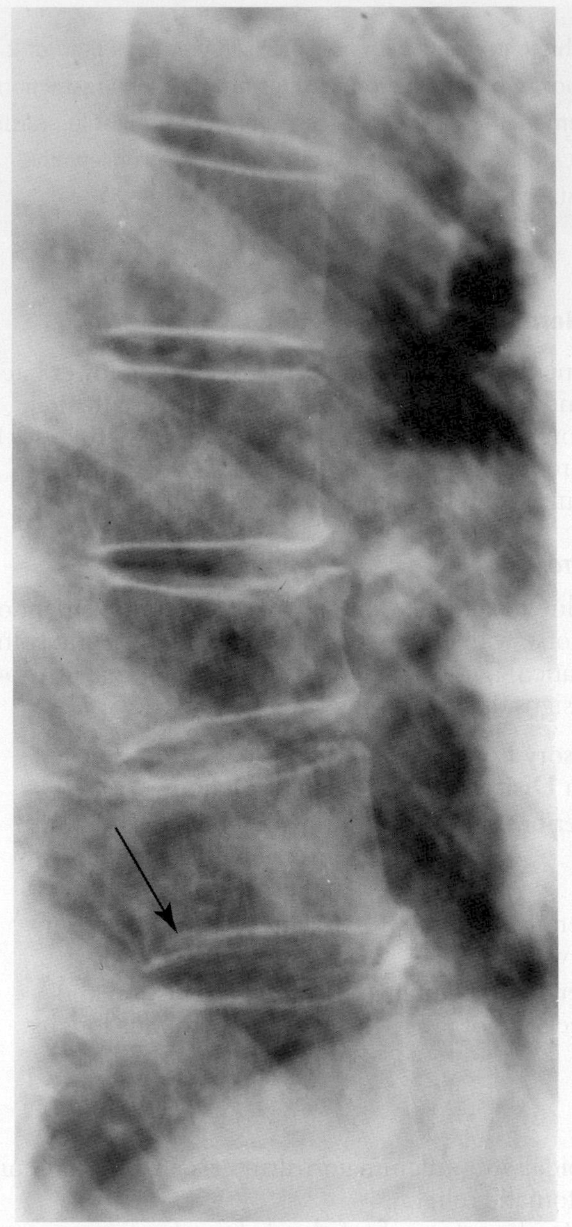

FIGURE 2.8-1. Compression fracture of osteoporosis.

Note the anterior collapse of the vertebra. (Reproduced, with permission, from Wilson FC, Lin PP. *General Orthopedics.* New York: McGraw-Hill, 1997: 489.)

DIAGNOSIS

- Plain radiographs of the lumbosacrum will not show compression fracture until there is loss of 25–30% bone height.
- Magnetic resonance imaging (MRI) and computed tomography (CT) are more sensitive.

Treatment

- Symptomatic relief with NSAIDs.
- Vertebroplasty:
  - Usually reserved for fractures with > 50% loss of bone height.
  - Consists of an orthopedic cement (polymethylmethacrylate) that is injected into the vertebral body.
  - Restores height and relieves pain.
- Prevention of osteoporosis:
  - Weight-bearing exercises.
  - Estrogen replacement therapy.
  - Calcium supplementation to ↑ bone mass.
  - Calcitonin to inhibit bone resorption.
  - Bisphosphonates to inhibit osteoclast activity.

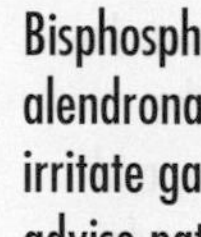

Bisphosphonates such as alendronate (Fosamax) irritate gastric mucosa, so advise patients to eat beforehand and stay upright for 30 minutes after taking it.

Spinal Metastasis and Cauda Equina Syndrome

- Metastatic lesions invade the spinal bone marrow, leading to compression of the spinal cord.
- Typically involves the thoracic spine.
- Cauda equina syndrome occurs when the compression occurs below spinal cord (which typically ends at around L1) at the lumbar and sacral nerve roots.
- The most common primary tumors involved include breast, lung, prostate, kidney, lymphoma, and multiple myeloma.

Spinal cord compression is an emergency. Missed diagnosis can lead to permanent paralysis.

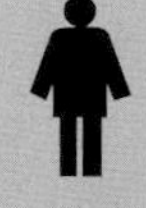

A multiple myeloma patient suddenly becomes incontinent of urine and has leg weakness. **Next step:** MRI and start steroids. Cord compression found: Get emergent neurosurgical and radiation consultation.

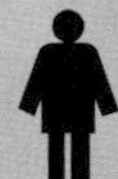

A 60-year-old man presents with severe back pain that has point tenderness. He says he has some numbness in his inner legs. **Next step:** Start steroids and send for emergent spine MRI.

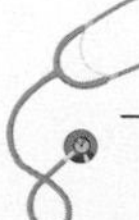

Any cancer patient who develops back pain should be investigated for spinal metastases.

Signs and Symptoms

- Back pain that is worse at night.
- **Lower extremity weakness.**
- Hyperreflexia.
- Upward Babinski sign.
- **Urinary incontinence.**
- ↓ rectal sphincter tone.
- Cauda equina syndrome classically has **saddle anesthesia** and bladder/bowel incontinence.

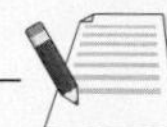

Common causes of spinal cord compression:

- **Multiple myeloma**
- **Lymphoma**
- **Metastatic lung, prostate, and breast cancer**

Diagnosis

MRI is the preferred imaging technique.

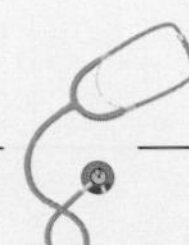

Saddle anesthesia: Loss of sensation over the buttocks, perineum, and thighs. Seen with cauda equina syndrome.

Treatment

Glucocorticoids are used to reduce inflammation and edema. Radiation therapy should be started as soon as possible. Surgery is indicated only if radiation fails to improve the symptoms or if compression is due to actual bone fragment (radiation will not shrink bone).

Osteoarthritis (OA)

- Degeneration of articular cartilage followed by new and abnormal bone formation; more common in women.
- Involves distal interphalangeal joint (DIP), proximal interphalangeal joint (PIP), thumb base, hip, knee, and spine.

Etiology

- Primary disease: Idiopathic.
- Secondary disease: Known underlying etiology such as trauma, metabolic (hemachromatosis, Wilson's disease), endocrine (acromegaly), or congenital (congenital hip dislocation).

Signs and Symptoms

- Joint pain worse with use and relieved with rest.
- Morning stiffness that resolves within 20 minutes.
- Painless nodules on the hand (see Figure 2.8-2):
  - **Heberden's nodes** at the DIPs.
  - **Bouchard's nodes** at the PIPs.
- Loss of range of motion (eg, ↓ internal rotation of hip).
- Joint effusions and crepitus.
- Periarticular muscle wasting and weakness from disuse.

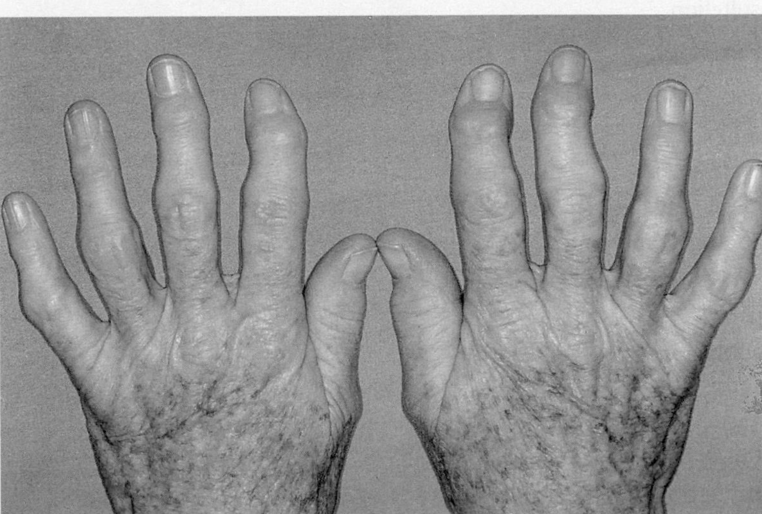

FIGURE 2.8-2. Heberden's and Bouchard's nodes of osteoarthritis.

(Reproduced, with permission, from Wilson FC, Lin PP. *General Orthopedics*. New York: McGraw-Hill, 1997: 413.)

Diagnosis

- Lab findings are normal.
- X-ray will show joint space narrowing, osteophyte formation, and subchondral cysts.
- Synovial fluid analysis shows noninflammatory picture (white cell count < 2000).

Treatment

- NSAIDs for symptomatic relief.
- Intra-articular injection of lidocaine, Hyaluronan, steroids provides temporary relief.
- Joint replacement as necessary.
- Weight loss.
- Strengthen periarticular muscles.

CONNECTIVE TISSUE DISORDERS

See Table 2.8-2 for synovial fluid characteristics.

Rheumatoid Arthritis (RA)

- A systemic inflammatory disease primarily affecting the synovial membranes.
- Pannus (granulation tissue) develops in the joint spaces and erodes into the articular cartilage and bone.

TABLE 2.8-2. Synovial Fluid Characteristics

	Noninflammatory (eg, OA)	Inflammatory (eg, RA, SLE, Gout, Pseudogout, Sarcoidosis)	Septic (eg, Bacterial)	Hemorrhagic (eg, Trauma, Tuberculosis, Coagulopathy)
Color	Clear/yellow	Yellow/white	Yellow/white	Red
Clarity	Transparent	Transluscent/ opaque	Opaque	Opaque
Viscosity	High	Variable	Low	Variable
WBC	< 2000	2000–100,000	> 100,000	Variable
Differential	< 25% PMN	> 50% PMN	> 95% PMN	NA
Culture	⊖	⊖	⊕	Variable

PMN, polymorphonuclear neutrophil; WBC, white blood cell count.

Common deformities in RA:
- **Ulnar deviation** of the digits.
- **Boutonniere deformity:** Hyperextension of the DIP and flexion of the PIP (Figure 2.8-3A).
- **Swan neck:** Flexion of the DIP and extension of the PIP (Figure 2.8-3B).

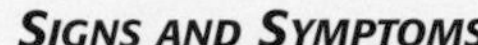

Signs and Symptoms

- Synovitis is characterized by joint swelling, warmth, erythema, and reduction in both active and passive range of movement.
- Early symptoms are nonspecific: Malaise, anorexia, fatigue, vague musculoskeletal complaints.
- Hypertrophy of synovial tissue.
- **Prolonged morning stiffness; pain worse in morning, too.**
- Joint pain—most common joints affected: PIP, metacarpophalangeal (MCP), wrist, knees, ankles.
- Joint subluxation results from ligament laxity and muscle weakness, causing deformity such as swan neck, Boutonniere, Z shape.
- Subcutaneous painless rheumatic nodules.
- Instability of cervical spine due to bone erosion.
- Extra-articular involvement also occurs. Common manifestations include vasculitis, pleuritis, pulmonary nodules, and secondary amyloidosis.

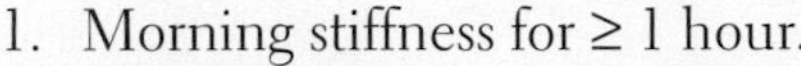

Diagnosis

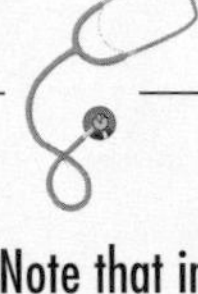

Note that in drug-induced SLE there is no kidney or central nervous system involvement.

At least four out of the following seven criteria must be present to diagnose rheumatoid arthritis; criteria 1 through 4 must have been present for ≥ 6 weeks:

1. Morning stiffness for ≥ 1 hour.
2. Arthritis of three or more joint areas.
3. Arthritis of hand joints (see Figure 2.8-3).
4. Symmetric arthritis.
5. Rheumatoid nodules.
6. ⊕ serum rheumatoid factor (see Table 2.8-3 for common serology of rheumatologic conditions).
7. Radiographic changes.

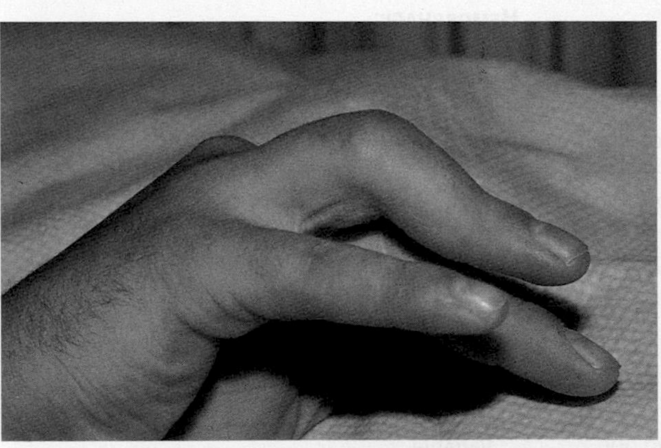

A

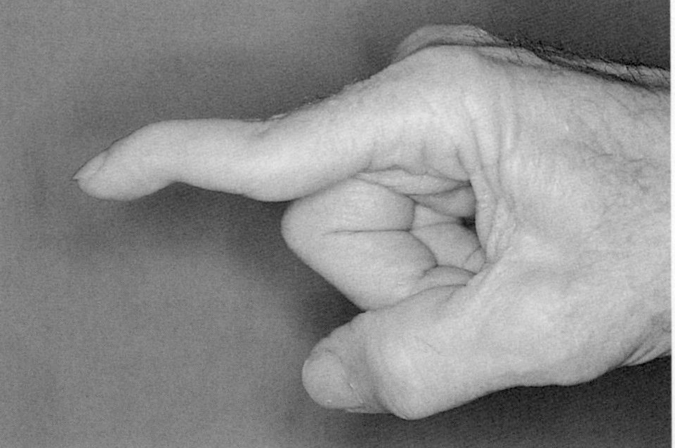

B

FIGURE 2.8-3. Boutonniere (A) and swan neck (B) deformities of rheumatoid arthritis.

(Reproduced, with permission, from Knoop KJ, Stack LB, Storrow AB, et al. *Atlas of Emergency Medicine*, 3rd ed. New York: McGraw-Hill, 2010: 384-385. Photo contributors: E. Lee Edstrom, MD and Cathleen M. Vossler, MD.)

TABLE 2.8-3. Common Serology of Rheumatologic Conditions

	Antibody	HLA
SLE	Anti-ds (60–70%) (indicates disease activity) Anti-SM (Smith) (25%) Anticardiolipin Lupus anticoagulant	DR2, DR3
DIL	Antihistone (sensitive, use to rule out DIL)	DR3
Sjögren's	Anti-SSA(Ro) Anti-SSB(La)	
Ankylosing spondylitis		B27
Reiter's		B27
MCTD		Anti-U_1 RNP
Poly/dermatomyositis	Anti-Jo (polymyositis) Anti-Mi2 (dermatomyositis) Anti-PM1	DR3
Systemic sclerosis	Anti-topoisomerase-1 (SCL-70) Antinucleolar	
CREST	Anticentromere	
RA	Rheumatoid factor	DR4 (associated with severe disease)
Behçet's		B5

CREST, calcinosis, Raynaud's phenomenon, esophageal dysmotility, sclerodactyly, and telangiectasia; DIL, drug-induced lupus; MCTD, mixed connective tissue disease; RA, rheumatoid arthritis.

Laboratory

- Rheumatoid factor (RF) is ⊕ in 80% of patients with RA.
- Anticyclic citrullinated peptide (anti-CCP): Sensitivity 50–75%; specificity 90–95%.
- Anemia of chronic disease.
- Elevated erythrocyte sedimentation rate (ESR).
- X-ray: Soft tissue swelling, juxta-articular osteopenia, subluxation, erosion.

Rheumatoid arthritis: Pain improves with use. **Osteoarthritis:** Pain worsens with use.

Treatment

- Once diagnosis is established, treatment with disease-modifying antirheumatic drugs (DMARDs; Table 2.8-4) should be initiated. DMARDs have been shown to slow or even reverse joint damage. They should be started within 3 months of diagnosis.
- NSAIDs, glucocorticoid injections, and/or low-dose steroids for symptomatic relief.
- Physical therapy to maintain strength and range of motion.

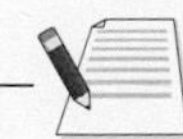

OA can cause morning stiffness but is it usually short-lived (in contrast to RA).

OA affects the **O**uter joints on the hand—the DIPs. RA affects the inner joints—MCPs and PIPs.

OA is not a systemic inflammatory disease; therefore, lab studies should be normal.

If the WBC count is low in an RA patient, think of **Felty's syndrome:**
- Rheumatoid arthritis
- Splenomegaly
- Leukopenia

TABLE 2.8-4. Disease-Modifying Antirheumatic Drugs (DMARDs)

Drugs	Toxicity	Monitoring Parameters
Methotrexate	Stomatitis, pneumonitis, hepatic fibrosis, marrow suppression	Blood counts (CBC), liver function tests
Leflunamide	Gastrointestinal disturbances, alopecia, mouth ulcers	Blood counts, liver function tests
Minocycline	Skin pigmentation (brown-black)	None
Gold	Rash, stomatitis, marrow suppression, proteinuria	CBC, urinalysis
Hydroxychloroquine	Retinal toxicity	Eye exam
Sulfasalazine	Marrow suppression, hepatitis	Blood counts, liver function tests
Cyclosporine	Hypertension, hirsutism, gingival hyperplasia, nephrotoxicity	Blood pressure, renal function
Azathioprine	Marrow suppression, hepatitis	CBC

Systemic Lupus Erytematosus (SLE)

- A chronic inflammatory disease that can affect virtually every organ system, including kidney, skin, joints, lungs, central nervous system (CNS).
- Classified as an autoimmune disorder with elaboration of characteristic autoantibodies.
- Can present with overlapping rheumatologic syndromes (though 90% have skin and joint involvement).
- Associated with HLA-DR2 and -DR3.

Epidemiology

- Female-to-male ratio: 9:1.
- People of African descent > whites.
- More common in African-Americans.

Signs and Symptoms

- Fever, fatigue, weight loss.
- Anemia (often Coombs' ⊕).
- Alopecia.
- Arthralgias (symmetric).
- Photosensitive rash.
- Raynaud's phenomenon.
- Serositis (pleuritic, pericarditis).
- Nephritis/nephrotic syndrome.
- Recurrent abortions (antiphospholipid syndrome).
- Purpura.

DIAGNOSIS

American College of Rheumatology (ACR) criteria: ≥ 4 of the following at any given time (sensitivity and specificity ~ 96%; mnemonic: **MD SOAP BRAIN**):

- Malar rash: "Butterfly" distribution; spares nasolabial folds.
- Discoid rash: Raised erythematous patches; scaling; may scar.
- Serositis: Pleuritis/pericarditis.
- Oral ulcers: Usually painless.
- Arthritis, systemic, more than two joints.
- Photosensitivity.
- Blood disorder: Any cell line can be affected.
- Renal disorder: Multiple types.
- Antinuclear antibody (ANA).
- Immunologic disorder: Autoantibodies, false-⊕ syphilis tests (rapid plasma reagin [RPR], Venereal Disease Research Laboratory [VDRL]).
- Neurologic disorder: Seizures, psychosis, "lupus cerebritis."

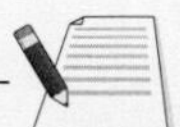

Ultraviolet light causes flare-ups, so many SLE patients are sensitive to sunlight.

LABS

- Autoantibodies:
  - **ANA**—present in about 95%.
  - **Anti-Smith (Sm)**—specific for SLE.
  - **Anti-dsDNA**—specific; associated with renal disease if high.
  - **Anticardiolipin** and **lupus anticoagulant**—associated with recurrent fetal loss, thrombocytopenia, heart disease; congenital heart block in the fetus. (*Note:* Lupus anticoagulant is a misnomer—it is a prothrombotic state, though it paradoxically causes an elevated partial thromboplastin time.)
- Flares can be associated with transaminitis, anemia, elevated ESR, proteinuria, hematuria, and granular casts in urine, Low complement C3, C4.

TREATMENT

- Avoid stress or medical procedure/surgery during flare (exacerbates SLE).
- NSAIDs.
- Antimalarials (chloroquines): Improves skin rash and arthritis.
- Glucocorticoids with severe disease/end-organ damage.
- Steroid-sparing threapy: Cyclophosphamide/azathioprine reserved for severe disease.
- Avoid drugs known to cause SLE-like syndrome.

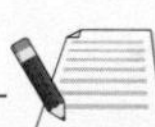

SLE mean survival rate (from diagnosis):

- 85% at 5 years
- 80% at 10 years
- 75% at 20 years

PROGNOSIS

- **Poorer prognosis:**
  - Hypocomplementemia C3, C4.
  - ⊕ anti-dsDNA.
  - Nephritis/nephrotic syndrome.
  - Hypoalbuminemia.
  - Cr > 1.5.
- **Better prognosis:** ⊕ antiU_1RNP.

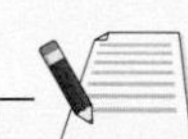

An SLE patient has arthritic pain despite being on NSAIDs. **Next step:** Start hydroxychloroquine.

Drug-Induced Lupus (DIL)

An entity distinct from SLE—it is an idiopathic reaction to certain drugs. Distinguished by:

- Complete resolution of disease once offending drug is discontinued.
- Presence of serum antihistone antibodies (very sensitive).
- Lack of renal or CNS involvement.

> ***Drugs associated with DIL–***
>
> ***H&P, IQ CAMP***
>
> **H**ydralazine
> **P**rocainamide
> **I**soniazid
> **Q**uinidine
> **C**hlorpromazine
> **A**lpha-interferon
> **M**ethyldopa
> **P**enicillamine
>
> Take H&P. If you're smart (in the high IQ CAMP), you'll discontinue these drugs in patients with a malar rash.

Etiology

- Procainamide: Most common offender—used in the treatment of atrial fibrillation in patients with Wolff-Parkinson-White syndrome.
- Hydralazine: Second most common offender—used to treat preeclampsia.
- Isoniazid: Used to treat tuberculosis (TB).
- Quinidine: Used to treat malaria and leg cramps.
- Methyldopa: Old antihypertensive drug, still used in obstetrics.
- Chlorpromazine: Antiemetic also associated with dystonic reactions.
- Penicillamine: Used to treat Wilson's disease.
- Alpha-interferon: Experimental, used to treat multiple sclerosis (MS) and other autoimmune and viral conditions.

Treatment

- Discontinue the offending drug.
- Supportive therapy.
- May need steroids for severe cases.

Scleroderma (Systemic Sclerosis)

An autoimmune disorder characterized by widespread small vessel fibrosis secondary to overproduction of collagen and other extracellular matrix proteins.

Signs and Symptoms

- Raynaud's phenomenon (vasospasm of arteries in hands in response to cold or emotional stress, resulting in discoloration of hands).
- Thickened, tight skin.
- Nailfold capillaries—giant loops formed by abnormal capillaries at nailfold.
- Dysphagia due to esophageal fibrosis especially the lower two-thirds.
- Renal artery fibrosis.
- Pulmonary hypertension and pulmonary fibrosis.
- Telangiectasias.
- Cardiac conduction disease/pericardial effusion.
- In the limited form of scleroderma, symptoms are generally limited to the **CREST syndrome:**
  - Calcinosis (calcium deposition forming nodules)
  - Raynaud's phenomenon
  - Esophageal dysmotility
  - Sclerodactyly (stiffness of skin of fingers)
  - Telangiectasias

Laboratory

- ANA ⊕ in 95%.
- Anti SCl-70 (topoisomerase antibody).
- Antibody to centromere—specific to CREST variant.

- Antibody to nucleolar Ag.
- Normochromic, normocytic anemia.
- Elevated ESR.
- ↓ vital capacity on pulmonary function tests (restrictive lung disease). May get ↓ DL_{CO} if pulmonary fibrosis.

TREATMENT

- Penicillamine—may inhibit collagen cross-linking.
- Captopril—helps control the renal hypertension.
- Calcium channel blockers—diminish the Raynaud's phenomenon.
- Steroids—rarely effective in altering the disease course.

Sarcoidosis

- A systemic illness with no known cause, primarily affecting the lungs.
- Characterized by noncaseating granulomas.
- More common among blacks and women.

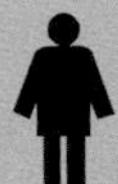

A 40-year-old black woman presents with dyspnea, malaise, visual disturbances, and a rash. Chest x-ray shows bilateral hilar adenopathy. *Think: Sarcoidosis.*

SIGNS AND SYMPTOMS

Almost any part of the body can be affected. Some typical extrapulmonary findings are:

- Skin—erythema nodosum (erythematous nodes on extensor surfaces of lower extremities, also seen in other conditions), lupus pernio on the face.
- Kidney—hypercalciuria (macrophages ↑ metabolism of vitamin D to 1,25-dihydroxyvitamin D).
- Eyes—uveitis (inflammation of uveal tract, iris, ciliary body, choroid).
- Cardiac—conduction defects.
- Nervous—Bell's palsy (self-limited 7th nerve palsy of unknown etiology).
- Lofgren's syndrome—triad of erythema nodosa, arthritis, and bilateral hilar lymphadenopathy (good prognosis).

STAGING

I: Bilateral hilar adenopathy.
II: Hilar adenopathy plus lung parenchymal involvement.
III: Lung parenchymal involvement alone.
IV: Pulmonary fibrosis.

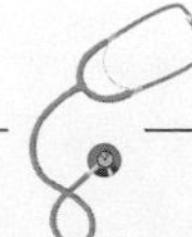

In sarcoidosis, remember, when you go from stage II to stage III, you actually lose the hilar adenopathy.

DIAGNOSIS

Requires transbronchial biopsy to prove existence **of noncaseating granulomas,** but not sufficient on its own to make diagnosis; requires clinical, laboratory, and radiographic adjuncts.

LABORATORY

Diagnosis cannot be made or excluded on the basis of laboratory findings alone. Common laboratory findings include:

- Lymphocytosis on bronchoalveolar lavage.
- Eosinophilia.
- False-⊕ RF and ANA.
- Elevated angiotensin-converting enzyme (ACE).
- Skin anergy to common antigens.
- **Kveim test:** Splenic tissue from a patient known to have sarcoidosis is injected intradermally to the patient being tested. The test is ⊕ if the patient develops a granulomatous reaction at the site and biopsy shows noncaseating granulomas.
- Elevated 24-hour urine calcium.
- Chest x-ray shows **bilateral hilar adenopathy** and perihilar calcifications (see Figure 2.8-4).
- Elevated ESR.

TREATMENT

Corticosteroids.

PROGNOSIS

- Most patients have resolution of their disease within 2 years.
- Death from pulmonary failure occurs in a minority of patients.

Sjögren's Syndrome

A lymphocytic infiltrate in salivary and lacrimal glands, causing ↓ secretions from these glands, usually in association with other rheumatological diseases (eg, RA).

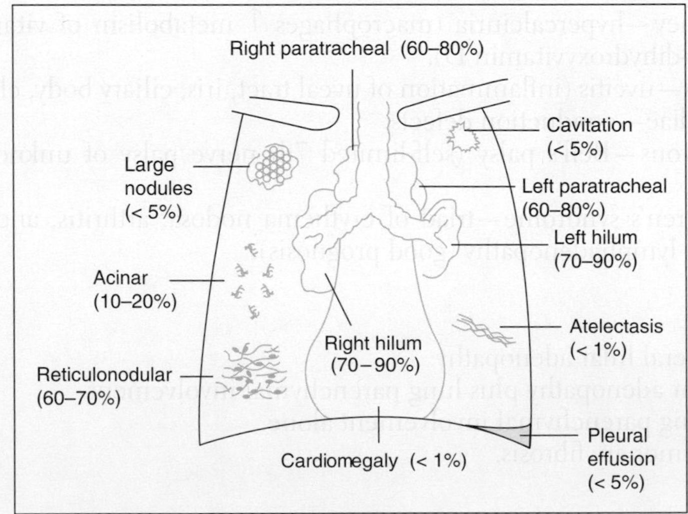

FIGURE 2.8-4. Abnormal CXR findings in sarcoidosis.

(Reproduced, with permission, from Fauci AS et al. [eds.]. *Harrison's Principles of Internal Medicine,* 14th ed. New York: McGraw-Hill, 1998: 1925.)

ETIOLOGY

- Autoimmune.
- Found in many with coexisting connective tissue diseases (any).

SIGNS AND SYMPTOMS

- Dry mouth, dry eyes (keratoconjuctivitis sicca).
- Can have any symptoms associated with other connective tissue disorders.

LABS

- ⊕ RF in 90%.
- ⊕ ANA in 70%.
- ⊕ La (SS_B) and Ro (SS_A).
- DR3 association.

DIAGNOSIS

- Biopsy of minor salivary glands would show sialadenitis with lymphocytic infiltration.
- Schirmer's test.
- Typical symptoms.

TREATMENT

- Treat symptoms with artificial tears, sialogogues (ie, sucking candies that increase saliva production). May use cyclosporine eye drops.
- Corticosteroids.

PROGNOSIS

Risk of lymphoma > 40%.

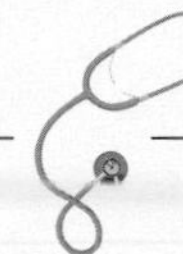

Both polymyositis and dermatomyositis are more common in women.

Seronegative arthritis—

PAIR

Psoriatic
Ankylosing spondylitis
Inflammatory bowel disease
Reiter's syndrome

Polymyositis and Dermatomyositis

- Connective tissue disease causing proximal muscle weakness.
- Associated with HLA-DR3.
- Dermatomyositis has similar manifestations to polymyositis plus skin involvement.

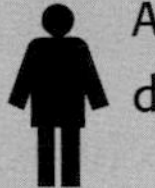

A 57-year-old woman complains of difficulty getting out of a chair and difficulty combing her hair. *Think: Polymyositis.*

ETIOLOGY

Unknown; many viruses implicated (coxsackie, influenza).

SIGNS AND SYMPTOMS

- Weakness first occurring in legs.
- Difficulty with squatting, kneeling, rising from chair, climbing stairs.
- Dysphagia, dysphonia.

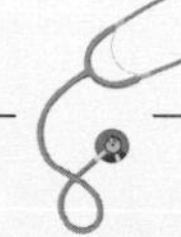

Polymyositis and dermatomyositis can be distinguished from myasthenia gravis by the lack of ocular involvement (ptosis).

- Abnormal ECG (with advanced disease).
- With dermatomyositis: Purple-red papular/scaly photosensitive rash on face, neck ("V sign," "shawl sign"); erythema, scaling on extensor surfaces of joints (Gottron's papules; very specific); periorbital edema, heliotropic rash.

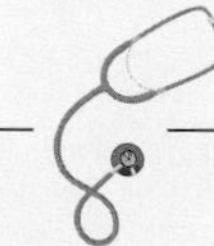

The rash of dermatomyositis involves the upper eyelids; the rash of SLE does not.

DIAGNOSIS

Four criteria:

1. Muscle weakness.
2. ↑ creatine phosphokinase (CPK)/aldolase.
3. Muscle biopsy showing T-cell infiltrate with myonecrosis.
4. Electromyogram (EMG) shows myopathy: Increased spontaneous activity, with low amplitude, short duration myopathic potentials on voluntary activation.

LABS

- ⊕ ANA.
- Elevated CPK, lactic dehydrogenase (LDH), aspartate transaminase (AST), aldolase.
- ESR is elevated in only ~50% of cases.
- One-third have **myositis-specific antibodies:**
  - **Anti-Jo**: One-third with pure myositis.
  - **Anti-Mi2**: Dermatomyositis specific.
  - **Anti-PM1.**
- CXR may show interstitial pulmonary disease.

Ankylosing spondylitis:
- Anterior uveitis
- Apical lung fibrosis
- Aortitis
- Aortic insufficiency
- Atrioventricular conduction defect
- Amyloidosis
- Achilles entesopathy

TREATMENT

- Glucocorticoids (for polymyositis or dermatomyositis): 80% respond within 6 weeks.
- If poor response to glucocorticoids, high suspicion of malignancy.
- Methotrexate, azathioprine if steroid resistant.

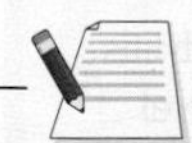

Both azathioprine and methotrexate suppress the bone marrow. Azathioprine is also hepatotoxic.

PROGNOSIS

- Approximately 15% have malignancy, especially with dermatomyositis.
- Insidious, progressive disease.

SERONEGATIVE ARTHRITIDES

- Includes ankylosing spondylitis, psoriatic arthritis, ulcerative colitis, and Reiter's syndrome.
- Many (not all) associated with HLA-B27 genotype.
- Unlike SLE, RA, and scleroderma, these have *asymmetric* arthritis and often have spinal involvement (sacroiliitis, spondylitis).

Ankylosing Spondylitis

Chronic systemic inflammatory disorder affecting primarily the axial skeleton, but can affect multiple organs.

SIGNS AND SYMPTOMS

- Peak onset of symptoms between ages 20 and 30.
- Affects men to women 3:1.
- Low back pain with reduced range of motion most common presenting symptom.
- Worse at night, better with exercise/worse with inactivity.
- Spinal ankylosis is a late manifestation of the disease.
- Highly variable disease course (may be self-limiting with spontaneous remission).
- Extra-articular involvement: Uveitis, neurological symptoms, pulmonary, renal, genitourinary (GU) abnormalities, gastrointestinal (GI), cardiac.

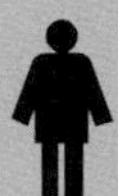

A young man presents with stiffness in the lower back that improves with exercise. *Think: Ankylosing spondylitis.*

DIAGNOSIS

- Pelvic radiograph: Sacroiliitis is the hallmark of ankylosing spondylitis.
- Osteitis and bone erosions at sites of osseous attachment of ligaments and tendons (enthesopathy).
- Spine radiograph: Syndesmophytes—vertical bridging between vertebrae and ossification of spinal ligaments seen in late disease ("bamboo spine"; see Figure 2.8-5).
- Elevated ESR, C-reactive protein (CRP).
- HLA-B27.

TREATMENT

- Exercise/physical therapy.
- Smoking cessation: Ankylosing spondylitis patients may develop costochondritis with restrictive pulmonary problems, worsened by development of chronic obstructive pulmonary disease (COPD).
- Avoid falls (high risk of vertebral fracture and cauda equina syndrome).
- NSAIDs.
- For advanced disease, sulfasalazine, DMARDs, and newer drugs such as anti–tumor necrosis factor therapy are being utilized.

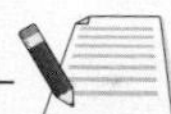

The brittle spine of ankylosing spondylitis is prone to fracture even with minimal trauma. Patients should be restricted from high-risk activities such as skydiving, bungee jumping, and contact sports.

Reactive Arthritis

An HLA-B27-associated syndrome involving the musculoskeletal, genitourinary, and ocular systems. Occurs in two forms:

1. Sexually transmitted (1–2 weeks after exposure); more common in men.
2. Post-dysentery (most commonly due to *Salmonella, Shigella, Yersinia*, and *Campylobacter*); more common in women and children.

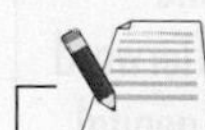

Reactive arthritis: "Can't see, can't pee, can't climb a tree."

SIGNS AND SYMPTOMS

- Conjunctivitis.
- Urethritis/cervicitis.
- Arthritis: Asymmetric, lower extremities.
- Oral ulcerations.
- Balanitis.

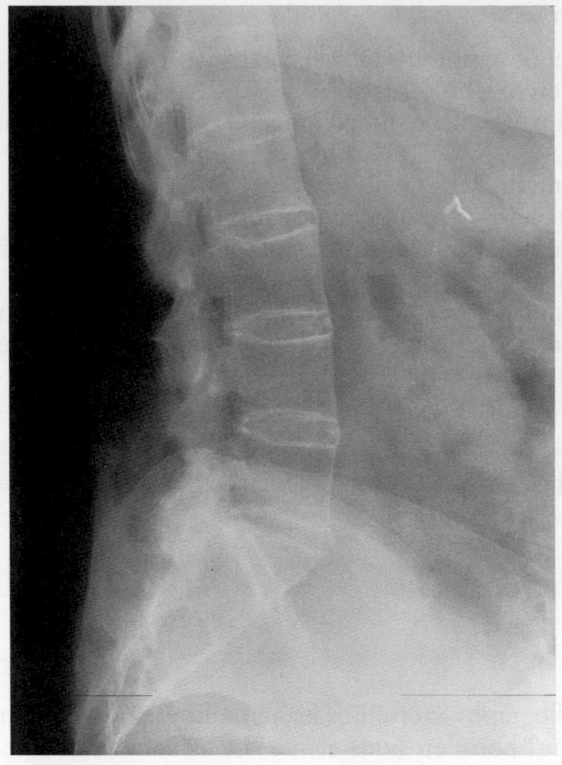

FIGURE 2.8-5. Bamboo spine of ankylosing spondylitis.

Note the bridging syndesmophytes. (Reproduced, with permission, from Wilson FC, Lin PP. *General Orthopedics.* New York: McGraw-Hill, 1997: 454.)

Laboratory

- Elevated ESR.
- Urethral culture may reveal *Chlamydia trachomatis.*

Treatment

- NSAIDs for arthritis.
- Doxycycline for urethritis/cervicitis.

Behçet's Syndrome

Autoimmune disease associated with HLA-B5, characterized by oral and genital ulceration and eye symptoms.

Behçet's syndrome: "Though I enjoyed the experience, I was afterward *beset* with oral and genital ulcers."

Signs and Symptoms

- Aphthous (oral) ulcers
- Genital ulcers
- Deep vein thrombophlebitis
- Arthritis (nondeforming)
- Uveitis
- Colitis
- Psychiatric disturbances

DIAGNOSIS

Must have recurrent oral ulcers plus two of the following:

- Recurrent genital ulcers.
- Eye lesions.
- Skin lesions.
- ⊕ pathergy test: Abnormal inflammatory skin reaction to scratch or intradermal saline injection.

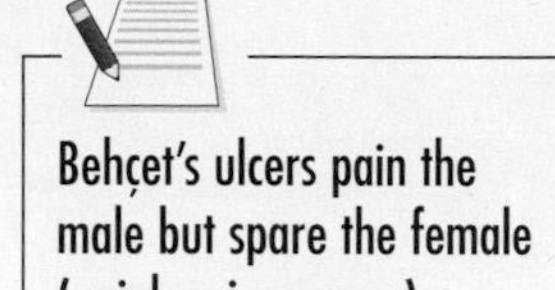

Behçet's ulcers pain the male but spare the female (painless in women).

LABORATORY

- Elevated ESR.
- Hypergammaglobulinemia.
- Cryoglobulinemia.
- **Pathergy test:** Inflammatory reaction of skin to any scratches.

TREATMENT

- Colchicine or interferon-α for arthritis.
- Aspirin or antiplatelet agents for thrombophlebitis.
- Steroids for uveitis and CNS manifestations.

Gonococcal Septic Arthritis

A disseminated gonococcal infection; more common in women than men.

ETIOLOGY

- *Neisseria gonorrhoeae.*
- More likely during pregnancy and menstruation.

SIGNS AND SYMPTOMS

- After 1–4 days of a **migratory polyarthritis,** 60% of patients develop a tenosynovitis and 40% a purulent monarthritis.
- Patients will sometimes have fever but, surprisingly, urethritis is rarely seen.
- Most patients develop a characteristic skin lesion—**small necrotic pustules**—over their extremities, usually the fingers and toes.

DIAGNOSIS

- Synovial fluid shows elevated WBCs.
- Gram stain and blood culture are ⊕ in < 50% of cases.
- Joint cultures are usually ⊖.

TREATMENT

- Very sensitive to antibiotic therapy (eg, ceftriaxone).
- Surgical drainage is not usually necessary.

VASCULITIS

Polyarteritis Nodosa (PAN)

Systemic necrotizing vasculitis of small and medium-sized muscular arteries.

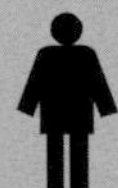

A 50-year-old woman complains of abdominal pain, fever, and joint pains. On lab work she is found to have acute renal failure with RBC casts in the urine. *Think: PAN (multisystem involvement).* **Next step:** Angiography. Biopsy shows characteristic vasculitis.

Signs and Symptoms

- Nonspecific symptoms predominate: Fever, weight loss, malaise.
- Specific symptoms depend on organ involved. Most common ones are:
  - Glomerulonephritis, arthritis, mononeuritis multiplex.
  - Other systems that may be involved are GI, skin, cardiac, GU, and CNS. Note conspicuous absence of pulmonary involvement.

Laboratory

- Red cell casts in urine.
- One-third of patients have hepatitis B antigenemia.
- Diagnosis is made by tissue biopsy of affected organ.

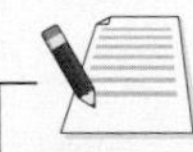

PAN—spares the lungs. **Churg-Strauss**—lung symptoms predominate.

Treatment

- Prednisone.
- Cyclophosphamide.

Churg-Strauss Disease

Medium-vessel arteritis, also known as allergic angiitis and granulomatosis; it is very similar to PAN except that the pulmonary findings predominate.

Signs and Symptoms

- Bronchospasm (asthma).
- Eosinophilia.
- Fever.
- Erythematous maculopapular rashes, palpable purpura, and cutaneous nodules.
- Red casts in urine.

Treatment

Steroids; if steroids fail, consider azathioprine and cyclophosphamide.

Wegener's Granulomatosis

Chronically relapsing small-artery vasculitis of upper and lower respiratory tracts and glomerulonephritis.

SIGNS AND SYMPTOMS

- Kidney: Glomerulonephritis.
- Lungs: Hemoptysis, pulmonary infiltrates.
- Nasopharynx: Sinusitis, otitis.
- Arthralgias/arthritis.
- Fever.
- Weight loss.

DIAGNOSIS

- Granulomatous vasculitis on lung biopsy.
- ⊕ circulating antineutrophil cytoplasmic antibody (c-ANCA) titer.
- Exclusion of Goodpasture's syndrome, tumors, and infectious disease.

TREATMENT

Steroids, cyclophosphamide.

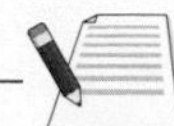

Goodpasture's is the other disease that involves both lungs and kidney. Its triad is:

- Glomerulonephritis
- Pulmonary hemorrhage
- Anti-GBM Ab

Takayasu's Arteritis

- An arteritis of unknown (possibly autoimmune) etiology that is seen commonly in young people of Asian descent.
- Usually affects medium and large-sized arteries.
- More common in women.

SIGNS AND SYMPTOMS

- Loss of pulses in arms and carotids bilaterally.
- Raynaud's phenomenon.
- Signs of transient brain ischemia such as blindness and hemiplegia.
- Abdominal pain, atypical chest pain.

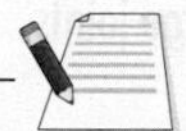

Takayasu's is also called *pulseless disease* and *aortic arch syndrome.*

DIAGNOSIS

- Arteriography shows narrowing of aorta +/– aneurysm.
- Magnetic resonance angiography (MRA) is helpful if arteriography is not available.

TREATMENT

- Steroids
- Methotrexate

Temporal Arteritis (Giant Cell Arteritis)

Inflammation of medium and large-sized arteries, commonly the temporal artery. See the Neurology chapter.

JOINT DISORDERS

Gout

- Inflammation and severe joint pain (arthralgia) secondary to urate crystal deposition.
- Caused by either overproduction or underexcretion of uric acid.

EPIDEMIOLOGY

- Men > women.
- Typical age of onset: 45.
- For serum urate > 9–10 mg/dL, incidence of attack 5%/year.

ETIOLOGY

- ↑ production of uric acid:
  - Idiopathic.
  - Leukemia/tumor lysis syndrome.
  - Hemolytic anemia.
  - Strenuous exercise.
  - Excessive fructose ingestion.
  - Glucose-6-phosphate dehydrogenase (G6PD) deficiency.
  - Lesch-Nyhan syndrome.
  - High-protein diet.
  - Nicotinic acid.
- ↓ excretion:
  - Aspirin
  - Chronic renal disease
  - Lead nephropathy
  - EtOH ingestion
  - DKA
  - Thiazide diuretics

Gout: *Small* joints, ⊖ birefringence, needle-shaped
Pseudogout: *Large* joints (eg, knee), ⊕ birefringence, rhomboid-shaped

SIGNS AND SYMPTOMS

- Rapid onset of extreme joint pain and swelling.
- Fifty percent of first attacks are in the great toe (podagra; see Figure 2.8-6).
- **Tophi:** Aggregates of urate crystals and giant cells, which may cause tissue erosion.

Fifty percent of first gout attacks involve first metatarsophalangeal joint.

DIAGNOSIS

- **Joint aspirate:**
  - Negatively birefringent needle-shaped urate crystals in joint aspirate.
  - Large number of PMNs (5000–7000).
  - ↓ viscosity of joint fluid (low hyaluronate).
- **Labs:**
  - ↑ WBC count, proteinuria, elevated ESR, elevated uric acid, isosthenuria.
  - Twenty-four-hour urinary uric acid level: > 750 mg indicates overproducer.

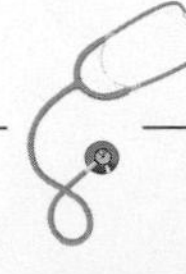

Aspirin is *contraindicated* in acute gout because it ↓ urate excretion.

TREATMENT

- **Acute attack:**
  - Colchicine: May be poorly tolerated secondary to GI effects, cytopenias.
  - NSAIDs, particularly indomethacin.
  - Steroids can be used if NSAIDS or colchicine are contraindicated.
- **Chronic:**
  - Initiate allopurinol and/or probenecid treatment only after acute attack is resolved; otherwise, may prolong or worsen attack.
  - Allopurinol: Use in overproducers and those with renal insufficiency.
  - Probenecid, sulfinpyrazone, uricosurics: ↑ excretion of uric acid. Do not use in patients with chronic renal insufficiency.

A man comes in with swollen, painful joint. What is the first step? Joint fluid aspiration and analysis.

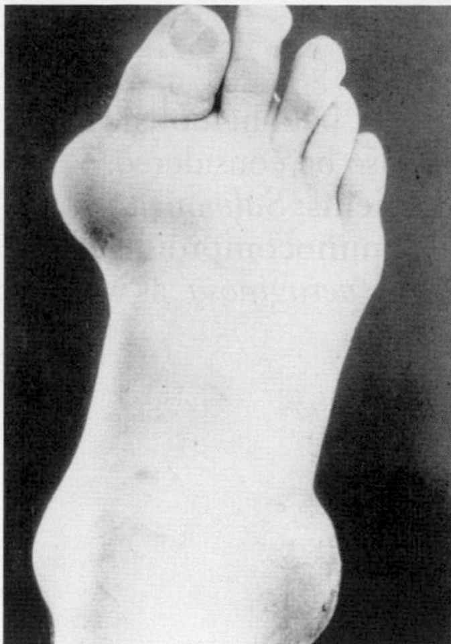

FIGURE 2.8-6. Podagra.

(Reproduced, with permission, from Fauci AS et al. [eds.]. *Harrison's Principles of Internal Medicine*, 14th ed. New York: McGraw-Hill, 1998: 2162.)

Pseudogout

Deposition of calcium pyrophosphate dihydrate (CPPD) crystals in joint spaces causing chondrocalcinosis.

Etiology

- Acute inflammatory reaction to the deposition of CPPD in joint spaces.
- Changes related to age that make the synovial fluid environment more hospitable to CPPD growth.
- Associated with hemochromatosis, hypothyroidism, hyperparathyroidism, diabetes mellitus.

Signs and Symptoms/Diagnosis

- Similar to gout: Affected joints are painful and red.
- Unlike gout:
  - Large joints are affected (knees, wrists, shoulder).
  - The crystals are rhomboid (gouty crystals are needle-shaped).
  - Radiographs demonstrate calcification in the articular cartilage.
  - There is ⊕ **birefringence** of crystals.

Treatment

- NSAIDs can alleviate symptoms.
- Aspirating synovial fluid shortens the duration of the attacks.
- No therapy is available to remove CPPD crystals.

Nongonococcal Septic Arthritis

- Nongonococcal septic arthritis is seen when there is previous joint damage or bacteremia.
- It is monarticular and affects the large joints (knee, hip, shoulder, and wrist).

ETIOLOGY

- **Young adults:**
  - *Staphylococcus aureus*, beta-hemolytic strep, and gram-⊖ bacilli.
  - Lyme disease must also be considered.
- **Sickle cell anemia patients:** *Salmonella* and *S aureus* (equal).
- **IV drug users and immunocompromised:** Gram-⊖ organisms such as *E coli* and *Pseudomonas aeruginosa*, as well as *S aureus*.

RISK FACTORS

- Rheumatoid arthritis
- Prosthetic joints
- Immunodeficiency
- Age
- IV drug abuse

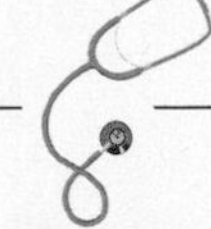

Nongonococcal septic arthritis: Patients will often describe previous **trauma** to the joint.

SIGNS AND SYMPTOMS

- Pain, swelling, and warmth over the joint.
- Limited range of motion.
- Fever.

DIAGNOSIS

- Blood cultures are ⊕ in 50% of cases.
- ESR and CRP will be elevated.
- Gram stain can pick up 75% of *S aureus* infections.
- **Arthrocentesis** is both diagnostic and therapeutic. Joint fluid will reveal an elevated white count (need > 50,000–100,000 cells/mm³), predominantly polymorphonucleocytes and a low glucose level. The arthrocentesis releases fluid, thereby lowering pressure within the joint capsule and alleviating pain. Arthrocentesis should be avoided if the overlying skin is infected or if there is bacteremia because the procedure introduces a portal of entry for bacteria into the joint.

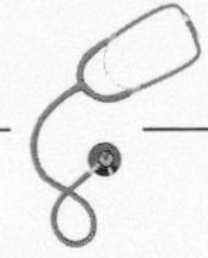

IV drug abuser with septic joint: Must do echo to rule out endocarditis.

TREATMENT

- Systemic antibiotics.
- Serial arthrocentesis may be necessary if synovial fluid rapidly accumulates.
- Surgical drainage is needed for septic hip and for septic joints that do not improve with intravenous antibiotics within 72 hours.

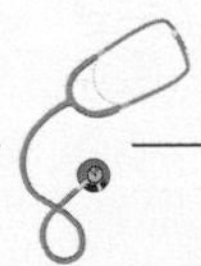

Arthrocentesis should never be attempted in hemophiliacs until the clotting disorder is corrected with the appropriate blood product.

Avascular Necrosis (AVN) of the Hip

The limited blood supply to the head of the femur makes this site particularly vulnerable to AVN.

ETIOLOGY

Seen with a variety of conditions such as trauma, long-term steroid therapy, excessive radiation, alcoholism, sickle cell disease, and Gaucher's disease.

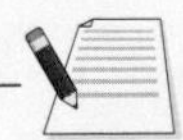

AVN of the hip in children is called Legg-Calvé-Perthes disease.

SIGNS AND SYMPTOMS

Pain, often referred to the **knee**, exacerbated by internal rotation of the hip.

DIAGNOSIS

MRI or bone scan is needed for early detection of the disease. Plain radiographs will be ⊕ only in the late stage.

TREATMENT

Total hip replacement.

Costochondritis

Painful swelling of the costochondral articulations at the anterior chest wall. Chest pain often confused with pulmonary embolism or myocardial infarction.

ETIOLOGY

Associated with:

- Recent upper respiratory tract infection.
- Trauma.
- Overuse.

SIGNS AND SYMPTOMS

- Typically affects the second through fifth costochondral joints.
- Pain is sharp, worse with deep breathing and movement; may radiate to the shoulders and arms.
- Pain is reproducible with palpation.

DIAGNOSIS

Diagnosis is clinical. Can do a chest x-ray to look for metastatic lesions to the sternal bone marrow, which can produce similar symptoms; however, chest x-ray is usually normal.

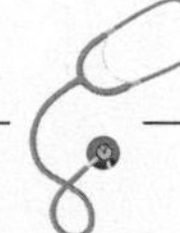

In patients with risk factors for MI, be sure to obtain ECG.

TREATMENT

- NSAIDs.
- Avoid overuse of muscles.

Carpal Tunnel Syndrome

- Painful compression of the median nerve as it passes through the carpal tunnel (see Figure 2.8-7).
- More common in women.

ETIOLOGY

- Anything that ↑ pressure within the carpal tunnel can cause it.
- Most common causes are trauma to carpal bones and flexor tenosynovitis.
- Can be secondary to systemic illnesses such as RA, sarcoidosis, acromegaly, hypothyroidism, diabetes.

SIGNS AND SYMPTOMS

- Muscle weakness and atrophy—mostly in the thenar eminence.
- **Phalen's sign:** Presence of paraesthesias along median nerve distribution after holding wrist flexed at 90 degrees for 30 seconds.
- **Tinel's sign:** Pain radiating down the fingers following percussion over the carpal tunnel.

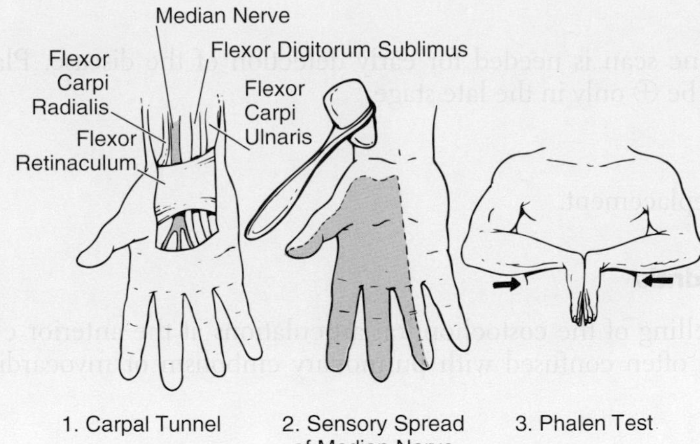

FIGURE 2.8-7. Carpal tunnel syndrome.

1. The flexor retinaculum in the wrist compresses the median nerve to produce hypoesthesia in the radial 3½ digits. 2. Percussion on the radial side of the palmaris longus tendon produces tingling in the 3½ digital region (Tinel's sign). 3. Phalen test. Hyperflexion of the wrist for 60 seconds may produce pain in the median nerve distribution; this is relieved by extension of the wrist. (Reproduced, with permission, from DeGowin DL, Brown DD. *DeGowin's Diagnostic Examination*, 7th ed. New York: McGraw-Hill, 2000: 720.)

TREATMENT

- Rest with wrist splint worn as much as possible and elevation of the hand to reduce inflammation.
- Steroids injected into carpal tunnel are suitable for temporary situations.
- Surgical division of the flexor retinaculum.

HIGH-YIELD FACTS IN

Neurology

STROKE

Abrupt onset of new neurologic deficits (see Table 2.9-1) caused by cerebrovascular disease, which can be ischemic or hemorrhagic in nature.

Types of Stroke

- **Stroke:** Cerebral vascular event resulting in infarcted cerebral tissue, regardless of the presence or absence of neurologic deficits.
- **Stroke in evolution:** Neurologic deficits continue to fluctuate or ↑ over time.
- **Completed stroke:** Neurologic deficits have remained stable for 24–72 hours.
- **Transient ischemic attack (TIA):** Neurologic deficit resolving completely in 24 hours (usually within 30 minutes) and resulting in no apparent infarcted tissue on magnetic resonance imaging (MRI).
- **Crescendo TIAs:** Two or more TIAs within 24 hours—highly predictive of impending stroke, constitutes a medical emergency.

Common Stroke Sequelae

- **Anosognosia:** The inability to identify body dysfunction—patients are unaware of their neurological deficits. From the Greek *nosos* (disease), *gnosis* (knowledge).
- **Aphasia:** A defect in comprehension or expression of spoken or written language.
- **Broca's aphasia:** A deficit in speech and written expression. Most typically occurs in Brodman's area 44 or 45—the left frontal region for 90% of the population (think: Broca's area = Broken expression).
- **Wernicke's aphasia:** Patients tend to articulate a fluent nonsense with natural rhythm, and comprehension is impaired. Results from injury to Brodman's area 22—posterior part of the superior temporal gyrus of dominant hemisphere. Patients are aware they are speaking, but they do not know what they are saying (Wernicke's is Wordy, Word salad).
- **Apraxia:** Disturbance in the ability to perform previously mastered motor tasks (ie, forgetting how to ride a bike = apraxia).
- **Dysarthria:** Disturbance in the articulation of speech. Possible injured areas are vast, including the trigeminal nerve motor branch (V), facial nerve (VII), glossopharyngeal nerve (IX), vagus nerve (X), and hypoglossal nerve (XII).
- **Dysphagia:** Difficulty swallowing.

Top 5 Leading Causes of Death in United States

"CORONers CAN STROKE POLEs ACCIDENTally"

1. **Coron**ary artery disease
2. **Can**cer
3. **CVA (Stroke)**
4. Chronic obstructive **"Pole"** munary disease
5. **Accident**s

Epidemiology (Sources: World Health Organization and American Stroke Association)

- **Worldwide:**
  - There were over 20.5 million strokes in 2001; 5.5 million of these were fatal.
  - High blood pressure contributes to over 12.7 million strokes.
- **United States:**
  - Stroke is the third leading cause of death, behind heart disease and cancer. It is the number one cause of long-term disability.
  - Each year, about 700,000 people suffer a stroke. About 500,000 of these are first attacks, and 200,000 are recurrent attacks.
  - At all ages, more women than men have a stroke.
  - African-Americans have a two- to threefold greater risk of ischemic stroke and are more likely to die of stroke.

TABLE 2.9-1. Neurological Deficits in Stroke

Artery Occlusion	Deficit	Other
Middle cerebral	■ Contralateral hemiparesis (face and hand more affected). ■ Contralateral hemisensory deficit. ■ Homonymous hemianopsia (blindness affecting the right or the left half of the visual fields of both eyes) opposite to occluded artery. ■ If dominant MCA affected (left side in 92–94% of people), patient will be aphasic. ■ If nondominant MCA affected, confusion, constructional apraxia, contralateral body neglect.	
Anterior cerebral (see Figure 2.9-1)	■ Contralateral weakness of leg or foot. ■ Broca's aphasia. ■ Incontinence. ■ Abulia (lack of motivation).	
Internal carotid	■ Presentation similar to MCA occlusion.	
Posterior cerebral (see Figure 2.9-2)	■ Homonymous hemianopsia of contralateral visual field (occipital cortex). ■ Other visual field defects including vertical gaze and oculomotor nerve palsy. ■ If dominant hemisphere affected, anomia (difficulty naming objects) or alexia (inability to read) may occur.	Pupillary reflexes spared.
Posterior inferior cerebellar	Clinical: Sudden onset of: ■ Nausea/vomiting. ■ Vertigo. ■ Hoarseness. ■ Ataxia. ■ Ipsilateral palate and tongue weakness. ■ Contralateral disturbance of pain and temperature sensation. ■ Dysphagia, dysarthria, and hiccup. ■ Ipsilateral Horner's syndrome (ptosis, miosis, hemianhidrosis, and apparent enophthalmos).	1. Motor system typically spared. 2. Lateral medullary (Wallenberg's) syndrome. Horner's syndrome: **HORNE** **H**—hemianhidrosis (loss of sweating). **O**—one eye (usually unilateral). **R**—relaxed eyelid (ptosis). **N**—narrow pupil (miosis). **E**—enophthalmos (sunken eyes).
Anterior inferior cerebellar	Definition: Infarction of lateral portion of pons. Clinical: ■ Ipsilateral facial weakness. ■ Gaze palsy. ■ Deafness. ■ Tinnitus.	No Horner's syndrome, dysphagia, or dysarthria.

(continued)

NEUROLOGY

TABLE 2.9-1. Neurological Deficits in Stroke *(continued)*

Artery Occlusion	Deficit	Other
Lacunar	Lenticulostriate branches of the middle cerebral artery (midbrain) become occluded as a result of chronic hypertension. ■ Symptoms may present gradually over several days. ■ CT or MRI may not detect stroke. Presentations: ■ Pure motor hemiparesis: Affecting face, arm, leg without other disturbances. ■ Pure sensory stroke: Hemisensory loss. ■ Ataxic hemiparesis: Pure motor hemiparesis combined with ataxia. ■ Clumsy hand dysarthria: Dysarthria, dysphagia, facial weakness, and weakness/clumsiness of contralateral hand.	

NEUROLOGY

Risk Factors for Ischemic Stroke—

"Ischemic strokes have only a* DASH *of tissue perfusion"

Diabetes
Atrial fibrillation
Smoking
Hypertension/
Hypercoagulability/
Hyperlipidemia/
Heart attack (recent)

- There is a high risk of a stroke within 6 years after a heart attack.
- Eight percent of ischemic strokes and 38% of hemorrhagic strokes result in death within 30 days.
  - **Ischemic penumbra:** The tissue surrounding an infarcted zone that is dysfunctional but not infarcted and that may recover full functionality if the hypoxic state resolves. The volume of the ischemic penumbra is often greater than that of the infarcted core, and thus its salvage can dramatically reduce the degree of permanent deficit.
- Almost a quarter of people who have an initial stroke die within a year.

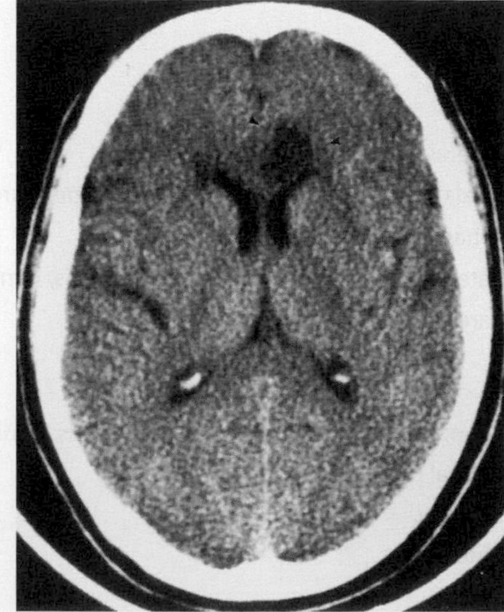

FIGURE 2.9-1. CT of ischemic stroke of the anterior cerebral artery (ACA).

Note that the lesion is hypodense. (Reproduced, with permission, from Johnson MH. CT evaluation of the earliest signs of stroke. *The Radiologist* 1(4): 89–199, 1994.)

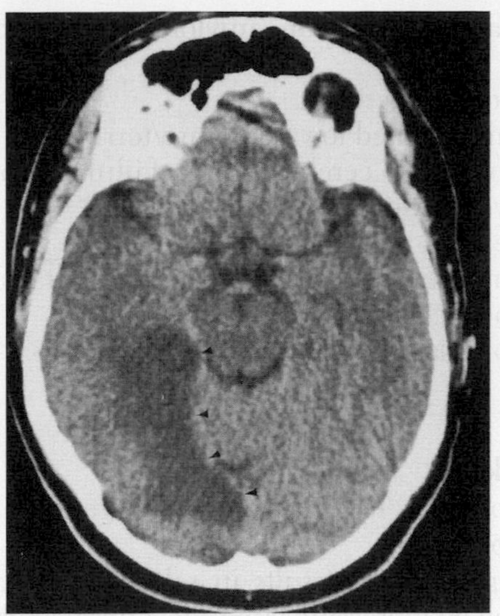

FIGURE 2.9-2. Low attenuation area within the cerebellum posteriorly on the right (arrowheads) suggestive of infarct in right PICA distribution.

Risk Factors

- **Ischemic:**
  - Hypertension (HTN)
  - Smoking
  - Diabetes mellitus (DM)
  - Dyslipidemia
  - Atrial fibrillation
  - Hypercoagulable state
  - Recent myocardial infarction (MI)
- **Hemorrhagic:**
  - Hypertension
  - Arteriovenous malformation (AVM)
  - Trauma
  - Ruptured aneurysm
  - Bleeding diathesis/anticoagulation

Classification and Etiology

- **Ischemic stroke:**
  - **Thrombotic:**
    - Large-vessel disease—atherosclerosis usually located at bifurcation of carotid, vertebrobasilar system, or middle cerebral artery. A disease process that starts with a **T** but does not Travel.
    - Small-vessel disease—microatheroma or lipohyalinosis usually due to HTN or DM, causing lacunar infarcts in subcortical tissues.
    - Similar pathophysiology to acute myocardial infarction, where a damaged vessel becomes occluded with thrombus.
  - **Embolic:** Usually of cardiac origin (60%), source often unknown, sometimes carotid (artery-to-artery embolus).
  - **Hypoperfusion:** Shock, etc.; most affect *watershed* areas (most commonly parasagittal strips of cortex).
- **Hemorrhagic stroke:**
  - **Subarachnoid:** Head trauma most common, aneurysms, AV malformations.

Risk Factors for Hemorrhagic Stroke–

"Hemorrhagic strokes leave you with a bloody HAT"

Hypertension
AVM/**A**neurysm/**A**nticoagulated
Trauma

For stroke: The strongest risk factor is **hypertension,** with **smoking** as a close second.

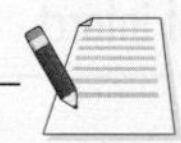

Watershed injury describes ischemic injury to brain tissue located at distal end of cerebrovascular tree, usually due to a low-flow state.

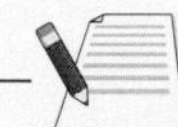

TIAs used to be defined as any stroke whose symptoms resolved completely within 24 hours. With the advent of MRI and the ability to detect "silent" infarctions, the definition has narrowed toward including only those cases with no detectable infarcts.

- **Intracerebral:** Hypertension, amyloid, bleeding disorders, trauma, tumors.
- **Metabolic stroke:**
  - Not necessarily related to vasculature/territories.
  - Usually secondary to cerebral energy failure (hypoglycemia).
  - Often resolves without deficits.
- **Venous stroke:**
  - Usually from thrombosis of cerebral veins/dural sinus.
  - Does not obey territories.
  - Often hemorrhagic.

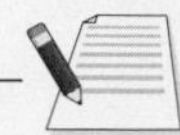
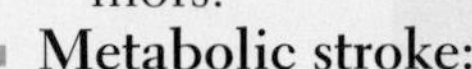

Risk of stroke after TIA:
- First month: 4–8%
- First year: 12–14%
- At 5 years: 24–29%

Pathophysiology

- **Ischemic stroke:**
  - Occlusion of artery feeding brain causes oxygen depletion and damage to neurons.
  - The ensuing ischemia results in release of inflammatory cytokines, which ↓ flow by increasing viscosity. These cytokines further damage neuronal function.
  - With reperfusion of ischemic area, oxygen free radicals are produced, which also damage neurons.
- **Hemorrhagic stroke** (see Figure 2.9-3): The extravasation of blood into the central nervous system (CNS) resulting from subarachnoid hemorrhage (SAH), HTN, or bleeding into a prior ischemic stroke.

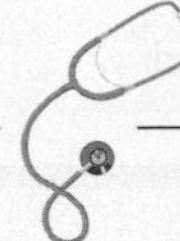

The initial CT should be done *without* contrast as fresh blood is radiolucent relative to old blood and normal cerebral tissue. Contrast-enhanced CT or MRI is useful subsequently to reveal regions of infarct.

Signs and Symptoms

- Thrombotic strokes often show relatively slow progressive onset, often during sleep.
- Embolic strokes present suddenly, often in discrete steps ("stuttering onset"), most often during waking hours.

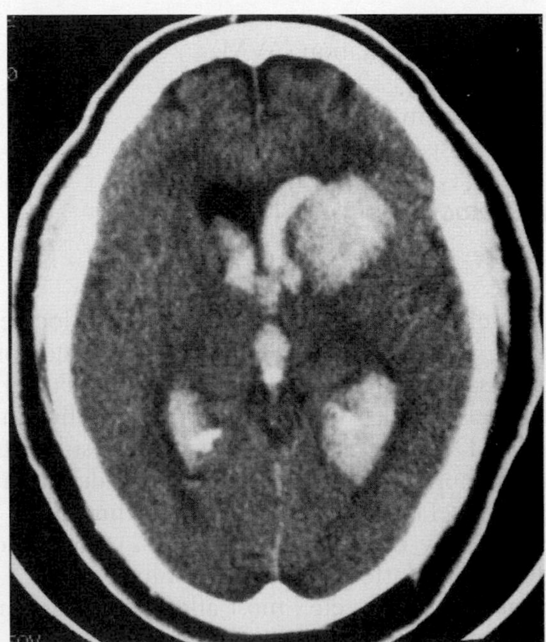

FIGURE 2.9-3. Head CT demonstrating intracerebral hemorrhagic.

- Hemorrhagic strokes evolve over minutes, invariably during waking hours.
- Twenty percent of stroke patients have a history of at least one TIA.

Diagnosis/Workup

- A noncontrast computed tomography (CT) scan is useful for quick diagnosis and localization. It can also be helpful to exclude hemorrhagic strokes. Will pick up ~ 90% of bleeds; the remaining 10% will be picked up with lumbar puncture.
- MRI/magnetic resonance angiography (MRA) for further study and follow-up.
- Carotid ultrasound to screen for carotid stenosis.
- Cardiac echocardiography may be used to screen for embolic source. Transesophageal echo (TEE) is most sensitive. A bubble study may be performed to evaluate for a patent foramen ovale (PFO). According to the American Stroke Association, PFO is present in up to 20% of the population, increasing the risk of cerebrovascular accident (CVA) by 25%. Also need to look for atrial/aortic thrombus or dilated atria.
- Electrocardiogram (ECG) to look for atrial fibrillation.

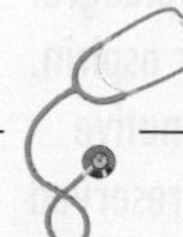

TIAs preceding thrombotic strokes tend to present with similar symptoms because the transient ischemia is locked to the distribution of the stenotic artery. Conversely, TIAs preceding embolic strokes tend to have more variable presentation.

Treatment

- **TIA:**
  - Main "treatment" involves assessment of risk factors, and diagnostic studies to see if there is a correctable cause for brain ischemia (eg, critical carotid stenosis).
  - Beyond that, patients should be started on a daily aspirin or alternative antiplatelet agent.
- **General measures for stroke:**
  - Correct hypoxemia (supplemental oxygen), hypoglycemia (D50), hypotension (IVF), and hyperthermia (acetaminophen).
  - Deep venous thrombosis (DVT) prophylaxis (compression stockings, low-molecular-weight subcutaneous injections).
  - Regular turning of comatose patients to prevent decubitus ulcers.
  - NPO initially, then parenteral feeding for those without intact gag reflex to avoid risk of aspiration. Of note, the gag reflex is absent (at baseline prior to CVA) in up to 25% of the population.
- **Ischemic stroke:**
  - Monitor blood pressure. Do not treat acutely unless other acute conditions such as concurrent MI, aortic dissection, hypertensive encephalopathy, congestive heart failure (CHF), or acute renal failure (ARF) are present.
  - Treat systolic blood pressure (SBP) > 220, diastolic blood pressure (DBP) > 110, or mean arterial pressure (MAP) > 130. Start with labetalol 10 mg IV. Do not ↓ the MAP more than 20%. MAP = (Systolic + 2 x Diastolic)/3.
  - For patients who present **within 3 hours** of symptom onset, IV tissue plasminogen activator (t-PA) is an FDA-approved option, currently considered standard of care. Patients must have a moderate-sized stroke and have no contraindications to thrombolytic therapy.
  - Investigational therapies include intra-arterial t-PA and mechanical clot retrieval via aspiration catheter introduced through the groin.
  - Anticoagulation is not indicated acutely; there is little evidence to support its use in any given case, although you will still see it being used. Often reserved for refractory cases and posterior circulation stroke.

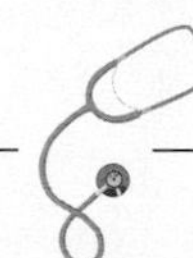

Remember, decreasing the systemic perfusion pressure (BP) causes a corresponding ↓ in cerebral perfusion pressure in ischemic stroke and can be detrimental, as it can extend the area of infarct. Be very careful when lowering BP in stroke.

- Aspirin or other antiplatelet agent both acutely and once daily following hospital discharge.
- **Hemorrhagic stroke:**
  - Elevate head of the bed 30 degrees.
  - Provide a quiet environment, analgesia, and sedation as needed.
  - Treat elevated intracranial pressure with hyperventilation, hyperosmolar agents (mannitol, glycerol), and steroids as needed.
  - Prevent straining (Valsalva) with antitussives and stool softeners as needed.
  - Nimodipine 60 mg for SAH (to reduce vasospasm).
  - BP control (more important in hemorrhagic than ischemic stroke).

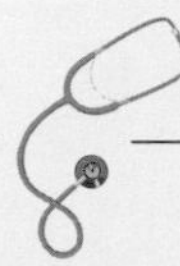

There has been no advantage shown of alternative antiplatelet agents such as clopidogrel or ticlopidine over aspirin. Use of these alternative agents should be reserved for those who have a true allergy to aspirin, or those who have had their stroke while on aspirin.

BRAIN HERNIATION

- The movement of brain tissue into a space that it does not normally occupy, which can lead to coma and death.
- It is usually caused by a mass/lesion; can be caused by a bleed.

CLASSIFICATION

- **Transtentorial herniation:** The upper thalamic region herniates downward through the tentorium.
  - *Uncal herniation* is a common type of transtentorial herniation in which the gyrus moves through the anterior section of the tentorial opening.
  - The third nerve is often affected by the brain tissue that is displaced.
  - Patients often present with an enlarged pupil on the ipsilateral side of the herniation as well as a contralateral hemiparesis.
  - This is often followed by coma.
- **Subfalcine herniation:** The cingulate gyrus herniates across the midline.
  - Clinically, this may compromise blood flow through the anterior cerebral artery and can present as a headache.
  - Anterior cerebral artery infarction is a complication of this type of herniation.
- **Central herniation:** The entire cerebral hemisphere herniates across the tentorium as a result of ↑ intracranial pressure.
- **Tonsillar herniation:**
  - Result of ↑ pressure in the posterior fossa, causing parts of the cerebellum to herniate through the foramen magnum.
  - This type of herniation results in compression of the lower brain stem, which contains the respiratory center and leads to central respiratory failure.

CNS INFECTIONS

Rabies

A rapidly progressing viral infection affecting the human nervous system; usually from raccoons or bats.

EPIDEMIOLOGY

- Fewer than 10 cases per year in the United States.
- Fifty percent of cases from raccoon bites.
- Other cases transmitted by dogs, skunks, foxes, coyotes, bats, and bobcats.
- Rare cases from tissue transplantation (cornea).
- First unvaccinated patient to survive a human rabies infection: Jeanna Giese in 2004.

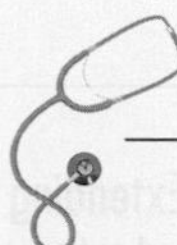

A patient with encephalitis, hydrophobia, and aerophobia should have rabies virus workup.

SIGNS AND SYMPTOMS

Two phases:

- *Prodromal phase:* Pain, paresthesias, gastrointestinal (GI)/respiratory symptoms, irritability, apprehension, **hydrophobia** (aversion to swallowing water because of pain), aerophobia (fear of fresh air).
- *Excitation phase:* Hyperventilation, hyperactivity, disorientation, and seizures. Patient becomes increasingly lethargic. Further involvement of cardiac and respiratory nerves leads to death.

RABIES

Respiratory failure
Aerophobia/
Apprehension/
Aversion to water
Bad pains
Irritability
Excitation
Seizures

DIAGNOSIS

- Fluorescent antibody staining, polymerase chain reaction (PCR).
- Presence of Negri bodies postmortem in brain tissue.

TREATMENT

- Wash affected area thoroughly with soap and water.
- No antiviral therapy available.
- Supportive treatment:
  - Rabies immunoglobulin (passive immunization).
  - Human diploid cell rabies vaccine (active immunization—because of long incubation period, early injections provide sufficient time for protective immunity).
  - Active and passive immunization are administered in different parts of body so that immunoglobulin (passive) does not neutralize the vaccine (active).
  - Isolation of patient.
  - Preexposure prevention with vaccine should be used for high-risk individuals like zookeepers and veterinarians.

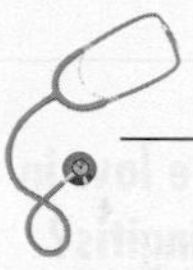

Rabies is universally fatal unless vaccine is given prior to the onset of symptoms. Immunize for:

- Raccoon bites
- Skunk bites
- Bat exposure (bite may be too small to see)
- Fox bites
- Bite from feral dog or cat

Bacterial Meningitis

Acute infection of the subarachnoid space and leptomeninges.

CAUSES (IN DESCENDING ORDER)

- *Streptococcus pneumoniae* (40–60%).
- *Neisseria meningitidis* (young adults).
- *Listeria monocytogenes* (immunocompromised hosts and very young or old). ("*Listeria* affects those with tumbling motility.")
- Gram-⊖ bacilli.
- *Haemophilus influenzae* (unimmunized adults). ("*Hae,* I was going to get vaccinated, but my chance *flu* by.")
- Group B strep (neonates). Penicillin is given to birthing mothers to treat this normal flora in 25% of women.

Kernig's sign: Extending the knee with the thigh at right angles causes pain in back and hamstring.

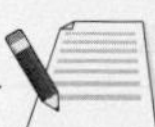

Brudzinski's sign: Forced neck flexion results in flexion at the knee and hip.

"*Neisseria* sucks down sugar and poops protein"
↓ Glucose ↑ Protein

Why is glucose low in bacterial meningitis?
Low glucose in CNS is caused mainly by bacterial inhibition of glucose transport into the CSF, less so by bacterial consumption. The value should be compared to a concurrently determined blood glucose level.

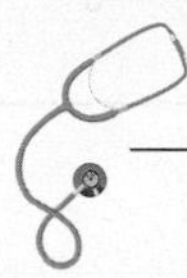

When meningitis is suspected on clinical grounds, do not wait for results of lab tests or imaging studies: Treat empirically!

PATHOPHYSIOLOGY

- Bacteria commonly colonize the nasopharynx, which can then enter the bloodstream.
- Via the blood, the bacteria make their way into the cerebrospinal fluid (CSF) through the choroid plexus.
- Most signs and symptoms are secondary to the body's own inflammatory response.
- Bacteremia, sinusitis, otitis, and direct trauma could predispose to meningitis.

SIGNS AND SYMPTOMS

- Triad of headache, stiff neck, and fever (95%).
- Mental changes such as confusion, lethargy, or coma in 80%.
- Seizures occur in 10–30%.
- Nausea, vomiting, and photophobia are common complaints.
- Look for classic maculopapular rash of meningococcemia—occurs on days 1–3 of illness in 30–60% of infected patients; prominent in areas of the skin subjected to pressure.

DIAGNOSIS

- Blood culture is ⊕ in 50–60%.
- Lumbar puncture (LP; see Table 2.9-2):
  - Neutrophil count, protein, and opening pressure ↑.
  - Monocytes may predominate in cases of *Listeria*.
- Glucose ↓.
- Check Gram stain for presence of microorganisms.
- Cerebrospinal fluid (CSF) culture ⊕ in 80%.
- CT before LP to rule out abscess as source of meningeal irritation/infection and mass effect. These pose risk of herniation during LP.

TREATMENT

- Good empiric coverage includes third-generation cephalosporin and vancomycin.
- Empiric treatment with antibiotics based on age. This is adjusted once the Gram stain or sensitivity results are completed.

TABLE 2.9-2. CSF Findings in Meningitis and Abscess

	WBCs	Diff.	Protein	Glucose	Opening Pressure
Bacterial meningitis	Very high	Polys	High	Low	High
Viral meningitis	High	Lymphs/monos	Norm	Norm	Norm/high
TB/fungal meningitis	High	Lymphs/monos	High	Low	High
Brain abscess	Norm/high	Polys	High	Low	Very high

- *Streptococcus pneumoniae:* Vancomycin + cefotaxime or ceftriaxone.
- *N. meningitidis:* Penicillin G or ceftriaxone.
- If patient is at risk for *Listeria* (old, young, or immunocompromised), you must add ampicillin.
- "Amp up" the coverage for those with tumbling motility.
- Add steroids before antibiotics if *S. pneumoniae* is the cause (↓ neurologic sequelae).

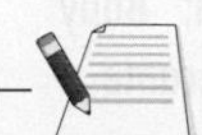

For CSF findings, remember: Viruses utilize proteins to replicate (low protein), utilize intracellular glucose (normal to high "extracellular" glucose), and are perceived as an immunological threat, (high lymphocyte count).

Viral Meningitis

- Also called aseptic meningitis.
- ↑ incidence in summer, early fall.
- Most commonly caused by enterovirus.
- More common than bacterial.
- Course is more benign.
- Signs and symptoms are similar to bacterial, but less pronounced (patient does not appear toxic).
- CSF shows normal to low protein, normal to high glucose, and lymphocytosis. Cultures and PCR can usually identify the cause.
- Treatment is supportive except in cases of varicella or herpes, in which antiviral therapy might be useful.

Botulism

A paralytic disease caused by the toxin of *Clostridium botulinum*, resulting in presynaptic destruction of neuromuscular junction.

Etiology

- Ingestion of improperly prepared home-processed foods, canned foods.
- Wound contamination.

Pathophysiology

- Toxin blocks the release of acetylcholine at the peripheral nerve endings.
- Usual incubation period is 18–36 hours.
- A **descending** paralysis ensues, leading to respiratory failure and death.

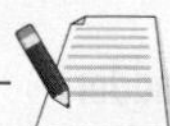

Descending weakness: Botulism; tick disease; and Guillain-Barré syndrome, Miller Fischer variant.

Signs and Symptoms

- **Neurologic:** Dry mouth, diplopia, dysphagia, dysarthria, **descending weakness** of the extremities and muscles of ventilation.
- **GI:** Nausea, vomiting, diarrhea, abdominal cramps.
- Patient will generally be afebrile.

Diagnosis

Detection of neurotoxin by serology, only in specialized labs.

Signs of Botulism—"5 Ds"

Dry mouth
Diplopia
Dysphagia
Dysarthria
Descending weakness

Treatment

- **Ingestion:**
  - Antitoxin.
  - Whole bowel irrigation (requires either alert patient or protected airway).
  - Toxic ingestion of substance not adsorbed to charcoal (charcoal has greateast utility only in iron, lead, lithium, and zinc [**Lead LiFe Zeal**ously]).

Botulinum spores in honey can replicate in the gut of a newborn (who does not have normal bacterial flora yet) and cause botulism. (Typically on exam: "Baby ate honey, then became hypotonic . . .")

- **Wound contamination:** Drainage of lesion, antitoxin, and penicillin.
- **For both:**
  - Intubation with ventilatory support.
  - Prevention.
  - The toxin can be inactivated after 10 minutes in boiling water. The spores, however, can withstand boiling temperatures for several hours.

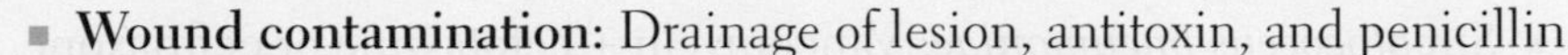

SEIZURE DISORDERS

NEUROLOGY

- **Seizure:** Abnormal and excessive neuronal discharge causing a transient disturbance of cerebral function.
- **Epilepsy:** Two or more unprovoked seizures.
- One percent of population has disease.
- A range of effects can be seen, from the asymptomatic to overt convulsions.

Classification

- **Partial:** Focal, only part of cortex involved.
- **Simple:** No loss of consciousness (LOC), no postictal state.
- **Complex:** Postictal state present, LOC may or may not be present.
- **Generalized:** Always associated with LOC, whole cortex is involved.
- **Absence (petit mal):** Brief episode of nonresponsiveness to external or internal stimuli; motor tone is preserved.
- **Tonic-clonic (grand mal):** Generalized convulsion—brief tonic phase (stiffening) followed by clonic phase (rhythmic jerking).
- **Status epilepticus:** A long continuous seizure lasting 30 minutes or two or more seizures in a row without a lucid interval. *Emergency:* must implement the ABCs (airway, breathing, and circulation) of cardiopulmonary resuscitation (CPR).

Etiology

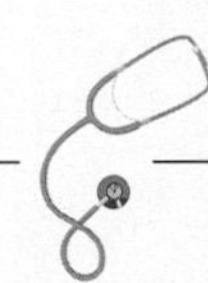

Loss of bowel or bladder function and tongue biting are important clues in the diagnosis of a seizure.

- Fever (affects 2–5% of 6- to 60-month-old kids); long-term risk 2.4% (baseline population risk of epilepsy = 1%).
- Idiopathic.
- Head trauma—an isolated seizure following trauma does not imply epilepsy. Risk of sequelae depends on severity of injury/hypoxia.
- Stroke.
- Mass lesions.
- Meningitis/encephalitis (infectious).
- Metabolic: Hypoglycemia, hyponatremia, hyperosmolarity, hypocalcemia, uremia, hepatic encephalopathy, porphyria, drugs, eclampsia, hyperthermia.
- Brain malformation/dysplastic cortex.

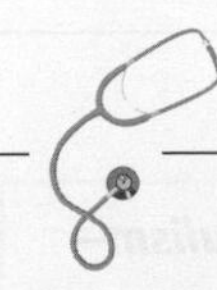

3-Hz spike and wave is the pathognomonic EEG pattern of absence seizures.

Diagnosis

- Electroencephalogram (EEG).
- CT or MRI to rule out any lesions.
- Routine blood tests and toxicology screen to rule out metabolic or drug-induced seizures.

TREATMENT

- Address underlying cause if appropriate.
- Anticonvulsant therapy: Check for therapeutic levels in known epileptics.
- Benzodiazepines to break ongoing seizure.
- Phenytoin, carbamazepine, and valproic acid are common preventive medications for seizure.

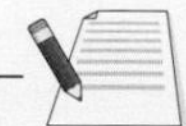

Isoniazid (INH) causes seizures refractory to anticonvulsant therapy. They are treated with pyridoxine (vitamin B_6).

BRAIN NEOPLASMS

See Table 2.9-3.

TABLE 2.9-3. CNS Tumors

TUMOR	DESCRIPTION
Astrocytoma	■ Most common neuroectodermal tumor (also **most common intracranial tumor** in general). ■ Those occurring in adults are usually high grade–poor prognosis. ■ **Glioblastoma multiforme (GBM)** is an aggressive anaplastic type.
CNS lymphomas	■ Originate from B cells that have entered the CNS. ■ Commonly affects eyes, spinal cord, or leptomeninges. ■ Presents with headache, vision problems, and behavioral/personality changes. ■ Diagnose by identifying malignant lymphocytes. ■ Treatment with chemotherapy, radiation, and steroids.
Oligodendrogliomas	■ Tend to calcify. ■ More benign and better prognosis than astrocytoma. ■ Epileptogenic.
Ependymoma	■ In adults, characteristically found in spinal canal. ■ In children, most common location in fourth ventricle. ■ With excision, 5-year survival rate is 80%.
Meningiomas	■ Most common mesodermal tumor. ■ Usually benign and slow growing, but usually discovered at large size. ■ Clinically, may present as a cranial nerve palsy.
Schwannomas	■ Most common cranial nerve tumor. ■ Vestibular (acoustic) neuromas are eighth cranial nerve tumors. Anyone with unilateral deafness should have this ruled out. ■ Associated with neurofibromatosis type 1 > type 2.
Pituitary tumors	See Endocrinology chapter.
Metastatic tumors to CNS	■ 80,000 per year. ■ More common than primary tumors. ■ Metastases common from lung, breast, and malignant melanoma.

ETIOLOGY

- Exposure to ionizing radiation.
- Hereditary syndromes (ie, neureofibromatosis—six or more café au lait spots; tuberous sclerosis—facial angiofibromas, subungual fibromas, and ash leaf spot).
- HIV (lymphoma is typically of the B-cell subtype).

EPIDEMIOLOGY

- Kills > 13,000 per year.
- Originates from brain, spinal cord, or meninges.
- Most common:
  - Glial origin (50–60%)
  - Meningiomas (25%)
  - Schwannomas (8%)

SIGNS AND SYMPTOMS

In migraines, prolonged headache may be followed several hours later by vomiting. In brain tumors, acute headache is followed immediately by vomiting.

- Headache (40%); usually the result of ↑ intracranial pressure:
  - Present upon awakening and disappears within 1 hour (but can take any form).
  - Can wake patient from sleep.
  - Worse while lying supine.
  - New headache in middle-aged or older person.
  - Change in headache character in person with chronic headaches.
- Nausea or vomiting especially on awakening.
- Irritability, apathy.
- Sometimes vision loss, weakness of extremities.
- Seizures, focal neurologic deficits.
- Lethargy, weight loss more common with metastatic disease (patients are cachetic secondary to the ↑ metabolic demands of the tumor).

DIAGNOSIS/WORKUP

- MRI/CT for detection of mass and preliminary diagnosis.
- Biopsy for histology and definitive diagnosis.
- Positron-emission tomography (PET) scans and EEG occasionally have some diagnostic role.

TREATMENT

- Corticosteroids to ↓ edema and intracranial pressure.
- Surgical resection, if possible.
- Radiation and perhaps chemotherapy for high-grade tumors.

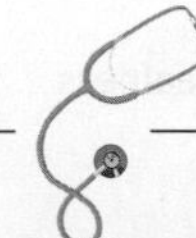

Forty to fifty percent of patients with ocular myasthenia gravis go on to develop generalized myasthenia gravis.

NEUROPATHIES

Myasthenia Gravis

PATHOPHYSIOLOGY

Autoimmune disease in which antibodies against the postsynaptic nicotinic acetylcholine receptor prevent acetylcholine from binding. Therefore, an end-plate potential is ↓ at the neuromuscular junction.

EPIDEMIOLOGY

- Two peaks of incidence:
  - Women ages 20–40.
  - Men older than age 60.
- Twenty percent have thyroid disease.
- Ten percent thymoma, 70% thymic hyperplasia.

SIGNS AND SYMPTOMS

- Muscular weakness and fatigue.
- Ptosis and diplopia (by affecting muscles of eye).
- Proximal muscle weakness.
- Intact reflexes.
- Nasal speech, dysphagia.
- Myasthenic crisis: Severe, life-threatening exacerbation, usually compromising respiratory status, and often requiring ventilatory support.
- Exacerbations in known patients may occur secondary to medication: aminoglycosides, ciprofloxacin, ampicillin, erythromycin, beta blockers, lithium, magnesium, procainamide, verapamil, quinidine, chloroquine, timolol.

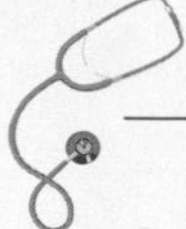

Symptoms worsen as day progresses. (This is the opposite of rheumatoid arthritis.)

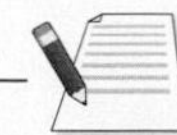

"E-DRO-PHONE-I-UM" ("ET phone home")
Imagine ET's "tensed" trembling index finger improve as his myasthenia gravis symptom is lessened by edrophonium.

DIAGNOSIS

- Myasthenia antibodies on serology.
- **Edrophonium (Tensilon™) test:** Edrophonium, which inhibits acetylcholinesterase, is given to the patient and a set of muscle groups is observed. In order for the test to be ⊕, the patient's muscle strength must improve, which is due to the ↑ availability of acetylcholine at the postsynaptic receptor (typically this test is used in acute setting).
- **Repetitive nerve stimulation** will display a quick reduction in the amplitude of the action potentials in myasthenic patients.
- CT of chest for thymoma/thymic hyperplasia (peak mass of thymus normally is puberty).

In myasthenia gravis, repetitive muscle use quickly induces fatigue, whereas in Eaton-Lambert syndrome, repetitive muscle use improves muscle strength.

LABS AND TESTS

- Antibody presence against acetylcholine receptor (AChR).
- Chest MRI to evaluate any thymus abnormalities.

TREATMENT

- Most patients are able to have normal lives.
- If mild, anticholinesterase drug.
- Thymectomy when indicated (most patients experience long-term improvement; curative for 35%).
- Prednisone as first-line therapy.
- Cyclosporine or azathioprine if prednisone is not effective.
- Plasmapheresis and immunoglobulin therapy can also be useful.
- Patients in crisis should get steroids, pulmonary function tests, ICU admission, but not acetylcholinesterase inhibitors until crisis is under control. (Patients in crisis are unable to clear their secretions, so giving cholinergic agonists may worsen the ability to maintain their airway.)

Anterio mediastinum differential (limited and worth knowing)–

The 4 Ts

Thymomas—slow growing, varying sizes
Teratoma—large, round, lobulated
Thyroid, parathyroid—causes tracheal deviation at thoracic outlet
"**T**errible" lymphoma—usually causes adjacent pleural effusion

Guillain-Barré Syndrome

Syndrome of transient immune-mediated **ascending paralysis** usually following a viral upper respiratory tract infection.

Etiology

- Most cases are preceded by a respiratory or GI infection.
- *Campylobacter jejuni*: Most frequently associated as molecular mimicry occurs between human gangliosides and *C jejuni* lipo-oligosaccharides (LOSs). First our immune systems fight the bacteria LOSs, then our own gangliosides!
- Other potential causes: Herpes simplex virus, cytomegalovirus, Epstein-Barr virus, and *Mycoplasma*.
- Vaccines have been implicated as a potential cause in the past (ie, influenza, rabies vaccines).

Pathophysiology

An immune-mediated demyelination of axons/axonopathy can also occur.

Signs and Symptoms

- Initial symptoms include paresthesias in the feet (or arms) and leg weakness, which progresses as an ascending motor paralysis, usually over several days.
- Distal muscle weakness is common soon afterward—may last a few weeks.
- Deep, aching pain in back and legs.
- Areflexia.
- Tachypnea.
- Quadriparesis and respiratory muscle paralysis occur in 30% of patients, and one-third of patients will need mechanical ventilation.
- Respiratory muscle paralysis can be fatal.
- Cranial nerves can be involved.

Diagnosis

- CSF shows ↑ protein, but no WBCs.
- Electromyography (EMG) shows signs of demyelination with marked ↓ in action potential conduction velocities.
- The diagnosis is usually made clinically since CSF and EMG testing are often normal in the early course of this syndrome.

Treatment

- Most patients will have to be hospitalized.
- Mechanical ventilation for respiratory muscle paralysis.
- Plasma exchange and IV immunoglobulin in selected patients.
- Reassurance. Most patients make a full recovery, although < 5% of patients die from respiratory failure.
- Most cases resolve spontaneously over the course of several weeks to months.

HEADACHE

Top 10 Causes of Headache

- Chronic headache syndromes (migraine, cluster, tension headaches).
- SAH.
- Meningitis.
- Hypertension.

- Mass lesion.
- Temporal arteritis.
- Trigeminal neuralgia.
- Brain abscess.
- Pseudotumor cerebri.
- Subdural hematoma.

Migraine Headache

Pathophysiology

- According to the vasogenic theory, cerebral vasoconstriction is followed by vasodilation.
- It is thought that there are genetic and hormonal components to migraines.

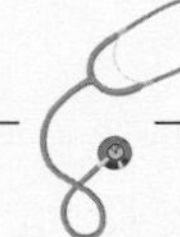

Triggers of migraines include: red wine, chocolate, monosodium glutamate (MSG), lack of sleep, menses, stress.

5-HT receptor agonists can cause coronary vasospasm.

Epidemiology

- Sixty percent have family history.
- Twelve percent in the United States affected.
- Females > males.

Signs and Symptoms

- **Migraine with aura** (classic, rarely seen): Patient suffers from aura approximately 1 hour before onset. The focal neurological dysfunction can include photophobia, sonophobia, nausea, vomiting, vertigo, dysarthria, tinnitus, diplopia, weakness, and ataxia. Patient may also complain of scintillating scotoma (65%) or homonymous hemianopsia.
- **Migraine without aura** (common): Photophobia and sonophobia are again noted, along with anorexia, nausea, vomiting, and general malaise. Specific visual findings are usually not involved.
- Both types have prodromal symptoms (60%) 1–2 days before attack. These include lethargy, food craving, depression, and fluid retention.
- Headache phase of migraine may last several hours. It is characterized by a unilateral, throbbing head pain.
- Paresthesias occur over 10–20 minutes, as opposed to those caused by CVA. A CVA produces paresthesias much more acutely. Never miss a stroke!

Treatment

- **Nonpharmacologic:** Avoidance of triggers; stress reduction; dark, quiet environment.
- **Acute treatment:**
  - Nonsteroidal anti-inflammatory drugs (NSAIDs).
  - Ergotamine derivatives.
  - 5-HT receptor agonists (sumatriptan—may cause malignant HTN).
  - Antiemetics (metoclopramide IV—watch for dystonic reaction, which is treated with diphenhydramine).
  - Valproic acid, tricyclics, gabapentin.
- **Prophylaxis:** Calcium channel blockers, beta blockers, tricyclics, and serotonergic drugs.

Tension Headache

SIGNS AND SYMPTOMS

- Muscular contractions causing bandlike pain located in head and neck.
- Neck stiffness.
- Usually bilateral.
- No prodrome.
- Worsens as the day progresses.

TREATMENT

- Aspirin or acetaminophen.
- Narcotics if severe.
- Prophylaxis with tricyclics such as amitriptyline.
- Relaxation.

Cluster Headache

A severe vascular headache that clusters in the same area of the head and time of day, usually lasting for several weeks.

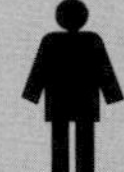

A 38 year-old-man believes he is having a cluster headache. He presents with drooling and right facial nerve paralysis. On exam, he has vesicular lesions on an erythematous base in the ear canal. *Think: "Ramsay Hunt Syndrome", Herpes Zoster infection of the 7th nerve.*

EPIDEMIOLOGY

- Greater incidence in males than females.
- ↑ incidence after alcohol, nitrates, or stress.

SIGNS AND SYMPTOMS

- Unrelenting unilateral facial pain, which tends to occur in clusters.
- Pain so severe it can lead to suicide.
- Headaches are often seasonal.
- Accompanied by ipsilateral autonomic signs, including conjunctival injection, lacrimation, rhinorrhea, nasal congestion, ptosis, miosis, eyelid edema, and facial sweating.

TREATMENT

- **Acute episodes:**
  - High-flow oxygen.
  - Intranasal lidocaine.
  - Ergotamine, sumatriptan, and antiemetics if the above fail.
- **Prophylaxis:** Verapamil, methysergide, high-dose prednisone followed by rapid taper, lithium, or indomethacin.

Headache of Temporal (Giant Cell) Arteritis

Idiopathic inflammation of medium and large arteries, usually the temporal artery, histologically characterized by giant multinucleated cells.

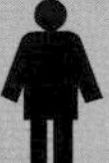

A 62-year-old woman presents with headache, pain when she chews, and scalp tenderness. *Think: Temporal arteritis.* **Next step:** Treat with steroids. This can save vision.

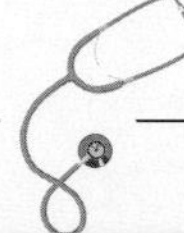

Causes of painful vision loss:

- Optic neuritis
- Giant cell arteritis
- Acute angle-closure glaucoma

ETIOLOGY

Thought to be part of a systemic vasculitis that has gone undetected except for the temporal and ophthalmic artery involvement.

EPIDEMIOLOGY

More common in women and persons older than age 60.

SIGNS AND SYMPTOMS

- Unilateral headache in distribution of temporal artery.
- Thickened, tender temporal arteries.
- Ipsilateral visual loss (ophthalmic artery).
- Claudication of the masseter, temporalis, and tongue muscles.
- Scalp tenderness.
- Pulsating temporal artery, also sometimes nodular.

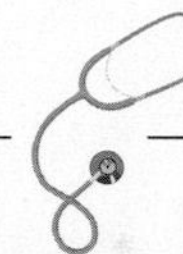

More than 50% of patients with temporal arteritis have polymyalgia rheumatica.

DIAGNOSIS

- Based on the 1990 American College of Rheumatology criteria for classification of temporal arteritis, at least three of the following five items must be present (sensitivity [⊕ in disease] 93.5%, specificity [absent in healthy] 91.2%):
  1. Age of onset > 50 years.
  2. New-onset headache or localized head pain.
  3. Temporal artery tenderness to palpation or reduced pulsation.
  4. Erythrocyte sedimentation rate (ESR) > 50 mm/h.
  5. Abnormal arterial biopsy (necrotizing vasculitis with granulomatous proliferation and infiltration).
- Definitive diagnosis by temporal artery biopsy.
- Anemia is frequently seen.

TREATMENT

- Corticosteroids as soon as suspected; *can lead to blindness if treatment is delayed.*
- NSAIDs for pain relief.

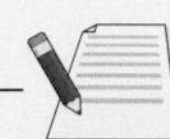

Closed-angle glaucoma can be exacerbated by anything that dilates eyes (ie, sympathomimetics, anticholinergics). Treat with timolol or pilocarpine drops or systemic acetazolamide. Avoid atropine and scopolamine!

NEUROLOGY

ACUTE VISION LOSS

See Table 2.9-4 for the differential diagnosis for acute vision loss.

TABLE 2.9-4. Differential Diagnosis for Acute Vision Loss

Differential Diagnosis	Description	Treatment
Central retinal artery occlusion	▪ Typically painless loss of vision. ▪ Causes ischemic stroke of retina. ▪ Cherry red spot on fovea.	Dissolve or dislodge embolus.
Retinal detachment	▪ Symptoms include flashes of light. ▪ Floaters. ▪ Vision loss.	Surgery or laser treatment.
Vitreous hemorrhage	▪ Caused by bleeding into vitreous humor. ▪ Common causes are diabetic retinopathy and retinal tears. ▪ Symptoms initially include floaters, which progress to vision loss.	Photocoagulation or vitrectomy.
Optic neuritis	▪ Painful, unilateral vision loss with partial resolution. ▪ Inflammation of optic nerve or absence of clinical findings. ▪ Caused by demyelination. ▪ Visual acuity at its worst in 1 week. ▪ Other symptoms include headache and eye pain with movement. ▪ Many patients have progression to multiple sclerosis.	Steroids.
Temporal arteritis	▪ See description under Headaches.	

Causes of painless vision loss:
- Central retinal artery occlusion (pallor and cherry red spot)
- Central retinal vein occlusion (thunderstorm)
- Retinal detachment (curtain)

Dementia

Loss of cognitive function with normal sensorium.

Etiology

- Stroke.
- Infection (particularly syphilis, AIDS, Creutzfeldt-Jakob disease).
- Epilepsy.
- Vitamin deficiency (folate [chemo, alcoholics], B_{12} [alcoholics, elderly] thiamine [Wernicke's], niacin [patients on pyridoxine therapy for tuberculosis]).
- Normal pressure hydrocephalus (NPH).
- Neurodegenerative disorders (Alzheimer's, Parkinson's, Huntington's, amyotrophic lateral sclerosis).
- Trauma.
- Toxins.
- Tumors.

Diagnosis/Workup

Dementia workup should include complete blood count (CBC), electrolyte panel, vitamin B_{12}, folate, rapid plasma reagin (RPR), and head CT.

Treatment

- Treat underlying disorder.
- Optimize sensory function (vision aids, hearing aids).
- Simplify activities of daily living (simplify floor plans, stairs).
- Ensure physical safety (bedrails, companions).

Causes of dementia—

VINCENT van Gogh was demented

Vitamin deficiency
Infection
NPH
CVA
Epilepsy
Neurodegeneration
Trauma/**T**umors/**T**oxins

Alzheimer's Disease

Slowly progressive dementia characterized by amyloid plaques and neurofibrillary tangles in the neurons of the cerebral cortex (mostly temporal lobe).

Epidemiology

- Older people.
- Family history (apolipoprotein E genotype).
- Higher incidence in patients with Down syndrome.
- Down's syndrome has ↑ incidence of four "A's": ALL (acute lymphocytic leukemia), ASD (atrial septal defect), Alzheimer's, and Atlantoaxial instability.

Signs and Symptoms

- Usually present with subtle onset of memory deficits accompanied by a progressive dementia.
- The earliest signs may include the inability to pay bills, go shopping, or other routine daily activities.
- Later on, patients will display aphasia, apraxia, confusion, and hallucinations.
- Patients may become incontinent and mute and require constant assistance with most tasks.

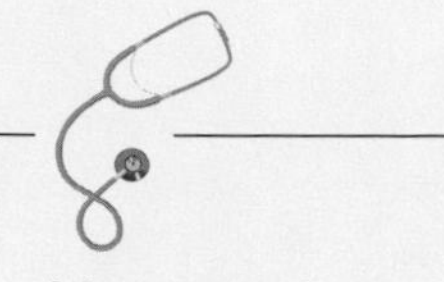

Alzheimer's is the most common cause of dementia.

Diagnosis

- Diagnosis is mainly clinical; other causes of dementia need to be ruled out.
- Cortical atrophy on CT or MRI (see Figure 2.9-4).
- EEG slowing later in disease.

Treatment

- Donepezil, tacrine, and selegiline may slow cognitive decline.
- Memantine, vitamin E, exercise, and mental activity may be protective.
- Behavioral symptoms can be treated with neuroleptics, anxiolytics, and antidepressants.

Parkinson's Disease

Complex progressive disorder involving movement and higher cognitive function.

Etiology

- Degeneration of neurons in the substantia nigra.
- May be secondary to toxins (manganese, carbon monoxide, designer drugs—"ecstasy") and encephalitis.

Epidemiology

Mean age is 55; more common in men (3:2).

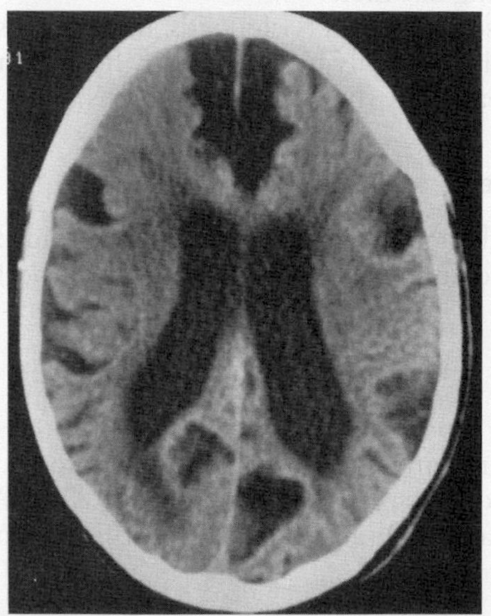

FIGURE 2.9-4. Alzheimer's disease.

Note the severe frontal atrophy. (Reproduced, with permission, from Lee SH, Rao K, Zimmerman RA [eds.]. *Cranial MRI and CT*. New York: McGraw-Hill, 1999: 194.)

NEUROLOGY

SIGNS AND SYMPTOMS

Signs and symptoms fluctuate:

- **Pill-rolling resting tremor** (thumb rubs fingers, most prominent at rest).
- **Cogwheel rigidity** (ranging the extremities is awkward, there are alternating moments of brief fluidity followed by coarse rigidity—actually thought to be a tremor of the entire limb).
- **Bradykinesia:** ↓ amplitude and slowing of movements, manifested as micrographia, hypomimia (mask facies), hypophonia.
- Shuffling gait, festinating gait.
- Depression, hallucinations (occurs in 25% of patients, partially secondary to dopaminergic agonist therapy).
- Impaired autonomic dysfunction (gastroparesis, orthostatic hypotension).
- Postural instability usually occurs 8 years into disease process.
- Cognitive decline is a late feature.

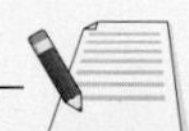

Remember: Parkinson's is marked by a resting tremor.

DIAGNOSIS

- Clinical presentation.
- Response to levodopa-carbidopa.

TREATMENT

- Amantadine (antiviral) may improve tremor and bradykinesia in early disease by blocking reuptake of dopamine into presynaptic neurons.
- Levodopa: Converted to dopamine in substantia nigra; co-administer with carbidopa (does not cross blood-brain barrier) to block metabolism of levodopa in peripheral tissues.
- Anticholinergics: Block cholinergic inhibition of dopaminergic neurons in substantia nigra; commonly trihexyphenidyl, benztropine mesylate.
- Selegiline: Selective monoamine oxidase MAO-B inhibitor, blocks central metabolism of dopamine.
- Dopamine receptor agonists such as bromocriptine, pergolide, pramipexole.

Normal Pressure Hydrocephalus (NPH)

A distinct clinical syndrome in the setting of hydrocephalus without ↑ intracranial pressure.

ETIOLOGY

Most patients have no clear cause; however, it can sometimes be seen after a CNS event (SAH, meningitis, trauma, tumor).

SIGNS AND SYMPTOMS

Classic triad ("Wet, Wild, and Wobbly"):

- Urinary incontinence.
- Dementia (most refractory to treatment).
- Gait disorder (most responsive to treatment).

DIAGNOSIS

- Normal pressure on lumbar puncture (LP).
- Enlarged ventricles on CT or MRI.
- Temporal horns are normally slitlike, their dilatation is a sensitive indicator of early of mild hydrocephalus.
- Clinical improvement after LP and removal of a volume of CSF.

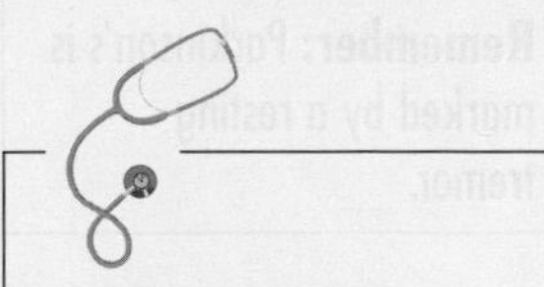

NPH is one of the few reversible causes of dementia.

TREATMENT

- CSF ventricular shunt.
- Choroid plexectomy in some cases.

FEATURES OF BRAIN DEATH

- Preserved cardiac function.
- No spontaneous respiratory function.
- No cranial nerve reflexes (especially pupils).
- No posturing (decerebrate [predominant extensors] or decorticate [flexors predominate, with fists clenched over the "core" muscles]).
- No evidence of hypothermia (rectal).
- No known reversibility of state (drugs).

HIGH-YIELD FACTS IN

Dermatology

> ***Rashes That Can Be Seen on Palms and Soles—***
>
> ***Mrs. E***
>
> **M**eningococcemia
> **R**MSF
> **S**yphilis
> **E**rythema multiforme

TOP CAUSES OF RASH WITH FEVER

- Rubella.
- Measles.
- Staphylococcal scalded syndrome.
- **Toxic shock syndrome.**
- Scarlet fever.
- **Meningococcemia.**
- **Disseminated gonococcal infection.**
- **Bacterial endocarditis.**
- **Rocky Mountain spotted fever (RMSF).**
- Kawasaki's disease.
- **Erythema nodosum.**
- **Hypersensitivity vasculitis.**

IMPORTANT QUESTIONS TO ASK IN ANY SKIN CONDITION

See Tables 2.10-1 and 2.10-2 for definitions of primary and secondary skin lesions and Table 2.10-3 for diagnostic procedures used in dermatology.

1. When did it start?
2. Where did it start?
3. Does it hurt? Itch? Other symptoms?
4. How has it spread?
5. How has each lesion changed over time?
6. What makes it worse (sun, heat, pregnancy, cold, medications, exposures)?
7. Previous treatments?

TABLE 2.10-1. Definitions of Primary Skin Lesions

Macule	A flat, nonpalpable area of skin discoloration (vitiligo, café au lait spot).
Papule	An elevated, palpable solid area of skin < 0.5 cm diameter (acne, lichen planus).
Plaque	An elevated area of skin > 2 cm diameter that has a larger surface area compared to its elevation above the skin (psoriasis, seborrheic keratosis).
Wheal	An elevated, rounded or flat-topped area of dermal edema that disappears within hours (urticaria).
Vesicle	A circumscribed, elevated, fluid-containing lesion of < 0.5 cm diameter (varicella-zoster).
Bullae	A circumscribed, elevated, fluid-containing lesion of > 0.5 cm diameter (pemphigus vulgaris).
Pustule	A circumscribed, elevated, pus-containing lesion (acne, disseminated gonococcal infection).
Nodule	An elevated, palpable solid lesion > 0.5 cm diameter (nodulocystic acne, erythema nodosum).
Petechiae	A red-purple nonblanching macule < 0.5 cm diameter, usually pinpoint in size (meningococcemia).
Purpura	A red-purple nonblanching macule > 0.5 cm diameter (Henoch-Schönlein purpura).
Telangiectasia	A blanchable dilated blood vessel (rosacea, cirrhosis, Osler-Weber-Rendu).

TABLE 2.10-2. **Definitions of Secondary Skin Lesions**

Scale	An accumulation of dead, exfoliating epidermal cells.
Crust	Dried serum, blood, or purulent exudate that accumulates on the skin surface (scab).
Erosion	A superficial loss of epidermis, leaving a denuded, moist surface; heals without scarring because doesn't penetrate through dermal-epidermal junction.
Excoriation	A linear erosion produced by scratching.
Ulcer	A loss of epidermis extending into dermis; heals with scarring because it penetrates into dermis.
Scar	Replacement of normal skin with fibrous tissue as a result of healing.
Atrophy	Thinning of skin.
Lichenification	Thickening of epidermis with accentuation of normal skin markings.

TABLE 2.10-3. **Diagnostic Procedures Used in Dermatology**

Diascopy	Pressing of a glass slide firmly against a red lesion will determine if it is due to capillary dilatation (blanchable) or to extravasation of blood (nonblanchable).
KOH preparation	Used to identify fungus and yeast. Scrape scales from skin, hair, or nails and treat with a 10% KOH solution to dissolve tissue material. Septated hyphae are revealed in fungal infections, and pseudohyphae and budding spores are revealed in yeast infections.
Tzanck preparation	Used to identify vesicular viral eruptions. Scrape the base of a vesicle and smear cells on a glass slide. Multinucleated giant cells will be identified in herpes simplex, herpes zoster, and varicella infections.
Scabies preparation	Scrape skin of a burrow between fingers, side of hands, axilla, or groin. Mites, eggs, or feces will be identified in scabies infection.
Use of Wood's lamp	Certain conditions will fluoresce when examined under a long-wave ultraviolet light ("black" lamp). Tinea capitis will fluoresce green or yellow on hair shaft.
Patch testing	Detects type IV delayed hypersensitivity reactions (allergic contact dermatitis). Nonirritating concentrations of suspected allergen are applied under occlusion to the back. Development of erythema, edema, and vesicles at site of contact 48 hours later indicates an allergy to offending agent.
Biopsy	Type of biopsy performed depends on the site of lesion, the type of tissue removed, and the desired cosmetic result. Shave biopsy is used for superficial lesions. Punch biopsy (3–5 mm diameter) can remove all or part of a lesion and provides tissue sample for pathology. Elliptical excisions provide more tissue than a punch biopsy and are used for deeper lesions or when the entire lesion needs to be sent to pathology.
Therapeutic modalities	Cryosurgery, curettage and electrodesiccation, phototherapy.

Urticaria, angioedema, anaphylaxis, and atopic dermatitis are examples of type I hypersensitivity reactions occurring in the skin.

Immediate Type I Hypersensitivity Reactions (IgE Mediated)

- Immunologic reaction mediated by immunoglobulin E (IgE) and mast cells, characterized by vasodilation and transudation of fluid.
- As the antigen binds to IgE on the mast cell surface, the mast cell degranulates and releases histamine and prostaglandin, causing vasodilation, ↑ capillary permeability, and smooth muscle contraction.
- **Urticaria** (hives/wheals): Leakage of plasma into the dermis causes a swelling after exposure to allergen. Wheals usually last < 24 hours and may recur on future exposure to the antigen.
- **Angioedema:** A deeper involvement of subcutaneous tissues with less demarcated swelling, usually characterized by swelling of the eyelids, lips, and tongue (see Figure 2.10-1). A deficiency of C1 esterase can cause hereditary angioedema.
- **Anaphylaxis** is the most severe systemic form of type I hypersensitivity reaction, characterized by bronchoconstriction and hypotension.

TREATMENT

- Antihistamines (H_1 and H_2 blockers).
- Corticosteroids.
- Airway protection (if needed).
- Epinephrine (for anaphylaxis).

Hypersensitivity (Leukocytoclastic) Vasculitis

- A group of vasculitides in which immune complexes lodge in small blood vessels, resulting in inflammation; fibrinoid necrosis; and painful, palpable purpura.
- Can be caused by drugs, infectious agents, or other sources.
- Gastrointestinal (GI) tract, kidney, and joints affected.

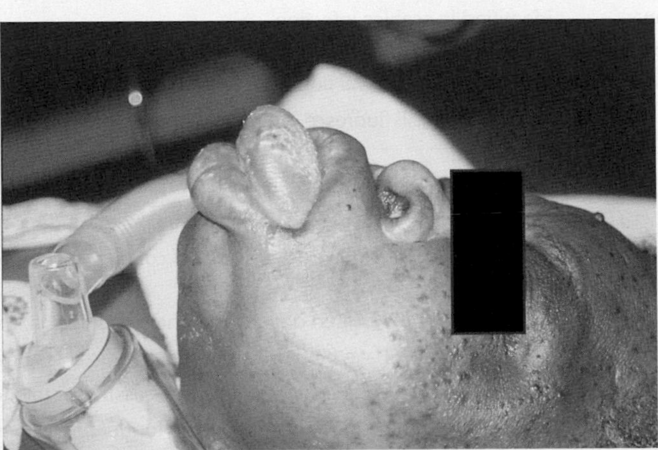

FIGURE 2.10-1. Angioedema.

Also see Color Insert. Note severe tongue, lip, and peri-orbital swelling. In addition, patient has a tracheostomy to maintain the airway. (Reproduced, with permission, from Knoop KJ, Stack LB, Storrow AB, et al. *Atlas of Emergency Medicine*, 3rd ed. New York: McGraw-Hill, 2010: 112. Photo contributor: W. Brian Gibler, MD.)

- Henoch-Schönlein is a classic example (associated with strep infection + penicillin; small-vessel vasculitis with purpura of lower extremities/ buttocks; IgA deposits in glomeruli).
- Common causes: Idiopathic, infection, sulfonamides and penicillin, neoplasms, connective tissue disorders (systemic lupus erythematosus [SLE], Sjögren's, rheumatoid arthritis, Wegener's granulomatosis).

Signs and Symptoms

- Pruritus and pain, associated with fever and malaise.
- **"Palpable purpura"**—multiple, scattered, nonblanchable red papules distributed over lower extremities, arms, and buttocks (see Figure 2.10-2).
- May be crusted due to necrosis of tissue overlying the blood vessel.

Diagnosis

Biopsy.

Treatment

- Eliminate and/or treat causative agent.
- Systemic corticosteroids/immunosuppressive agents.

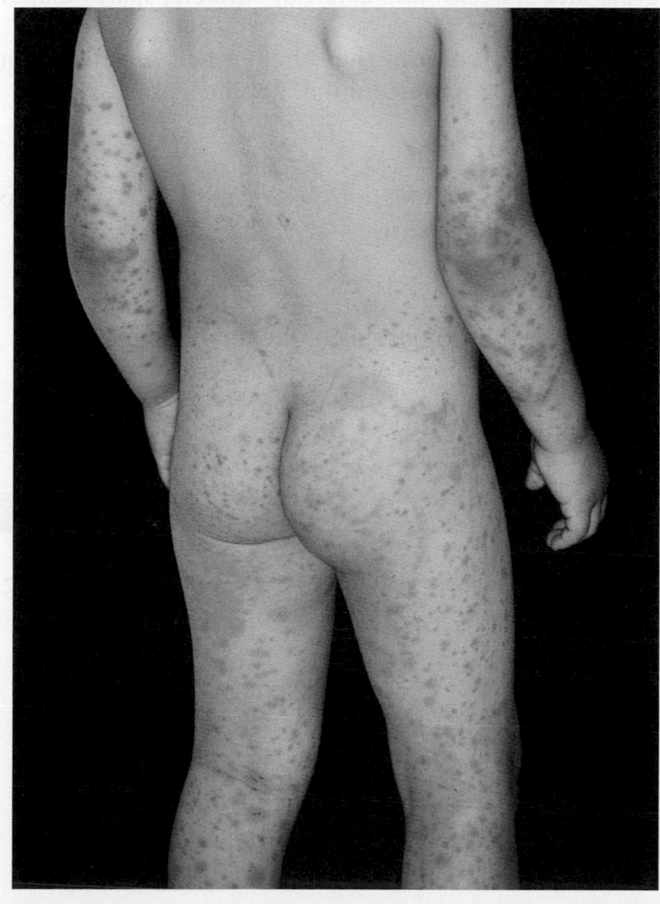

FIGURE 2.10-2. Henoch-Schönlein purpura.

Also see Color Insert. (Reproduced, with permission, from Knoop KJ, Stack LB, Storrow AB, et al. *Atlas of Emergency Medicine*, 3rd ed. New York: McGraw-Hill, 2010: 361. Photo contributor: Kevin J. Knoop, MD, MS.)

ATOPIC DERMATITIS/ECZEMA

An acute or chronic relapsing pruritic type I (IgE) immediate hypersensitivity inflammatory reaction where scratching and rubbing → further lichenification of skin (often described as the "itch that rashes").

Risk Factors

- Family history
- Lots of allergies
- Asthma
- ↑ IgE
- **Exacerbating factors:**
    - Scratching, **stress,** infection, wool, skin dehydration, pregnancy, menstruation, and foods (milk, eggs); symptoms are usually worse in winter.
    - Usually improves with age.

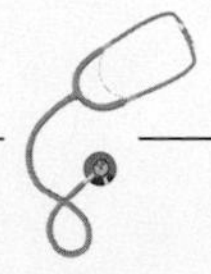

Allergic triad:
- **Atopic dermatitis**
- **Allergic rhinitis**
- **Asthma**

Signs and Symptoms

- Pruritus.
- **Infantile eczema:** Red, exudative, crusty, and oozy lesions primarily affecting the face (cheeks) and extensor surfaces; spares diaper area; may clear by 2 years of age.
- **Juvenile and adult eczema:** Dry, lichenified pruritic plaques distributed over flexural areas (antecubital, popliteal, neck).

Atopic dermatitis: Affected areas—**FACE**
Flexor surfaces get **A**dults.
Children get **E**xtensor surfaces.

Complications

Secondary bacterial and viral infections with *Staphylococcus*, herpes simplex virus, and molluscum contagiosum.

Treatment

- Topical corticosteroids (mainstay of therapy).
- Avoid scratching (will provoke the rash).
- Lubricate dry skin.

ALLERGIC CONTACT DERMATITIS

Dermatitis resulting from skin contact with a substance causing a delayed (type IV) hypersensitivity immune response.

Triggers

- Poison ivy, oak, sumac.
- Nickel (jewelry).
- Formaldehyde.
- Rubber.
- Chemicals in shoes.

Signs and Symptoms

Intensely pruritic rash with linear, papular, erythematous lesions with **indistinct margins in the distribution of the exposure** (if allergic to watch band, there is a bandlike rash in the same spot around wrist).

Diagnosis

History and physical usually enough; can biopsy.

Treatment

- Avoid exposure.
- If severe, use topical or systemic steroids/antihistamines.

IRRITANT CONTACT DERMATITIS

Dermatitis resulting from exposure to substances that cause physical, mechanical, or chemical irritation to the skin.

Triggers

Common exposures after daily repetitive use of soapy water, cleansers, rubbing alcohol.

Signs and Symptoms

- Erythematous pruritic chapped skin, dryness, fissuring.
- Most commonly affects hands.

Diagnosis

History and physical, but patch testing may be necessary to differentiate from allergic contact dermatitis.

Treatment

Goal is to restore normal epithelial barrier and then protect.

- ↓ exposure to soap and water.
- Emollients.
- Severe cases: Topical corticosteroids.

MISCELLANEOUS INFLAMMATORY CONDITIONS

Pityriasis Rosea

- A common self-limiting eruption of a single **herald patch** (see Figure 2.10-3) followed by a generalized secondary eruption within 2 weeks.
- The rash lasts around 2–6 weeks.

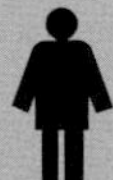

A young person presents with a pruritic, spotted rash on the trunk that began as one solitary larger patch. *Think: Pityriasis rosea.*

Etiology

Herpes simplex virus type 7 is suspected.

DERMATOLOGY

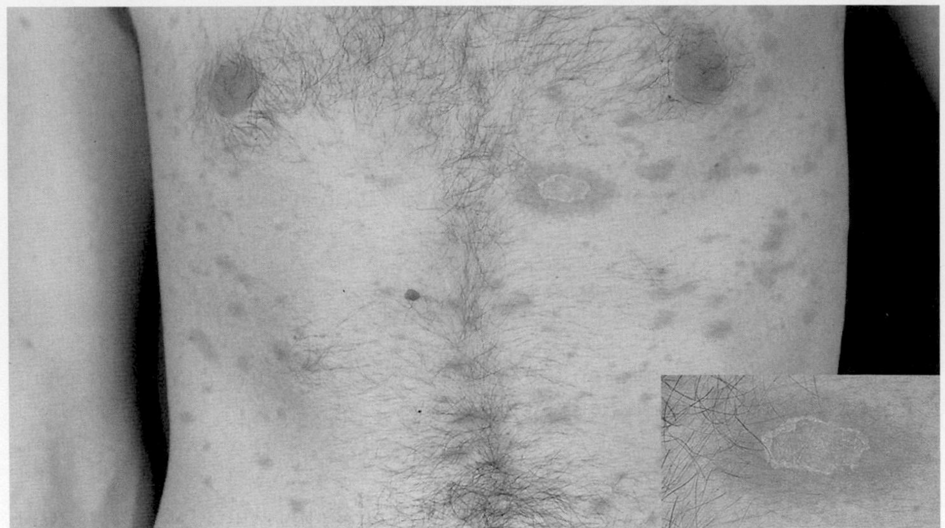

FIGURE 2.10-3. Pityriasis rosea.

Also see Color Insert. Papules and small erythematous plaques; note herald patch, an erythematous plaque with scale in central portion of lesion and collarette on border. (Reproduced, with permission, from Wolff K, Johnson RA, Suurmond D. *Fitzpatrick's Color Atlas & Synopsis of Clinical Dermatology*, 5th ed. New York: McGraw-Hill, 2005: 119.)

Epidemiology

- Affects children and young adults, primarily ages 10–40.
- Clusters of cases in spring and fall.

Signs and Symptoms

- Mild pruritus (present in 75% of cases).
- A 2- to 10-cm solitary, oval erythematous **herald patch** with a collarette of scale precedes the generalized eruption in 80% of patients.
- Within days, multiple smaller pink oval scaly patches appear over trunk and upper extremities.
- Secondary eruption occurs in a **Christmas tree** distribution, oriented parallel to the ribs.

Treatment

- Symptomatic.
- No treatment shortens disease course.
- Can use topical steroids, antihistamines if needed.
- Ultraviolet B (UVB) phototherapy or sunlight can help.

Psoriasis

- Chronic, noninfectious hyperproliferative inflammatory disorder characterized by thick adherent scales.
- Often presents with multiple exacerbations and remissions.

A 35-year-old man presents with salmon-colored papules covered with silvery white scale on his scalp, elbows, and knees. *Think: Psoriasis.*

Pathophysiology

↑ epidermal cell proliferation, forming thick adherent scales.

Risk Factors

- Trauma.
- Infection.
- Emotional stress.
- Drugs (lithium, beta blockers, iodine, and antimalarials).

Signs and Symptoms

- Mild pruritus.
- Well-demarcated, thick, **"salmon-pink" plaques** with an adherent silver-white scale.
- Distributed bilaterally over **extensor surface** of extremities, often on elbows and knees, and trunk and scalp.
- Nails are commonly involved: Pitting of nails, oil spots (yellow-brown spots under nail plate), onycholysis (separation of distal nail plate from nail bed), subungual hyperkeratosis (thickening of epidermis under nail plate).
- Can occur at site of injury **(Koebner phenomenon).**
- Pinpoint capillary bleeding occurs if scale is removed **(Auspitz sign).**

Complications

Psoriatic arthritis, a destructive arthritis of the distal interphalangeal joints of hands and feet **(rheumatoid factor ⊖).**

Treatment

- **Mild psoriasis:** Topical meds (tar, anthralin, steroids, calcipotriene).
- **Severe:** Systemic therapy—usually phototherapy or immunosuppressants (UVB phototherapy, PUVA [psoralin + UVA], retinoids, methotrexate, cyclosporine, infliximab).

Erythema Nodosum

An inflammatory disorder of subcutaneous fat (panniculitis) characterized by painful erythematous nodules on lower legs; likely immune reaction.

A 23-year-old woman presents with a cough, and a chest x-ray shows mediastinal lymphadenopathy. She has painful skin nodules on the skin of the tibia. *Think: Erythema nodosum* as a manifestation of sarcoidosis.

Etiology

- Idiopathic.
- Drugs (sulfonamides, oral contraceptives).
- Infection (strep, tuberculosis, histoplasmosis, coccidiomycosis).
- Autoimmune (sarcoid, inflammatory bowel disease).

Signs and Symptoms

- Nodules scattered over lower legs, bilaterally but not symmetrically (see Figure 2.10-4).
- Can be associated with fever, malaise, arthralgias.

Treatment

Removal/treatment of cause; steroids if necessary.

Erythema Multiforme

A general name used to describe an immune complex–mediated hypersensitivity reaction to different causative agents.

Note: Erythema multiforme, Stevens-Johnson syndrome, and toxic epidermal necrolysis are considered by many to be part of the same spectrum of disease.

Causes

- **Drugs** (penicillins, sulfonamides, barbiturates, nonsteroidal anti-inflammatory drugs [NSAIDs], thiazides, phenytoin).
- **Viruses** (usually herpes simplex virus, but also hepatitis A and B).
- **Bacteria** (*Streptococcus, Mycoplasma*)
- Fungi.
- Malignancy, radiotherapy, pregnancy.

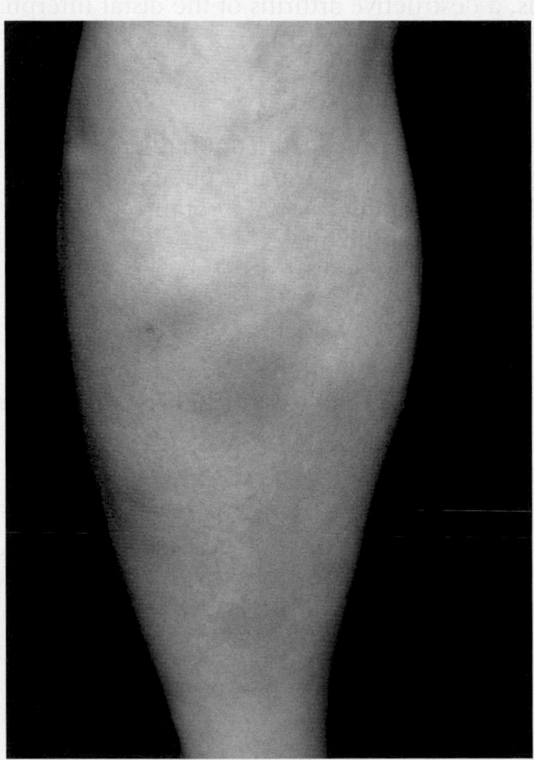

FIGURE 2.10-4. Erythema nodosum.

Also see Color Insert. (Reproduced, with permission, from Wolff K, Johnson RA, Suurmond D. *Fitzpatrick's Color Atlas & Synopsis of Clinical Dermatology*, 5th ed. New York: McGraw-Hill, 2005: 149.)

DERMATOLOGY

SIGNS AND SYMPTOMS

Although characterized by **target lesions,** multiforme refers to the wide variety of lesions that may be present, including papules, vesicles, and bullae (see Figure 2.10-5). Affected sites include dorsa of hands, palms and soles, penis (50%), feet, and face.

TREATMENT

Discontinue offending agent and treat any underlying infections (eg, oral acyclovir to prevent herpes outbreak).

Stevens-Johnson Syndrome

- Erythema multiforme with systemic illness (fever, malaise) and multiple mucous membrane involvement (oral, vaginal, conjunctival) (see Figure 2.10-6).
- Extensive target-like lesions and mucosal erosion covering < 10% body surface area.
- Ocular involvement may result in scarring, corneal ulcers, or uveitis; 5% mortality.
- May evolve to toxic epidermal necrolysis.

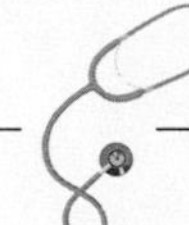

Stevens-Johnson syndrome and toxic epidermal necrolysis are severe variants of erythema multiforme that are potentially life threatening.

Toxic Epidermal Necrolysis

Widespread full-thickness necrosis of skin covering > 30% body surface area.

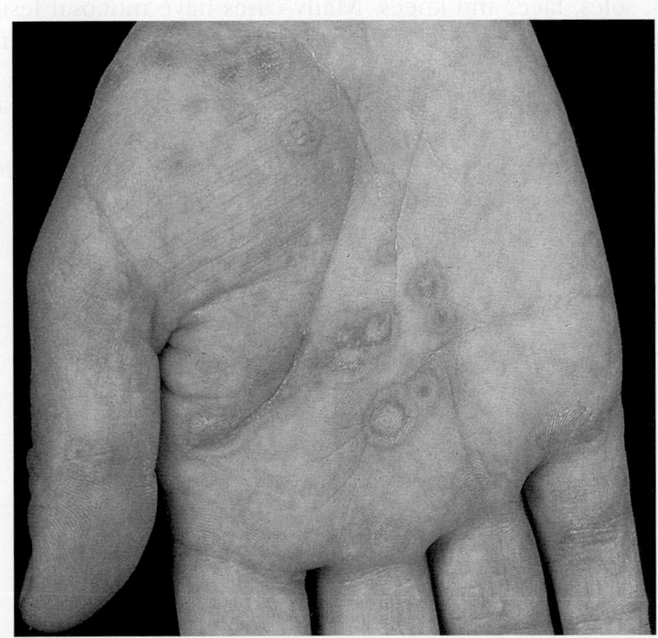

FIGURE 2.10-5. Erythema multiforme.

Also see Color Insert. (Reproduced, with permission, from Wolff K, Johnson RA, Suurmond D. *Fitzpatrick's Color Atlas & Synopsis of Clinical Dermatology*, 5th ed. New York: McGraw-Hill, 2005: 141.)

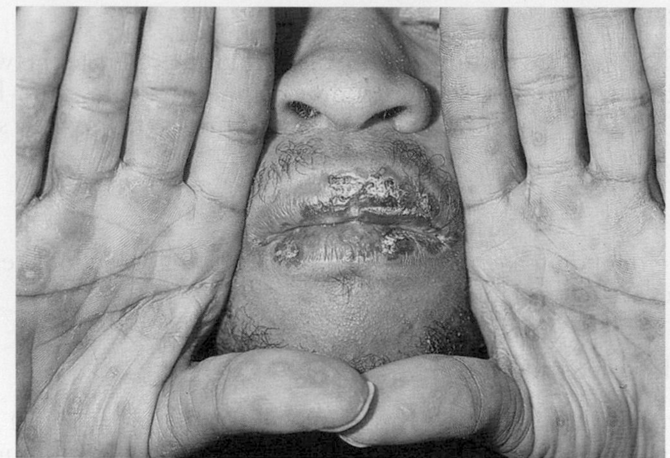

FIGURE 2.10-6. Stevens-Johnson syndrome.

Also see Color Insert. (Reproduced, with permission, from Knoop KJ, Stack LB, Storrow AB, et al. *Atlas of Emergency Medicine.* 3rd ed. New York: McGraw-Hill, 2010: 344. Photo contributor: Alan B. Storrow, MD.)

Stevens-Johnson syndrome and toxic epidermal necrolysis are severe variants of erythema multiforme that are potentially life threatening

Signs and Symptoms

- Prodrome of fever and influenza-like symptoms.
- Pruritus, pain, tenderness, and burning.
- Classic target-like lesions symmetrically distributed on dorsum of hand, palms, soles, face, and knees. Many cases have mucosal lesions—painful erythematous erosions on lips, buccal mucosa, conjunctiva, and anogenital region.
- Initial **target lesions** can become confluent, erythematous, and tender, with bullous formation and subsequent loss of epidermis.
- Epidermal sloughing may be generalized, resembling a second-degree burn, and is more pronounced over pressure points.
- ⊕ **Nikolsky's sign** (sloughing of skin with gentle pressure).

Diagnosis

Biopsy.

Complications

- Secondary skin infections.
- Fluid and electrolyte abnormalities.
- Dehydration.
- Death (30% mortality).

TREATMENT

- Removal and/or treatment of causative agent (suppressive therapy with acyclovir to prevent recurrences of herpes simplex virus).
- Hospitalization for severe disease, fluids (like burn victims) and steroids.

Decubitus Ulcers

Any pressure-induced ulcer that occurs secondary to external compression of the skin, resulting in ischemic tissue necrosis; may extend to underlying subcutaneous tissue, muscle, joints, or bones. Many patients who develop these are in the hospital.

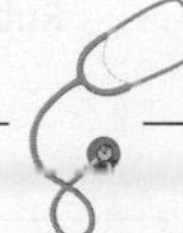

Decubitus ulcers develop over bony prominences: sacrum, ischial tuberosities, iliac crests, greater trochanters, heels, elbows, knees, occiput. Can develop at any site that can be compressed against a hard surface.

RISK FACTORS

Immobility, malnutrition, elderly, diabetes, ↓ level of consciousness.

STAGES

- I—nonblanching erythema of intact skin.
- II—partial-thickness skin loss involving epidermis and/or dermis (superficial ulcer).
- III—full-thickness skin loss involving epidermis and dermis (deep, crateriform ulcer). May involve damage to subcutaneous tissue, extending down to but not through fascia.
- IV—full-thickness skin loss with extensive damage to muscle, bone, or other supporting structures.

COMPLICATIONS

Osteomyelitis, bacteremia, sepsis.

TREATMENT

- **Prophylaxis:**
  - Mobilizing patients as soon as possible.
  - Repositioning patients every 2 hours.
  - Pressure-reducing devices (foam, air, or liquid mattresses).
  - Correction of nutritional status.
- **Local wound care:**
  - Proper cleansing with mild agents.
  - Moisturizing to maintain hydration and promote healing.
  - Polyurethane, hydrocolloid, or absorptive dressings, and topical antibiotics for wound.
  - Necrotic tissue may require surgical debridement, flaps, and skin grafts.
  - Antibiotics if infection.

SKIN DISEASES DUE TO INFECTIOUS AGENTS

See Table 2.10-4 for commonly tested infectious causes of fever and rash.

TABLE 2.10-4. Fever and Rash—Commonly Tested Infectious Causes

Disease	Etiology	Skin Finding(s)	Rash Characteristics	Other Clinical Findings
Measles	Paramyxovirus	Blanching erythematous maculopapular rash that becomes confluent.	Rash starts at hairline and behind ears → centrifugally to face → neck/trunk, extremities.	Koplik's spots, fever, cough, coryza, conjunctivitis.
Rubella	Rubella virus	Similar to measles but patient doesn't look as "sick."	By second day, facial exanthem fades.	Prominent postauricular, posterior cervical lymph nodes.
Varicella (chickenpox)	Varicella-zoster virus	Pruritic vesicular lesions in successive crops; vesicles evolve to pustules and crust over time.	First lesions begin on face/scalp → trunk/ back.	Herpes zoster (shingles): Painful vesicular lesions; does **not** cross midline.
Erythema infectiosum (fifth disease)	Parvovirus B19	Erythematous macules and papules giving lacy "reticulated" appearance.	"Slapped cheek" in children.	
Roseola infantum ("exanthem subitum")	HHV-6, HHV-7	Multiple blanchable macules and papules trunk → extremities (after high fever prodrome).	Rash spares face.	Primarily in infants. High fever 3–4 days prior to appearance of rash.
Infectious mononucleosis	Epstein–Barr virus	Generalized maculopapular rash in 100% of patients with administration of ampicillin/ amoxicillin.		Splenomegaly.
Scarlet fever	Group A *Streptococcus*	Coarse, erythematous, blanching rash; circumoral pallor; strawberry tongue; linear petechiae in skin folds (Pastia's lines).	Rash fades in several days → desquamation of skin.	Rash appears 1–3 days after strep pharyngitis.
Acute rheumatic fever	Group A *Streptococcus*	Erythema marginatum (transient macular rash with central clearing found on proximal extremities).	Subcutaneous nodules on bony prominences.	

Erysipelas

- Erysipelas, erysipeloid, and necrotizing fasciitis are variants of cellulitis.
- An acute onset of superficial spreading cellulitis, arising in inconspicuous breaks in skin (see Figure 2.10-7).

Etiology

Group A beta-hemolytic *Streptococcus pyogenes.*

Signs and Symptoms

- Pain.
- An **erythematous, shiny area** of warm and tender skin with a well demarcated and indurated advancing border.
- **Face is most commonly involved,** but can affect any area, especially sites of chronic edema.

Diagnosis

Gram stain reveals gram-⊕ cocci in chains.

Treatment

Penicillin: If allergic, use vancomycin or macrolide.

Cellulitis

An acute deep infection of dermis and subcutaneous tissue characterized by erythema, tenderness, and warmth of involved area.

Etiology

- *Staphylococcus aureus.*
- Group A beta-hemolytic *Streptococcus pyogenes.*
- *Haemophilus influenzae.*

Risk Factors

Abrasion, burn, surgery, bites, neuropathy, immunocompromise.

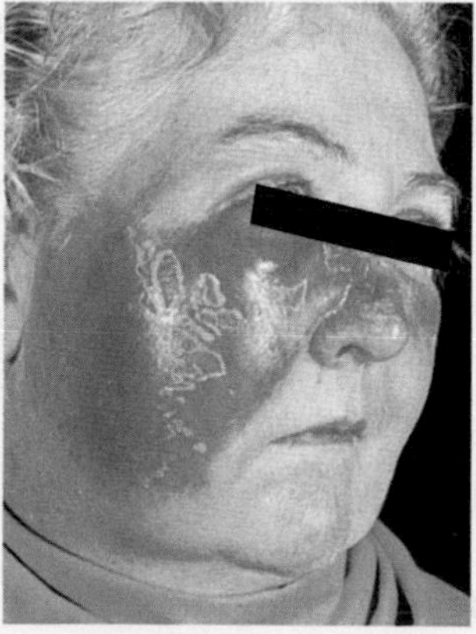

FIGURE 2.10-7. Erysipelas.

Also see Color Insert. (Reproduced, with permission, from Fauci AS et al [eds]. *Harrison's Principles of Internal Medicine,* 17th ed. New York: McGraw-Hill, 2008: 885.)

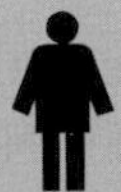

A 54-year-old man with insulin-dependent diabetes presents with a warm, erythematous, slightly tender rash with poorly demarcated borders that began on his calf yesterday and has now spread up his leg. *Think: Cellulitis.*

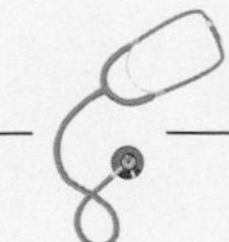

A detailed history is particularly important to reveal the portal of entry in cellulitis.

SIGNS AND SYMPTOMS

- Warmth and tenderness of infected site.
- Erythematous, edematous, **shiny area of warm and tender skin** with poorly demarcated, **nonelevated** border.

TREATMENT

- Penicillin: If penicillin allergic or methicillin-resistant *S aureus* (MRSA), use vancomycin.
- For *H influenzae*, use third-generation cephalosporin.

Toxic Shock Syndrome (TSS)

A toxin-mediated disease characterized by acute onset of fever, hypotension, diarrhea, and generalized skin and mucous erythema, followed by failure of multiple organ systems.

EPIDEMIOLOGY

- Ages 20–30.
- ↑ incidence in women using high-absorbency tampons and in patients with burns, ulcers, surgical wounds, and nasal packs.

ETIOLOGY

S aureus producing TSS toxin-1 (TSST-1) or group A beta-hemolytic streptococci (rare).

SIGNS AND SYMPTOMS

- Acute onset of fever, hypotension, tingling sensation in hands and feet, myalgia, headache, confusion, disorientation, and diarrhea.
- A generalized erythematous macular eruption occurs most intensely at affected site followed by desquamation of palms and soles 1–2 weeks after onset of illness with edema of face, hands, and feet.
- Erythema of oral mucosa, bulbar conjunctiva, vagina, and tympanic membrane.

TREATMENT

- Admission to intensive care unit.
- Removal of potential foreign bodies.
- Antibiotics (anti-staph) and supportive care.

Meningococcemia (*Neisseria* Meningitis)

A potentially fatal disease resulting from meningococcal bacteremia, usually affecting children 6 months to 1 year old, asplenic, or compliment-deficient patients.

Signs and Symptoms

- Acutely ill patient often with discrete **pink macules, papules,** and **petechiae,** which can be distributed over trunk, extremities, and palate (see Figure 2.10-8) (see Table 2.10-1 for definitions of primary skin lesions).
- With fulminant disease, patients have **purpura,** ecchymosis, and confluent area of gray-black necrosis.
- Signs of meningeal irritation (eg, nuchal rigidity).

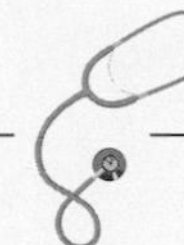

Meningococcemia is fatal if untreated. Treat empirically prior to completion of tests if suspected on clinical grounds.

Diagnosis

- Blood cultures reveal meningococci.
- Cerebrospinal fluid (CSF) culture is usually ⊕.

Complications

- Meningitis (50–90%).
- **Waterhouse-Friderichsen syndrome** (fulminant meningococcemia with adrenal hemorrhage).

Treatment

- Admission to intensive care unit.
- Vancomycin and ceftriaxone IV at first clinical suspicion of meningococcemia.

Rocky Mountain Spotted Fever (RMSF)

A potentially life-threatening disease due to *Rickettsia rickettsii,* transmitted via female *Dermacentor* tick (American dog tick in the eastern United States or the Rocky Mountain wood tick in the western United States).

Epidemiology

Mostly in children, southeastern states.

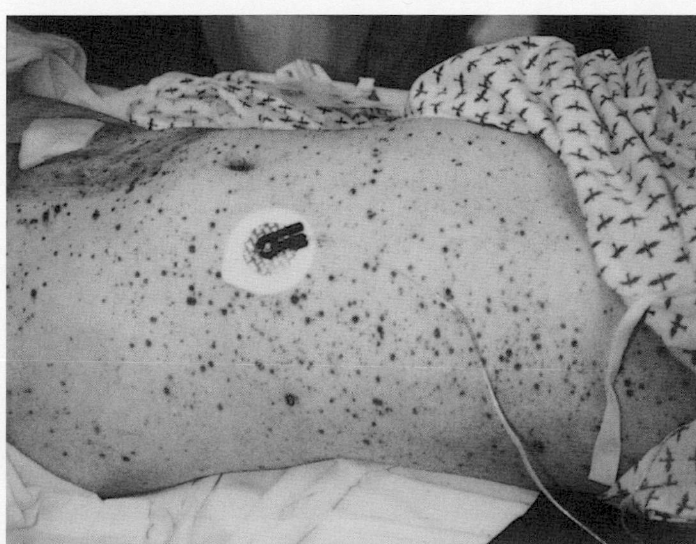

FIGURE 2.10-8. Meningococcemia.

Also see Color Insert. (Reproduced, with permission, from Knoop KJ, Stack LB, Storrow AB, et al. *Atlas of Emergency Medicine,* 3rd ed. New York: McGraw-Hill, 2010: 423. Photo contributor: Kevin J. Knoop, MD, MS.)

Signs and Symptoms

- Sudden onset of high **fever** (> 102°F), myalgia, severe headache, rigors, nausea, and photophobia within first 2 days of tick bite.
- Rash within a few days, consisting of small, pink **blanchable macules** that **first appear peripherally** on wrists, forearms, ankles, **palms,** and **soles** (see Figure 2.10-9) and then **spread centrally to trunk,** proximal extremities, and face. Finally evolve to deep red papules.

Diagnosis

Indirect fluorescent antibody (IFA) assay.

Complications

Some patients develop long-term sequelae lasting > 1 year, including paraparesis; hearing loss; peripheral neuropathy; bladder/bowel incontinence; and cerebellar, vestibular, and motor dysfunction.

Treatment

- **Doxycycline** is considered the drug of choice.
- **Chloramphenicol** for pregnant patients, children younger than 8 years (due to concern of staining the teeth), and severe disease.

Herpes Zoster

- An acute dermatomal viral infection caused by reactivation of latent varicella-zoster virus that has remained dormant in a sensory root ganglion.
- The virus travels down the sensory nerve, resulting initially in dermatomal pain, followed by skin lesions.
- Usually occurs in people > 50 or immunocompromised.
- Skin lesions are vesicles unilaterally along dermatome that ultimately crust over.

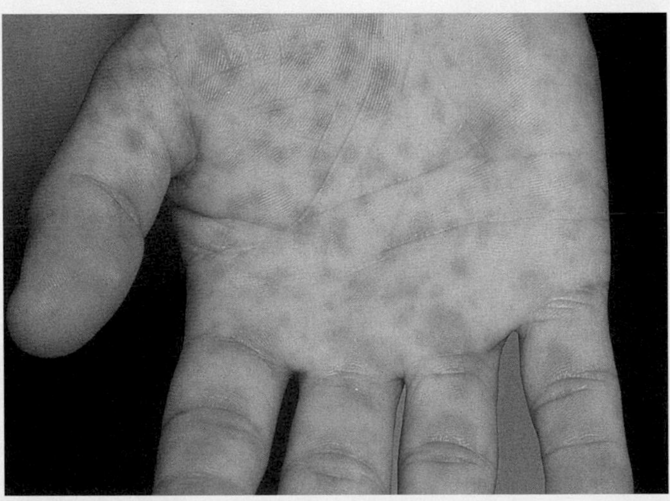

FIGURE 2.10-9. Rocky Mountain spotted fever.

Also see Color Insert. (Reproduced, with permission, from Knoop KJ, Stack LB, Storrow AB, et al. *Atlas of Emergency Medicine.* 3rd ed. New York: McGraw-Hill, 2010: 372. Photo contributor: Daniel Noltkamper, MD.)

Signs and Symptoms

See Figure 2.10-10.

Diagnosis

Confirmed by **Tzanck preparation** revealing multinucleated giant cells, and culture of lesions.

Complications

- **Postherpetic neuralgia** (more common in the elderly and may persist for weeks to years after infection).
- **Herpes zoster ophthalmicus:** Lesions on nasal tip or eye indicate zoster involvement of nasociliary branch of ophthalmic nerve, resulting in uveitis, conjunctivitis, retinitis, optic neuritis, or glaucoma. An ophthalmic consult is necessary.
- **Ramsay Hunt syndrome:** Lesions on external surface of ear or auditory canal indicate zoster involvement of facial and auditory nerve, resulting in facial paralysis, hearing loss, changes in taste perception, ear pain, and vertigo.
- **Herpetic whitlow is HSV of fingers** (see Figure 2.10-11). Occurs in medical personnel exposed to patient's secretions (even without clinical herpes; virus may be shed in saliva). Treat with wet-to-dry dressing. Do not open vesicles or infection will spread.

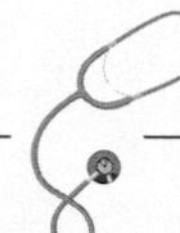

Patients with zoster can infect nonimmune contacts with chickenpox. Exposed nonimmune contacts should be treated with varicella-zoster immune globulin (VZIG).

Treatment

Antivirals (valacyclovir, famcyclovir); analgesia.

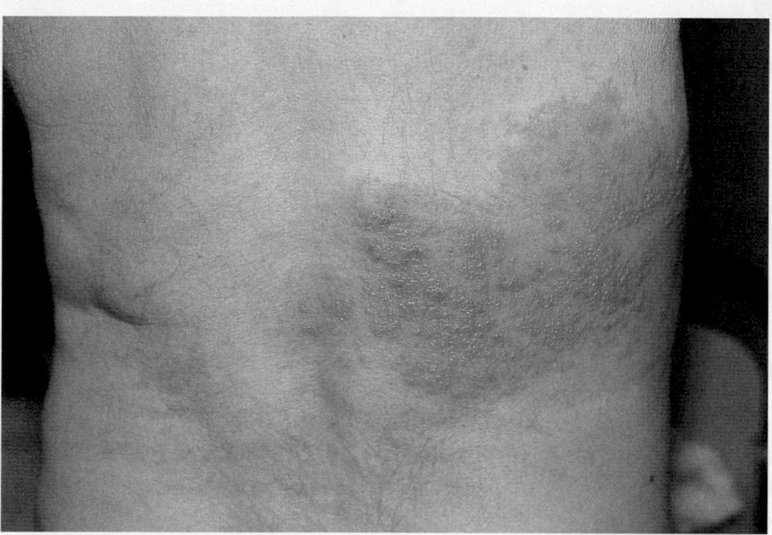

FIGURE 2.10-10. Varicella-zoster virus infection: herpes zoster in T8–T10 dermatome.

Note typical dermatomal distribution of rash. **Also see Color Insert.** (Reproduced, with permission, from Wolff K, Johnson RA, Suurmond D. *Fitzpatrick's Color Atlas & Synopsis of Clinical Dermatology*, 5th ed. New York: McGraw-Hill, 2005: 823.)

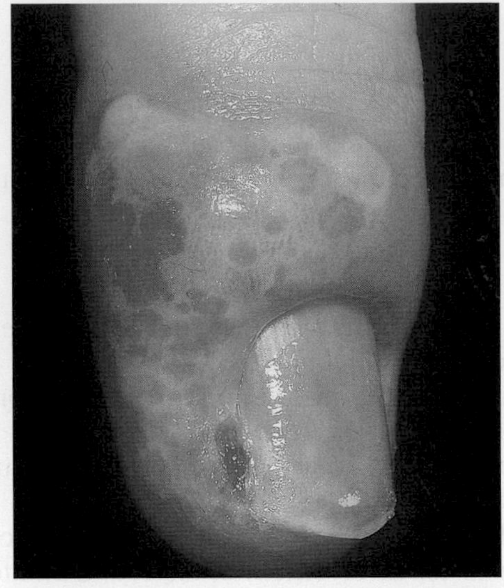

FIGURE 2.10-11. Herpes simplex virus infection: herpetic whitlow.

Also see Color Insert. (Reproduced, with permission, from Wolff K, Johnson RA, Suurmond D. *Fitzpatrick's Color Atlas & Synopsis of Clinical Dermatology,* 5th ed. New York: McGraw-Hill, 2005: 805.)

A 24-year-old medical student working in the ICU held a patient's endotracheal tube with his ungloved hand to keep it from falling out. Two weeks later he has a vesicular lesion on an erythematous base that is extremely painful. *Think: Herpetic whitlow.*

CUTANEOUS FUNGAL INFECTIONS

See Table 2.10-5.

Lyme Borreliosis (Lyme Disease)

- A multisystem disease transmitted by the bite of an *Ixodes* genus deer tick infected with a spirochete *Borrelia burgdorferi.*
- Characterized by three stages of disease: localized, disseminated, and chronic.
- Occurs more in summer, northeastern United States.

Signs and Symptoms

- Acute onset of fever, chills, myalgia, weakness, headache, and photophobia.
- **Erythema chronicum migrans** (ECM) develops at site of tick bite in most patients within 1 month (an expanding erythematous annular plaque with a central clearing) (see Figure 2.10-12).

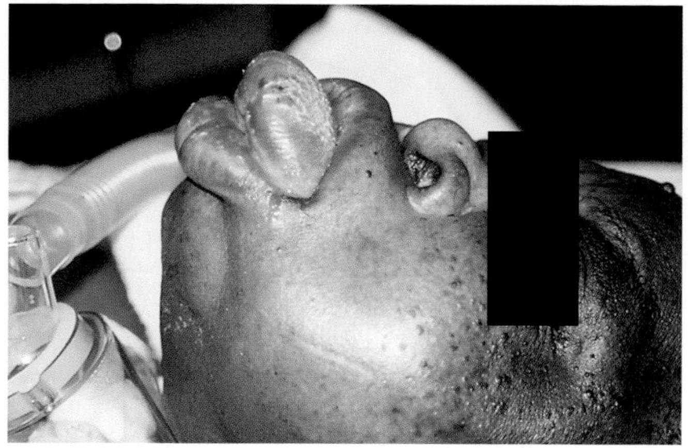

FIGURE 2.10-1. Angioedema.

(Reproduced, with permission, from Knoop KJ, Stack LB, Storrow AB, et al. *Atlas of Emergency Medicine*, 3rd ed. New York: McGraw-Hill, 2010: 112. Photo contributor: W. Brian Gibler, MD.)

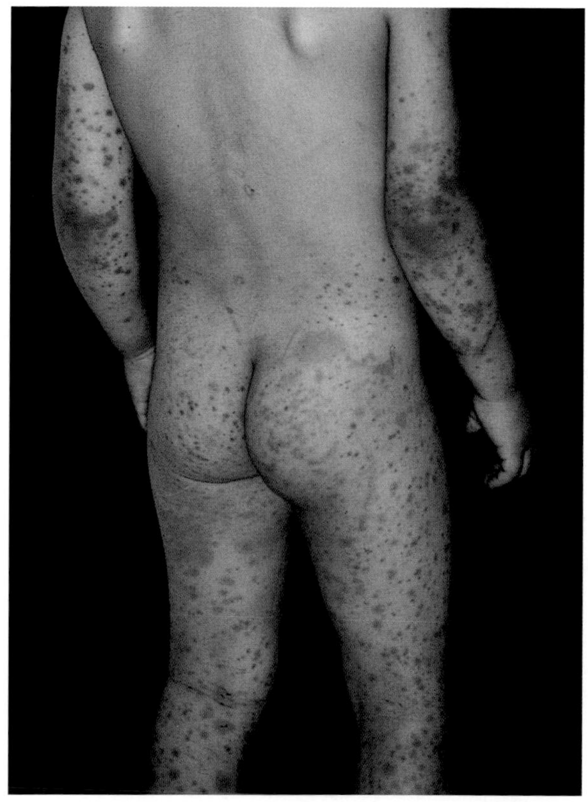

FIGURE 2.10-2. Henoch-Schönlein purpura.

(Reproduced, with permission, from Knoop KJ, Stack LB, Storrow AB, et al. *Atlas of Emergency Medicine*, 3rd ed. New York: McGraw-Hill, 2010: 361. Photo contributor: Kevin J. Knoop, MD, MS.)

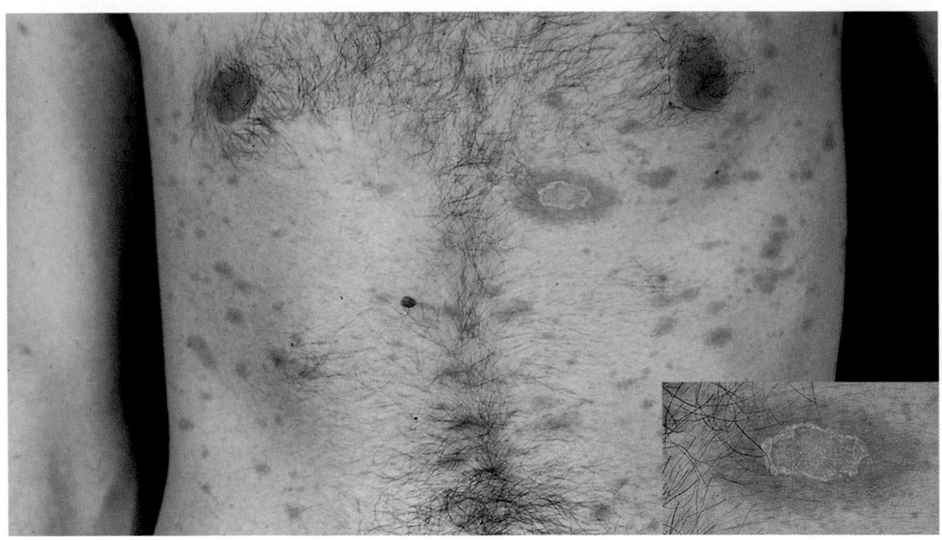

FIGURE 2.10-3. Pityriasis rosea.

Papules and small erythematous plaques; note herald patch, an erythematous plaque with scale in central portion of lesion and collarette on border. (Reproduced, with permission, from Wolff K, Johnson RA, Suurmond D. *Fitzpatrick's Color Atlas & Synopsis of Clinical Dermatology*, 5th ed. New York: McGraw-Hill, 2005: 119.)

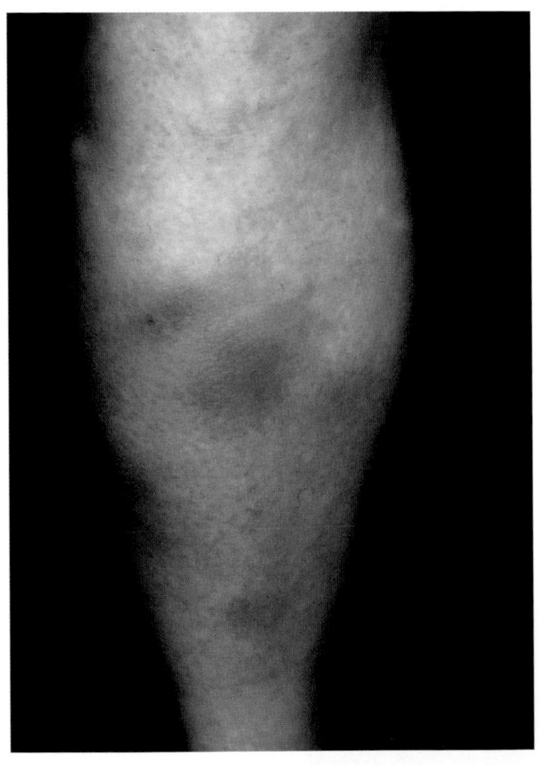

FIGURE 2.10-4. Erythema nodosum.

(Reproduced, with permission, from Wolff K, Johnson RA, Suurmond D. *Fitzpatrick's Color Atlas & Synopsis of Clinical Dermatology*, 5th ed. New York: McGraw-Hill, 2005: 149.)

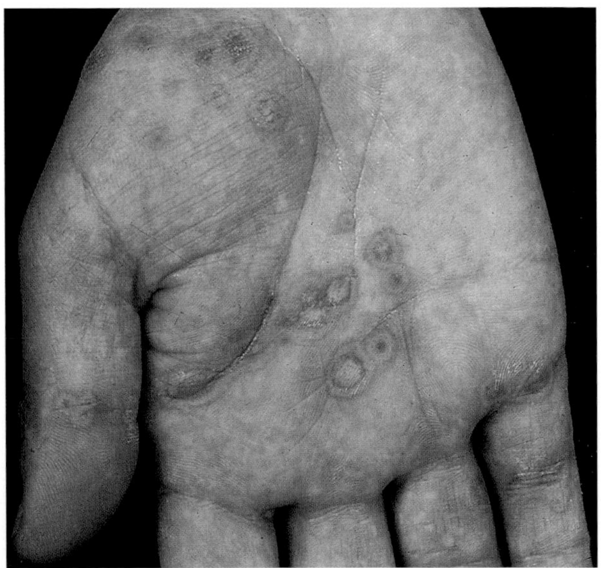

FIGURE 2.10-5. Erythema multiforme.

(Reproduced, with permission, from Wolff K, Johnson RA, Suurmond D. *Fitzpatrick's Color Atlas & Synopsis of Clinical Dermatology*, 5th ed. New York: McGraw-Hill, 2005: 141.)

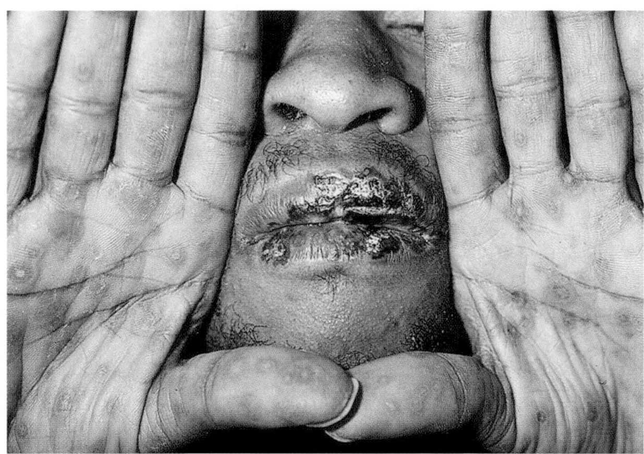

FIGURE 2.10-6. Stevens-Johnson syndrome.

(Reproduced, with permission, from Knoop KJ, Stack LB, Storrow AB, et al. *Atlas of Emergency Medicine.* 3rd ed. New York: McGraw-Hill, 2010: 344. Photo contributor: Alan B. Storrow, MD.)

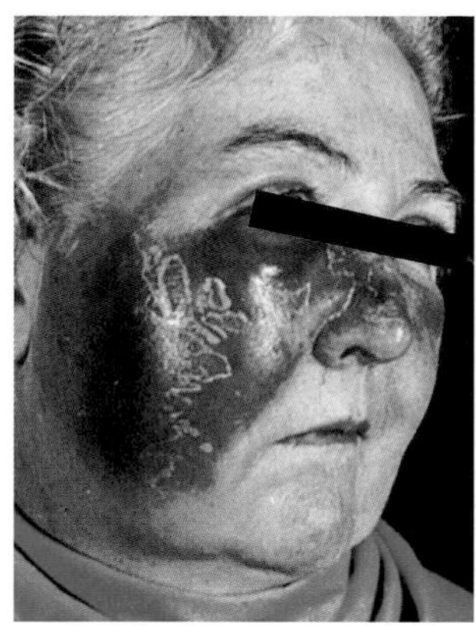

FIGURE 2.10-7. Erysipelas.

(Reproduced, with permission, from Fauci AS et al [eds]. *Harrison's Principles of Internal Medicine,* 17th ed. New York: McGraw-Hill, 2008: 885.)

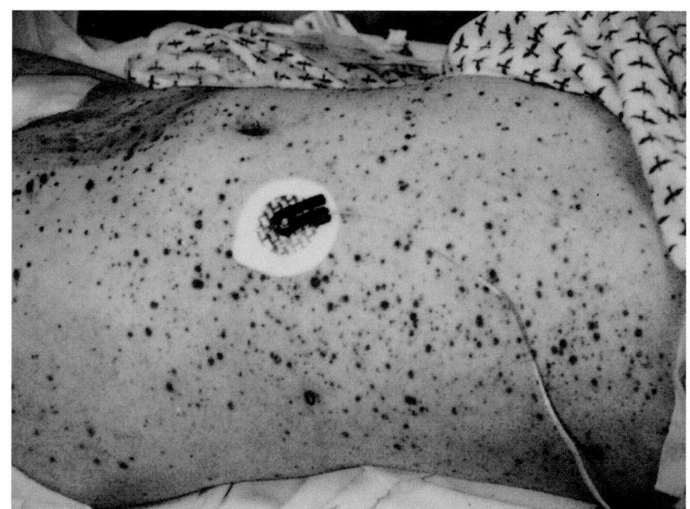

FIGURE 2.10-8. Meningococcemia.

(Reproduced, with permission, from Knoop KJ, Stack LB, Storrow AB, et al. *Atlas of Emergency Medicine,* 3rd ed. New York: McGraw-Hill, 2010: 423. Photo contributor: Kevin J. Knoop, MD, MS.)

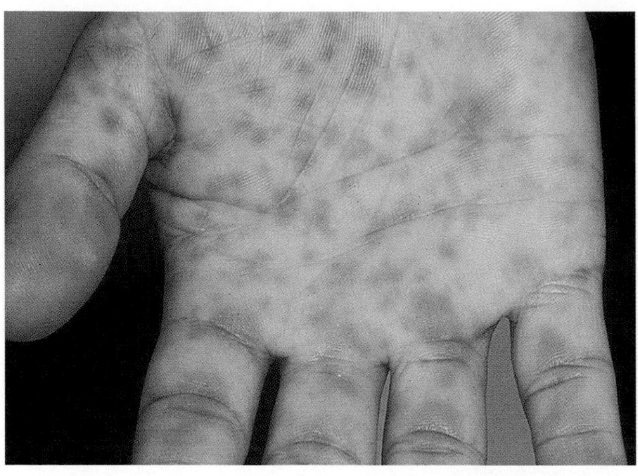

FIGURE 2.10-9. Rocky Mountain spotted fever.

(Reproduced, with permission, from Knoop KJ, Stack LB, Storrow AB, et al. *Atlas of Emergency Medicine.* 3rd ed. New York: McGraw-Hill, 2010: 372. Photo contributor: Daniel Noltkamper, MD.)

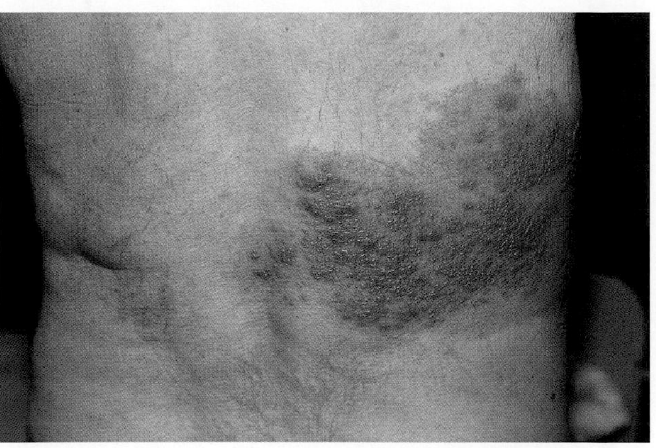

FIGURE 2.10-10. Varicella-zoster virus infection: herpes zoster in T8–T10 dermatome.

Note typical dermatomal distribution of rash. (Reproduced, with permission, from Wolff K, Johnson RA, Suurmond D. *Fitzpatrick's Color Atlas & Synopsis of Clinical Dermatology,* 5th ed. New York: McGraw-Hill, 2005: 823.)

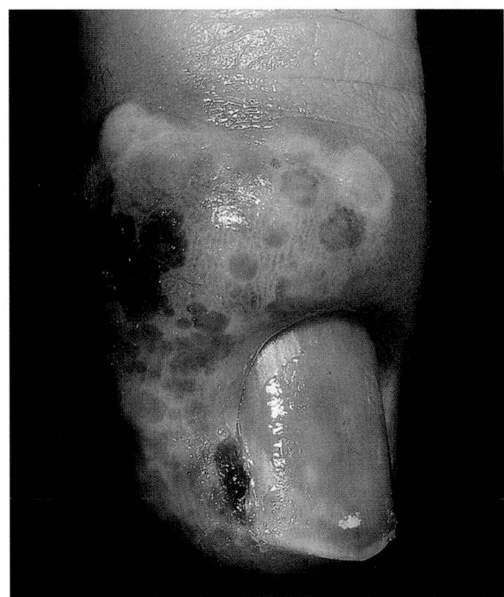

FIGURE 2.10-11. Herpes simplex virus infection: herpetic whitlow.

(Reproduced, with permission, from Wolff K, Johnson RA, Suurmond D. *Fitzpatrick's Color Atlas & Synopsis of Clinical Dermatology,* 5th ed. New York: McGraw-Hill, 2005: 805.)

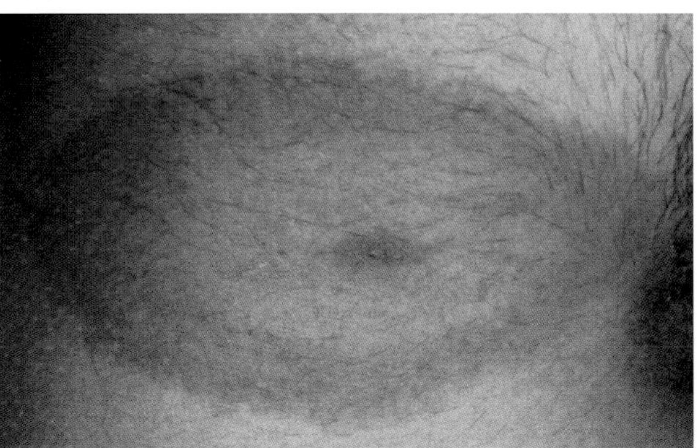

FIGURE 2.10-12. Erythema chronicum migrans rash of Lyme disease.

(Reproduced, with permission, from Fauci AS et al. [eds.]. *Harrison's Principles of Internal Medicine,* 17th ed. New York: McGraw-Hill, 2008: 1056.)

TABLE 2.10-5. Cutaneous Fungal Infections

	Dermatophytes	Candidiasis	Pityriasis (Tinea) Versicolor
Definition	Group of noninvasive fungi that infect keratinized tissue of epidermis, nails, and hair resulting in tinea infection.	Superficial yeast infection found on mucosal surfaces typically in moist occluded areas.	Chronic asymptomatic scaling condition characterized by well-demarcated patches with variable pigmentation usually on the trunk.
Etiology	*Trichophyton*, *Microsporum*, and *Epidermophyton*.	*Candida albicans* (most often). **Predisposing factors:** Diabetes, obesity, heat, maceration, steroid use (systemic and topical); invasive disseminated candidiasis in immunocompromised hosts.	*Plasmodium ovale* (aka *Malassezia furfur*).
Types	■ Tinea pedis (athlete's foot). ■ Tinea cruris (jock itch). ■ Tinea corporis (ringworm). ■ Onychomycosis (nail infection).	■ Genital (balanitis, vulvovaginitis). ■ Diaper dermatitis. ■ Oropharynx (thrush). ■ Nail (chronic paronychia). ■ Intertrigo.	
Diagnosis	■ **KOH → multiple septated hyphae.** ■ **Wood's lamp** → bright green fluorescence in hair shaft (tinea capitis).	**KOH → pseudohyphae** (elongated yeast without true septations).	KOH → round yeast and elongated pseudohyphae **("spaghetti and meatballs").**
Treatment	■ Prevention (well-ventilated, cotton clothing). ■ Topical antifungals (not for hair or nails). ■ Systemic antifungals (if no response to topicals).	■ Keep areas dry. ■ Topical antifungals (nystatin, azole, imidazole creams), oral antifungals for recurrent infections.	Topical agents (selenium sulfide shampoo, azole creams).

Diagnosis

- Serology: IgM titers are elevated in acute disease and peak 3–6 weeks after exposure.
- IgG levels peak when arthritis develops.
- May have false-⊖ results in first 4 weeks and false-⊕ results with other spirochetal infection and in patients with some autoimmune disorders (systemic lupus erythematosus, rheumatoid arthritis).

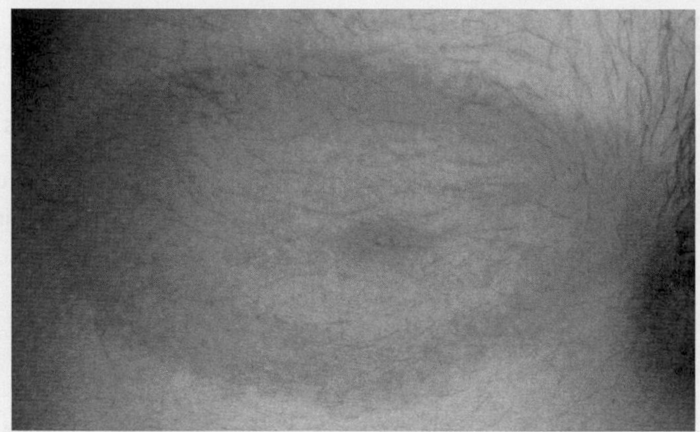

FIGURE 2.10-12. Erythema chronicum migrans rash of Lyme disease.

Also see Color Insert. (Reproduced, with permission, from Fauci AS et al. [eds.]. *Harrison's Principles of Internal Medicine,* 17th ed. New York: McGraw-Hill, 2008: 1056.)

COMPLICATIONS

- Sixty percent of untreated cases with disseminated infection develop arthritis (mediated by immune complex formation) 4–6 weeks following tick bite.
- May also develop **neurologic** (meningitis, encephalitis, or Bell's palsy) and cardiac involvement (carditis, atrioventricular block).

TREATMENT

Amoxicillin or doxycycline.

Acne Vulgaris

- Inflammation of pilosebaceous units of certain areas of the body including face, trunk, upper arms, and upper back caused by *Propionibacterium acnes* within the follicle.
- Typically seen in adolescents and up to 25 years.
- **Comedones** are the result—open (blackheads) and closed (whiteheads).
- Nodules or cysts are seen in more severe cases.

TREATMENT

- Goal is to remove plugging and treat infection (combination treatment is best).
- **Mild:** Topical antibiotics (clindamycin, erythromycin), benzoyl peroxide, topical retinoids.
- **Moderate:** Consider adding oral antibiotic (eg, minocycline) or oral contraceptives in females.
- **Severe:** Isotretinoin (Accutane).

Seborrheic Keratosis

- The most common benign tumor of the elderly.
- Develop from proliferating epidermal cells.
- Appear as waxy, stuck-on, tan-brown, verrucous lesions.

- **Sign of Leser-Trelat** is the association of multiple seborrheic keratoses with internal malignancy, usually adenocarcinoma of the gastrointestinal tract. No treatment is necessary.

SKIN CANCERS

Basal Cell Carcinoma

- The **most common** type of skin cancer due to a malignancy of the epidermal basal cells.
- Basal cells invade locally but almost never metastasize.
- Usually affect ages > 40 years.
- Whites generally affected.
- Risks are fair skin with chronic sun exposure, or radiation therapy.
- Diagnosed with biopsy and treated with excision.

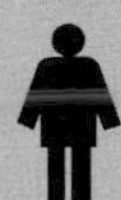

A 47-year-old white man presents with pearly, painless, ulcerated nodules with **overlying telangiectasias**. *Think: Basal cell carcinoma.*

FINDINGS

- **Nodular type:** A single translucent, **"pearly,"** waxy nodule or papule with **telangiectasias** and a **rolled border,** distributed on face and neck.
- **Superficial spreading type:** Multiple erythematous scaly plaques with a well-defined border distributed primarily on trunk; no relation to sun exposure.
- **Sclerosing type:** Yellowish white sclerotic waxy plaques with poorly defined borders, resembling scar tissue or morphea.
- **Pigmented type:** May have any of the above characteristics with pigmentation and is easily confused with malignant melanoma.

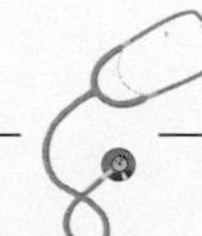

Dysplastic nevus is a premalignant precursor to malignant melanoma.

Squamous Cell Carcinoma

- A tumor of malignant keratinocytes accounting for the second most frequent type of skin cancer.
- Growth may be an **actinic keratosis** or de novo.
- Related to sun exposure, radiation exposure, immunosuppression, human papillomavirus, and xeroderma pigmentosum.

FINDINGS

- An erythematous scaling plaque that may be eroded or ulcerated with crust.
- Usually on sun exposed area of lips, cheeks, ears, scalp.
- **Biopsy:** Reveals malignant keratinocytes invading the dermis with keratin pearls.

TREATMENT

Excision or radiation if surgery can't be done.

Malignant Melanoma

- Melanoma is the malignant proliferation of melanocytes (pigment cells).
- It is the deadliest skin cancer.
- It may arise from normal-appearing skin (70%) or from a preexisting melanocytic nevi (mole) (30%).
- **Prognosis is based on the thickness of the primary tumor,** measured histologically according to the depth of invasion from the surface to the deepest part of the tumor (Breslow's classification) or according to the depth of penetration in relation to the different layers of the dermis (Clark's classification).
- Risks are sun exposure, fair skin and family history.

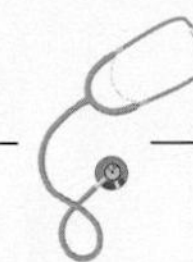

Melanomas can be brown, black, white, or blue.

CLINICAL VARIANTS

- **Superficial spreading melanoma:** Accounts for 70% of melanomas; characterized by horizontal growth. May develop as a new mole or as a change in a preexisting mole. It appears as an elevated plaque with irregular borders and variegated colors, but evolves into a nodule with bleeding and ulceration.
- **Nodular melanoma:** Characterized only by a vertical growth. Develops as a blue, gray, or black papule or nodule that may ulcerate or bleed. Associated with a poor prognosis because it metastasizes early.
- **Lentigo maligna melanoma:** Accounts for 10% of melanomas and occurs on sun-exposed areas of the skin in elderly patients. A slow-growing macule that gradually forms irregular borders, indistinct edges, or variable shades of color. May be present for years as a macule (lentigo maligna) before development of melanoma.
- **Acral lentiginous melanoma:** Accounts for $< 5\%$ of melanomas, and is common in black and Asian people. Develops as a flat, variably pigmented macule on the palms, soles, and nail beds that enlarges peripherally during its and then becomes nodular.

Suspicious features of malignant melanoma include the **ABCDEE**'s:
Asymmetry
Border (irregular)
Color (variegated and mottled)
Diameter ($>$ 0.6 cm)
Elevation
Enlargement

TREATMENT

- Surgical excision with margins of at least 1 cm, depending on depth of lesion for local disease.
- Interferon may be added in high risk as adjuvant therapy.

PROGNOSIS

Deep tumors and node involvement are high risk.

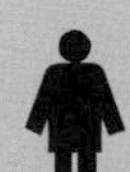

On exam, a patient is found to have an asymmetrical, variegated 7-mm lesion with an irregular border. *Think: Malignant melanoma.* **Next step:** Biopsy. **Treatment:** Resection.

HIGH-YIELD FACTS IN

Health Maintenance and Evidence-Based Medicine

Leading Causes of Death in the United States

1. Heart disease (26.6%).
2. Cancer (22.8%).
3. Stroke (5.9%).
4. Chronic obstructive pulmonary disease (COPD; 5.3%).
5. Unintentional injury (4.8%).
6. Diabetes mellitus (3.1%).

Note: Death rates for 2005. *National Vital Statistics Reports* 56(10): 2008.

Annual Exams

History and Counseling

- **Health maintenance:**
  - Nutrition.
  - Exercise (recommend 30 minutes of aerobic exercise 3×/wk).
  - Weight gain/loss.
- **Accident prevention:**
  - Safety belt/helmet use.
  - Smoke detectors.
  - Firearm safety.
- **Toxic habits:**
  - Alcohol consumption (CAGE criteria; see Alcohol section).
  - Tobacco use.
  - Illicit drug use.
- **Sexuality:**
  - Contraception.
  - Sexually transmitted disease (STD) prevention.
- **Domestic violence:**
  - Elder abuse.
  - Spousal abuse.

Tests and Exams

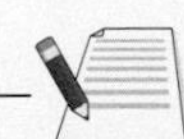

The only cancer screenings that are effective:

- Breast cancer (mammogram).
- Cervical cancer (Pap smear).
- Colon cancer (sigmoidoscopy/colonoscopy).
- Prostate cancer (prostate-specific antigen [PSA]—controversial).

- **Breast cancer screening protocol:**
  1. Ages 20–39 years:
     - Monthly breast self-exam (BSE).
     - Clinical breast examination (CBE) every 1–3 years.
  2. Ages 40–49 years:
     - Monthly BSE.
     - CBE every year.
     - Mammogram every 1–2 years.
  3. Ages 50–64 years:
     - Monthly BSE.
     - CBE every year.
     - Mammogram annually.
  4. Age 65 years and over:
     - Monthly BSE.
     - CBE every year.
     - Mammogram every 2 years.

- **Cervical cancer screening protocol:**
  - Perform Pap smear beginning within 3 years of first sexual activity or 18 years of age until the age of 65.
  - Perform every 2–3 years if three consecutive ⊖ Pap smears.
- **Colon cancer screening:**
  - Rectal exam yearly after age 50 years.
  - Occult blood in stool yearly after age 50 years.
  - Flexible sigmoidoscopy every 5 years after age 50 years, or colonoscopy every 8–10 years.
- **Prostate screening (controversial!):**
  - PSA and digital rectal exam yearly starting at age 50.
  - No screening after age 75.
- **Cardiovascular:**
  - Lipid profile starting at 25 years, every 5 years.
  - Blood pressure every 2 years.

Classification of Hypertension in Adults

- Normal: < 120/80 mmHg.
- Prehypertension: 120–139/80–89 mmHg.
- Stage 1 hypertension: 140–159/90–99 mmHg.
- Stage 2 hypertension: > 160/100 mmHg.

Age-Related Changes

- Height: ↓ as bone mass is lost with age.
- Vision and auditory screening at 65 years and older.

Adult Vaccinations

- **Tetanus:**
  - *Who:* Everyone.
  - *When:* Diphtheria, tetanus, and acellular pertussis (DTaP) series in childhood, booster every 10 years (or if > 5 years with a dirty wound).
- **Hepatitis A:**
  - *Who:* Travelers to countries with high /intermediate endemicity, men who have sex with men, illicit drug users, chronic liver disease, occupational risk, food handlers, clotting disorders.
  - *When:* Two doses 6–12 months apart, first dose takes 4 weeks to work effectively (any age).
- **Hepatitis B:**
  - *Who:* Everyone.
  - *When:* One series of three injections (time 0, 1 month, and 6 months) (any age).
- **Influenza:**
  - *Who:* Health care workers, age > 65, the chronically ill, and household contacts of these people.
  - *When:* Annually, autumn (new vaccine each year based on prediction of prevalent strains).
- **Pneumococcal (streptococcal) pneumonia:**
  - *Who:* Age > 65 or chronically ill.
  - *When:* Once every 5 years up to two doses.

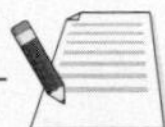

Vaccinations for AIDS patients:
- Influenza
- Hepatitis B
- *Haemophilus influenzae*
- Childhood vaccines, if missed

- **Measles, mumps, rubella (MMR):**
  - *Who:* All persons born after 1956 who lack evidence of immunity to measles.
  - *When:* First one at age 12–15 months, second one between 4 and 6 years, then a booster during adulthood if not previously received or not immune.
- **Varicella:**
  - *Who:* Healthy adults with no history of varicella infection or previous vaccination.
  - *When:* Two doses of varicella vaccine delivered 4–8 weeks apart are recommended.
- **Human papillomavirus:**
  - *Who:* Females 49 years and younger.
  - *When:* 0, 2, and 6 months.

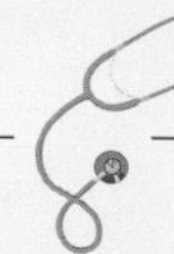

Raloxifene mimics estrogenic effects on osteoclasts but has no effect on breast, endometrium, or lipid profile. Useful for prevention of osteoporosis in women at high risk for breast cancer. Other benefits are lost.

HEALTH PROMOTION IN WOMEN

Hormone Replacement Therapy (HRT)

- Indicated in women with moderate to severe postmenpausal symptoms including vasomotor and urogenital symptoms.
- **Benefits:** ↓ risk of:
  - Osteoporosis.
  - Senile dementia.
  - Urinary incontinence, urinary tract infections (UTIs), and vaginal atrophy (local estrogen also effective).
  - Reduces hot flashes.
- **↑ risks:**
  - Coronary artery disease and stroke: Recent trials (Heart and Estrogen/Progestin Replacement Study [HERS and HERS II]) show ↑ risk.
  - Endometrial cancer: Associated with unopposed estrogen use. Can be prevented by using estrogen-progestin combination.
  - Breast cancer: Women with estrogen receptor–⊕ breast cancer worsen with HRT. Increases risk as well.
  - Venous thromboembolism.

Estrogen:
- Inhibits osteoclast bone resorption.
- Elevates high-density lipoprotein (HDL), lowers low-density lipoprotein (LDL), but raises triglycerides.

Domestic Violence

Epidemiology

- Lifetime prevalence 20% for women.
- In the United States, ~ 2000 women die each year as a direct result of injuries.

Signs and Symptoms

- Frequent or unexplained injuries.
- Depression.
- Suicide attempts.
- Anxiety.
- Chronic pain.
- Substance abuse.
- Headaches.

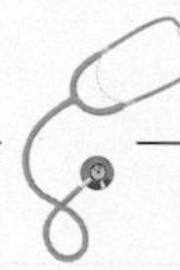

How to ask about domestic violence:
- "Have you ever been hit, hurt, or threatened by your partner?"
- "Have you ever been a victim of domestic violence?"
- "Many of my patients with your symptoms have experienced physical violence. Has this happened to you?"

Screening

- Women should be routinely asked about domestic violence due to its high prevalence.
- Routine screening of women by physicians is thought to yield ⊕ results in about half of all cases.

Treatment

- Treat medical conditions.
- Assess safety of patient's current situation.
- Provide information (shelters, social agencies).
- Reassure patient that no one deserves to be abused.

Differential diagnosis of depression:

- Bereavement
- Substance abuse
- Hypothyroidism
- Medication side effect
- Organic brain disease

Depression

Epidemiology

- Debilitating mood disorder that has a lifetime prevalence of about 15%.
- Incidence higher in women.
- Mean age is 40 years.

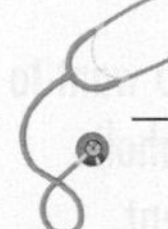

How to ask about depression:

- "Have you been feeling overwhelmingly sad lately?"
- "Have you lost pleasure in the things you used to enjoy?"

Risk Factors

- Family history of depression, suicide, substance abuse.
- Presence of chronic disease.
- Personal history of substance abuse.
- Lack of support system.

Signs and Symptoms

- Depressed mood with sadness.
- Weight loss.
- Guilt.
- Fatigue.
- Insomnia or hypersomnia.
- Anhedonia.
- Psychomotor agitation or retardation.
- Difficulty concentrating or suicidal ideation, for at least 2 consecutive weeks.

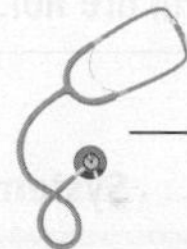

How to ask about suicidal intent:

- "Have you ever thought that life was not worth living?"
- "Have you ever thought about killing yourself?"
- "Have you ever made a plan to kill yourself?"

Treatment

- All patients should be asked specifically about suicidal intent.
- Patients who are actively suicidal require inpatient evaluation by a psychiatrist.
- Evaluate for antidepressant medication.

SUBSTANCE ABUSE

Alcohol Abuse

- Associated with failure to fulfill work or social obligations, physical danger because of alcohol use, or recurrent legal problems due to alcohol use.

Cancers due to alcohol use:
- Head and neck cancers
- Esophageal and gastric cancers
- Pancreatic cancer
- Liver cancer
- Breast cancer

What order do you want to give a chronic alcoholic vitamin replacement therapy to prevent neurologic deterioration? Thiamine, then glucose and folate.

Alcohol and benzodiazepine withdrawal are **life threatening.** Opioid and cocaine withdrawal are not.

- Alcohol dependence is at least three of the following: tolerance, withdrawal, taking more than intended, desire to cut down, time spent obtaining alcohol, aspects of life sacrificed.

Screening

CAGE questions:

1. Have you ever tried to Cut down your drinking?
2. Have you ever been Angry/Annoyed when people ask about your drinking?
3. Have you ever felt Guilty about your drinking?
4. Have you ever had an Eye-opener (drink on waking up in the morning)?

Systemic Effects

See Table 2.11-1.

Withdrawal Syndrome

- Can range from mild anxiety and tremor to alcohol withdrawal seizures and delirium tremens.
- **Alcohol withdrawal is life threatening.**
- Treat with benzodiazepine taper.
- Usual onset is 12–48 hours after last drink.

Delirium Tremens

- Tachycardia, fever, hallucinations.
- Five to thirty percent mortality if untreated.
- Treatment: Sedation with benzodiazepines and intensive care.

TABLE 2.11-1. Systemic Effects of Alcohol Abuse

	Acute	Chronic
Central nervous system (CNS)	CNS depression, amnesia, fragmented sleep.	Peripheral neuropathy, Wernicke's and Korsakoff's syndromes (thiamine deficiency), cerebellar degeneration, alcoholic dementia.
Cardiovascular system	Decreased myocardial contractility, peripheral vasodilation.	Hypertension, cardiomyopathy, ↑ HDL cholesterol.
Gastrointestinal system	Esophageal and gastric inflammation, acute pancreatitis.	Mallory-Weiss tear, esophageal varices, portal hypertension, chronic pancreatitis.
Liver	Impaired gluconeogenesis.	Alcohol-induced hepatitis, cirrhosis.
Hematopoietic system	Macrocytosis.	Thrombocytopenia, hypersplenism, ↓ platelet aggregation.
Genitourinary system	Erectile dysfunction.	Testicular atrophy, amenorrhea, ovarian atrophy, ↑ risk of spontaneous abortion, fetal alcohol syndrome.

Tobacco Use

- Single largest cause of preventable death in the United States.
- About 450,000 people in the United States die each year from tobacco-related disease:
  - 40% cardiovascular
  - 35% due to cancer
  - 20% respiratory
  - 5% cerebrovascular

TOBACCO-RELATED DISEASE

Smoking:

- Promotes atherosclerosis, thrombosis, arrhythmias.
- Reduces oxygen-carrying capacity of the blood.
- Reduces elasticity in the lungs and causes COPD and emphysema.
- During pregnancy associated with increased risk of spontaneous abortion, fetal death, and sudden infant death syndrome.
- Smokeless tobacco products cause oral and head and neck cancers.

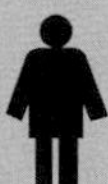

A 50-year-old man complains of pain in legs with walking. Straight leg raising test indicates claudication. **Next step:** Smoking cessation counseling.

SMOKING CESSATION

Counseling should be a primary focus of all physician encounters with smokers:

- Identify all smokers and tobacco users by routine questioning during history.
- Instruct all tobacco users to stop, giving personalized advice and support (eg, " If you stop smoking, your cough will improve").
- Evaluate each patient for readiness and motivation. If the patient is not motivated, reinforce that support for smoking cessation will be available when the patient is ready.
- Formulate a plan with the patient, including a quit date, nicotine replacement or other pharmacologic therapy, and follow-up appointment for support.
- **Pharmacotherapy:**
  - Nicotine patches are associated with a 40% quit rate.
  - Bupropion is associated with a 55% quit rate.
  - Chantix (varenicline): Oral preparation works by partially activating the nicotine receptors in the brain. Typically given for 12 days.
  - Combination is associated with a 66% quit rate.
  - Ongoing counseling may improve abstinence.

Types of Tobacco-Related Cancer—

CANCER PLUS

Colon
A
Neck
Cervix
Esophagus
Renal
Pancreas
Lung
Urogenital (bladder)
Stomach

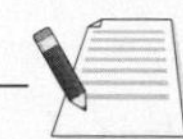

The most effective way to extend life expectancy in a healthy patient is smoking cessation.

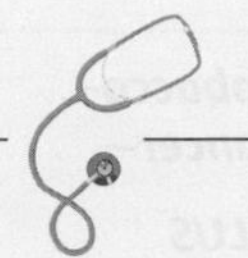

A patient on opioids for true pain control has little risk of developing opiate dependence.

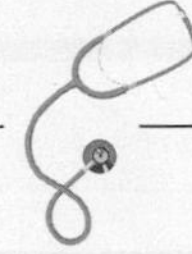

A significant percentage of patients presenting with cocaine chest pain will have biochemical evidence for a myocardial infarction.

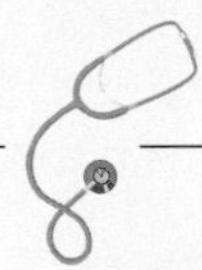

Beta blockers are relatively contraindicated in patients with cocaine use due to the risk of unopposed alpha-adrenergic tone, which may worsen vasoconstriction.

Opioid Use

Signs and Symptoms of Use and Overdose

- Depressed mental status.
- Respiratory depression.
- Pupillary constriction (or dilation with profound respiratory depression).
- Overdose can cause death.

Treatment of Overdose

- Naloxone is an opioid antagonist that rapidly reverses toxicity, but is short acting (< 30 min).
- Use is both diagnostic and therapeutic.
- Respiratory support if respiration is depressed.

Opiate Withdrawal Syndrome

- Not life threatening, except in very young and very old, but may → relapse, using street drugs, and exposure to needle sharing with its attendant risks such as acquisition of HIV and hepatitis C.
- **Signs and symptoms:** Nausea, vomiting, diarrhea, mydriasis, piloerection, muscle pain.
- **Treatment of withdrawal and addiction:**
  - Symptomatic relief for withdrawal.
  - Long-acting opioid (eg, methadone) for treatment of addiction.

Sympathomimetics (Cocaine and Speed)

Signs and Symptoms

Syndrome of catecholamine excess: Agitation, tachycardia, hypertension, hyperthermia, psychosis, seizures, chest pain.

Treatment

- Benzodiazepines to control excess sympathetic discharge and anxiety.
- Cooling measures to control hyperthermia.
- Nitroglycerin and heparin to control chest pain.

INJURY PREVENTION

Motor Vehicle Injuries

- Statistics:
  - Cause 30% of all deaths between ages 15 and 25.
  - Disproportionately affect the young, so responsible for more years of life lost than any other single cause.
  - Alcohol is implicated in 44% of all traffic fatalities.
  - Seatbelt use is associated with an 89% reduction in mortality, and concurrent airbag use further reduces mortality.
  - Motorcycle use is associated with a fatality rate 20 times greater than that of passenger cars.
  - Helmet use reduces motorcycle fatalities by 37% and reduces the incidence of head injury by 67%.

- Screening:
  - Ask all patients about seatbelt use, airbag availability, helmet use, child safety seat use, and alcohol use.
  - Intervene when patients show behaviors that put others in danger (eg, adult does not provide toddler with a child safety seat).

Falls

Most common cause of injuries.

Risk Factors

- Elderly
- Disabled
- Alcohol

Prevention

- Assess gait of each patient.
- Assess vision of each patient.
- Provide corrective devices or referral for identified impairment.
- Counsel alcohol cessation.

NUTRITIONAL DISORDERS

Malnutrition

- Marasmus: Starvation.
- Kwashiorkor: Protein deficiency.
- Essential fatty acids: Linoleic and linolenic acids.

Risk Factors

- Low socioeconomic class.
- Nursing home and hospitalized patients.

Complications

- Anemia.
- Anasarca.
- Poor wound healing.
- Decubitus ulcer.
- Infection.
- Death.

Obesity

Body mass index (BMI) > 30 kg/m^2.

Complications

- Atherosclerosis.
- Metabolic syndrome.
- Type 2 diabetes.
- Sleep apnea.
- Osteoarthritis.
- Gout.

- Venous stasis.
- Biliary disease.
- Endometrial cancer.
- Postmenopausal breast cancer.

TREATMENT

- Behavior modification, exercise.
- Low-calorie diet with < 25% of calories from fat.
- Goal: 10% weight loss over 6 months.
- If the above fail, consider:
  - Pharmacologic therapy.
  - Bariatric surgery (for BMI > 40 m² or > 35 m² with comorbid disease).

Vitaminoses

See Table 2.11-2.

TABLE 2.11-2. Syndromes of Vitamin Deficiency and Excess

VITAMIN	DEFICIENCY	EXCESS
Vitamin A	▪ **Early:** Night blindness. ▪ **Late:** Keratomalacia, blindness.	**Acute:** Gastrointestinal symptoms, headache, papilledema. **Chronic:** Joint pain, hair loss, fissured lips, anorexia, weight loss, hepatomegaly.
Vitamin C	**Scurvy:** Petechial hemorrhage, ecchymoses, gum bleeding, poor wound healing, anemia.	Uricosuria, kidney stones.
Vitamin E	Areflexia, decreased proprioception, gait abnormality.	Potentiates oral anticoagulants.
Vitamin K	Prolonged bleeding time.	Attenuates oral anticoagulants.
Niacin	**Pellagra:** Chronic wasting, dermatitis, dementia, diarrhea.	Gastrointestinal symptoms, flushing, pruritus, hepatotoxicity.
Thiamine (vitamin B_1)	▪ Beriberi (dry). ▪ Peripheral neuropathy. ▪ Wernicke' s encephalopathy (horizontal nystagmus followed by lateral rectus palsy, fever, ataxia, encephalopathy, death). ▪ Korsakoff' s syndrome (retrograde amnesia, confabulation).	
Pyridoxine (vitamin B_6)	▪ Seizures. ▪ Glossitis, cheilosis. ▪ Gastrointestinal symptoms. ▪ Weakness. ▪ Peripheral neuropathy.	

ENVIRONMENTAL EXPOSURES

Heat Exhaustion

- Normal core temperature, symptoms due to dehydration and salt loss.
- Characterized by headache, nausea and vomiting, weakness, irritability, and cramps.
- Treat with oral or IV hydration with salt-containing fluids, and patient should rest in a cool environment.

Heatstroke

- Failure of thermoregulation.
- Associated with elevated core temperature and central nervous system (CNS) dysfunction such as altered mental status, focal deficits, hemiplegia, and posturing.
- Exertional heatstroke is a result of exercise or physical labor in a high-heat-index environment.
- Classic or nonexertional heatstroke is usually seen in elderly or nonacclimated patients during summer heat waves.
- **Treatment:** Rapid cooling by cooling blanket, evaporation, ice packs to axilla and groin, or gastric or peritoneal lavage is critical to prevent rhabdomyolysis, multiorgan failure, and death.

Cold-Related Illness

Risk factors: Overwhelming cold exposure, extremes of age, intoxication, homeless, chronic illness, iatrogenic.

FROSTBITE

- Caused by exposure of the skin to freezing temperatures; usually seen on the extremities, nose, and ears.
- As the body reduces cutaneous blood flow in freezing temperatures to maintain the core body temperature, capillary blood becomes more viscous, and ice crystals form in the extracellular space. This causes direct tissue injury and osmotic pressures that cause intracellular dehydration.

TREATMENT

- Rapid rewarming with clean water at 40–42°C.
- Tetanus prophylaxis.
- Debridement of tissues and prophylactic antibiotics remains controversial.

HYPOTHERMIA

Core (rectal) temperature:

- Mild: 32–35°C.
- Moderate: 28–32°C.
- Severe: < 28°C.

SIGNS AND SYMPTOMS

- Shivering.
- Poor judgment.
- Paradoxical undressing.

What would a hypothermic patient show on electrocardiogram? Osborn wave

- Cardiac dysrhythmias.
- Osborne wave: A convex, upward deflection of the J point on electrocardiogram.

Treatment

- **Rewarming** by:
  - Warming blanket.
  - Warm packs to groin and axillae.
  - Infusion of **warmed IV fluid.**
- For severely hypothermic or pulseless patients: Warm-fluid lavage of bladder, stomach, peritoneum, and pleural space.

MEDICAL ETHICS

See Table 2.11-3.

TABLE 2.11-3. Principles of Medical Ethics

Principle	Definition
Autonomy	▪ Ability to function independently and to make decisions about one's care free from the undue influence or bias of others. ▪ All patients are considered autonomous if they have the ability to understand the situation as evaluated with competency examination by psychiatrist (capacity) and are not a danger to self or others (suicidal, homicidal, demented, delirious).
Nonmalfeasance	▪ The principle of *primum non nocere,* or first, do no harm.
Beneficence	▪ The principle of doing good. ▪ The practice of doing whatever is best for the patient without the consideration of the patient's wishes is called *paternalism.*
Distributive justice	▪ The principle of equal and fair allocation of benefit. Patients of different race, gender, and disability should be treated differently only on the basis of medical need and projected benefit.
Advance directives	▪ Oral or written instructions from a patient to family members and health care professionals about health care decisions. ▪ May include living wills, designation of a health care proxy, specific instructions about which therapies to accept or decline including intubation, surgery or medical treatments, and Do Not Resuscitate (DNR) orders. A DNR order applies only to advanced cardiac life support (ACLS) resuscitation, and does not include intubation and ventilation unless specifically addressed.

- Practice of incorporating the best available evidence from the medical literature for a diagnostic test or treatment into daily patient care.
- Best evidence obtained from randomized clinical trials.

STEPS

1. Identify a clinical problem.
2. Formulate a question.
3. Search for the best evidence.
4. Appraise the evidence.
5. Apply the information to the clinical problem.

SOURCES OF MEDICAL EVIDENCE

- **Randomized controlled clinical trial:** *This is the strongest type of evidence.* The selected population is randomized to receive either the treatment in question or a placebo (or the current standard of care), and the outcome is measured. The ideal randomized controlled trial is triple-blinded, meaning that the treating physician, the patient, and the investigators do not know which treatment has been given until the analysis is complete. These studies can establish cause and effect.
- **Cohort study:** The selected population is identified as being exposed or not exposed, and is monitored for subsequent effects. These studies are used when the exposure cannot be assigned for logistical or ethical reasons.
- **Case control study:** Populations with and without a given outcome are selected, and historical (retrospective) data is collected on exposure to a given agent or treatment.
- **Meta-analysis:** Evaluates the data of many trials that address the same question, and attempts to combine the information. These studies are best used when the clinical problem is infrequent and large randomized trials cannot be done.

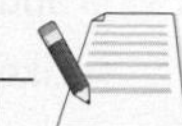

If a disease has a high incidence with a low prevalence, it is a disease that causes rapid fatality. If a disease has a high prevalence with a low incidence, it is a chronic disease with a low fatality.

Statistical Concepts

See Table 2.11-4 for statistical concepts and Table 2.11-5 for sensitivity and specificity vs. positive and negative predictive value.

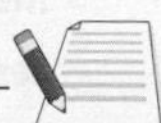

By screening a population, the death rate of a cancer dropped from 1% to 0.4%. How many people are needed to screen to save one life? NNT = 1 / (control rate – experimental rate); 1 / (0.01 – 0.004) = 167

Types of Prevention

- **Primordial:** Deals with underlying conditions → exposure to causative factors.
- **Primary:** Deals with limiting the incidence of disease by controlling causes and risk factors.
- **Secondary:** The detection and amelioration of disease in a preclinical and presymptomatic stage.
- **Tertiary:** Prevention of future negative effects of the existing disease.

TABLE 2.11-4. Statistical Concepts

CONCEPT	DEFINITION
Sensitivity	▪ Measures the ability of a test to accurately detect true-positive results: TP / (TP + FN) (true positive test results/all patients with the disease). ▪ The more sensitive a test, the less likely the test is to fail to detect a positive result. This is sometimes called a true-positive rate (TPR).
Specificity	▪ Measures the ability of a test to accurately detect true-negative results: TN / (FP + TN) (true negative test result/all patients without the disease). ▪ The more specific a test, the less likely the test is to fail to detect a negative result. This is sometimes called a true-negative rate (TNR).
Positive predictive value	▪ Measures the chance that a patient with a positive test result in truth has the disease: TP / (TP + FP) (true positives/test positives). **Depends on disease prevalence.**
Negative predictive value	▪ Measures the chance that a patient with a negative test result in truth does not have the disease: TN / (TN + FN) (true negatives/test negatives). **Depends on disease prevalence.**
Likelihood ratio	▪ Measures the fixed relationship between the chance of given test result in a patient with the disorder and the chance of the same test result in a patient without the disorder. ▪ Likelihood ratio for a positive test result is expressed as: sensitivity/(1-specificity) or true-positive rate (TPR)/false-positive rate (FPR). ▪ Likelihood ratio for a negative test result is expressed as: (1-sensitivity)/specificity or false-negative rate (FNR)/true-negative rate (TNR). ▪ A test with known likelihood ratios can help a clinician with decision making; the pretest likelihood that a patient has a disease can be either improved with a high positive likelihood ratio (< 2) or reduced with a low negative likelihood ratio (> 0.5).
Confidence interval	▪ Range around a sample mean that contains the true population mean to any desired degree of probability (frequently 95%).
Number needed to treat	▪ Measures the number of patients with a given disease that a clinician would need to treat with the tested therapy in order to see one beneficial event or prevent one adverse event. **Calculating numbers needed to treat NNT:** Number needed to treat = 1 / (control group rate – experimental group rate)
Prevalence	▪ Number of individuals with a given disease in a population at one point in time (number with disease/ number in population).
Incidence	▪ Number of new events (new cases of disease) over a specific period of time (number of new events/ number in population).

TABLE 2.11-5. Sensitivity and Specificity vs. Positive and Negative Predictive Value

	Disease Present	Disease Absent	
Test Positive	True Positive (TP)	False Positive (FP)	Positive predictive value = TP / (TP + FP)
Test Negative	False Negative (FN) Sensitivity = TP / (TP/FN)	True Negative (TN) Specificity = FP / (FP + TN)	Negative predictive value = FN / (FN + TN)

SECTION III: CLASSIFIED

Awards and Opportunities for Students Interested in Medicine

- General Awards
- Research Awards
- Summer Externships
- Year-Long Fellowships
- For Minority Students
- Ethnic
- For Women
- Awards and Links to Medical Subspecialty Societies
- Evidence-Based Medicine Links

The Columbia University College of Physicians and Surgeons web site has an excellent web site with a list of resources for medical students, which is a great place to start your search for opportunities: *www.cumc.columbia.edu/dept/ps/affairs/subject1.html.*

The Paul & Daisy Soros Fellowships for New Americans

The fellowships are grants for $20,000 for up to 2 years of graduate study in the United States. The recipients are chosen on a national competitive basis. Thirty fellowships will be awarded each year.

A New American is an individual who (1) is a resident alien (i.e., holds a green card) or (2) has been naturalized as a U.S. citizen or (3) is the child of two parents who are both naturalized citizens.

The purpose of The Paul & Daisy Soros Fellowships for New Americans is to provide opportunities for continuing generations of able and accomplished New Americans to achieve leadership in their chosen fields. The program is established in recognition of the contributions New Americans have made to American life and in gratitude for the opportunities the United States has afforded the donors and their family. *Contact:* 400 West 59th Street, New York, NY 10019. Phone: 212-547-6926; fax: 212-548-4623; *www.soros.org/initiatives/map.*

AMERICAN ASSOCIATION FOR THE HISTORY OF MEDICINE OSLER MEDAL

The medal is awarded for the best unpublished essay on a medico-historical subject written by a student in a school of medicine or of osteopathy in the United States or Canada. Essays appropriate for consideration by the committee may pertain either to the historical development of a contemporary medical problem or to a topic within the health sciences of a discrete past period. The essay should demonstrate either original research or an unusual appreciation and understanding of the problem or situation discussed. Winner will receive $500 in travel money to deliver paper at the American Association for the History of Medicine.

Coe Memorial Scholarship

For medical students who are from the Auburn, New York, area. *Contact:* Norstar Trust Company, Coe Memorial Scholarship Fund, 120 Genesee St., Auburn, NY 13021.

Country Doctor Scholarship Program

$10,000 annually, $40,000 aggregate

Georgia residents qualify for funding to obtain primary care medical degrees such as internal medicine, general surgery, OB/GYN, pediatrics, and family practice. In return, the student must practice in a Georgia board-approved town of 15,000 or less population. *Contact:* Joe B. Lawley, PhD, State Medical Education Board, 270 Washington St. SW, 7th Floor, Room 7093, Atlanta, GA 30334.

ILLINOIS HOSPITAL ASSOCIATION SCHOLARSHIP

$500 award for students who are Illinois residents with demonstrated financial need and academic acheievement. *Contact:* Scholarship, The Illinois Hospital Association, Center for Health Affairs, 1151 East Warrenville Rd., P.O. Box 3015, Naperville, IL 60566.

New York Academy of Medicine: David E. Rogers Fellowship Program

The David E. Rogers Fellowship Program is national fellowship for medical students in support of a project initiated during the summer between the first and second years of medical school. Ten fellowships of $2,500 will be awarded. The fellowship is meant to enrich the educational experiences of medical students through projects that couple medicine with the needs of underserved or disadvantaged patients or populations. For more information, contact the Rogers Fellowship at *rogers@nyam.org* or the New York Academy of Medicine. Contact your school's financial aid office for more info.

DoctorsCare Internationale Foundation Scholarships

DoctorsCare is an independent nonprofit organization created to promote scientific research, education, and medical health programs that contribute toward improving the health of mankind. The foundation has funds for annual grants for needy men and women in the field of medicine. Applications may be obtained by sending a self-addressed, stamped envelope to: Grants Department, Doctors Care Internationale Foundation, P.O. Box 1111, Houston, TX 77251-1111.

WILDERNESS SOCIETY CHARLES S. HOUSTON AWARD

Award for a project proposal that is likely to result in a substantive contribution to the field of wilderness or environmental medicine. The applicant will conduct his project during the calendar year and present results at the Annual Meeting of the Society. Award: $1,500; *www.ddcf.org/page.asp?pageId=12.*

U.S. Department of Health and Human Services Innovations in Health Award

An annual competition for innovative proposals for health promotion and disease prevention. The proposal must be concerned with disease prevention or health promotion. It could describe a community risk-reduction effort; a project for a whole community or a special population group, such as the aged or children; a health promotion program at the worksite; or a preventive approach for community education, such as primary and secondary school programs. Awards range from $250 to $3,000; *www.medicalreservecorps.gov/HomePage.*

Life and Health Insurance Medical Research Fund Medical Scientist Scholarship

A 5-year scholarship program for an MD/PhD student who will have completed 2 years of medical school before July and is usually not already funded. $16,000 per year; *http://mstp.uci.edu/currentstudents/fellowships.php.*

AMERICAN ACADEMY OF MEDICAL ETHICS WILLIAM LILEY ESSAY CONTEST

An essay contest for medical students and residents on a topic designated by the Academy. $250–2,000 prizes; *http://ps.cpmc.columbia.edu/affairs/awards/awrd0087.html.*

Paul W. Mayer Scholarship in Medicine and Biology

Sponsored by the Alliance for Engineering, this is a scholarship to encourage student excellence in the field of biomedical engineering. Grant is $200. Contact your school's financial aid office for more info.

Jerry L. Memorial Pettis Scholarship

Sponsored by the American Medical Association Education and Research Foundation, this scholarship will be awarded to a junior or senior medical student with a demonstrated interest in the communication of science. Financial need of nominees will not be a consideration. *Contact:* American Medical Association Education and Research Foundation, 515 North State Street, Chicago, IL 60610. Phone: 312-464-5357; fax: 312-464-5973; *www.ama-assn.org/medsci/erf/toc.htm.*

STUDENT PAPER COMPETITION IN MEDICAL INFORMATICS

Students are invited to submit papers expressing original ideas in the broad areas of medical informatics and computer applications in medical care for the SCAMC (Symposium on Computer Applications in Medical Care). Awards consist of the Martin N. Epstein Award of $1,000 and two cash prizes of $600 and $400 for second and third place. Contact your school's financial aid office for more info.

American College of Legal Medicine Schwartz Award

Each year the ACLM presents the Schwartz Award for the outstanding paper on legal medicine. The award provides a $1,000 honorarium, transportation, accommodations, and meals at the ACLM annual meeting. Contact your school's financial aid office for more info.

Medical History Society of New Jersey Stephen Wickes Prize in the History of Medicine

Any currently enrolled undergraduate, graduate, or professional student is eligible to submit an original essay on a historical subject in the medical or allied fields. The topic may be historical aspects of a current problem, or it may deal with a specific subject in a defined period of the past. Prize: $100. Contact your school's financial aid office for more info.

NORTHEASTERN OHIO UNIVERSITY COLLEGE OF MEDICINE WILLIAM CARLOS POETRY COMPETITION

The Human Values in Medicine at Northeastern Ohio Universities College of Medicine is sponsoring this annual poetry-writing competition for students attending schools of medicine or osteopathy in the United States. Prize: $100–$300. Contact your school's financial aid office for more info.

New York Academy of Medicine: The Paul Klemperer Fellowship in the History of Medicine and the Audrey and William H. Helfand Fellowship in the Medical Humanities

Each year the New York Academy of Medicine offers the Paul Klemperer Fellowship and the Audrey and William H. Helfand Fellowship to support work in history and the humanities as they relate to health, medicine, and the biomedical sciences. The Klemperer Fellowship supports research using the Academy Library as a historical resource. It is intended specifically for a scholar in residence in the collections of the Academy Library.

The Helfand Fellowship more broadly supports work in the humanities, including both creative projects dealing with health and the medical enterprise, and scholarly research in a humanistic discipline—other than history of medicine—as applied to medicine and health. Although residence is not obligatory, preference in the selection process will be given applicants whose projects require use of the resources of the Academy Library and who plan to spend time at the Academy. The Helfand Fellowship and the Klemperer Fellowship each provide stipends of up to $5,000 to support travel, lodging, and incidental expenses for a flexible period between June 1, 2001, and May 31, 2002. Besides completing research or a creative project, each Fellow will be expected to make a presentation at the Academy and submit a final report on the project. Applications are accepted from anyone—regardless of citizenship, academic discipline, or academic status—who wishes to use the Academy's collections for historical research or for a scholarly or creative project in the medical humanities. *Contact:* Fellowship Program Coordinator, New York Academy of Medicine, 1216 Fifth Avenue, Room 612, New York, NY 10029. Phone: 212-822-7204; fax: 212-996-7826.

Agency for International Development Internship

Sponsoring Agency: A.I.D.

Two-week educational program (over Christmas holiday) for graduate students from the Caribbean and South and Central America, which may lead to summer placement in transnational corporations over summer. Program focuses on U.S. foreign policy and Latin American indebtedness. Travel costs to seminar in Baton Rouge paid.

ALPHA OMEGA ALPHA ESSAY AWARD

The purpose of these $500–$750 awards is to stimulate medical students to address general topics in medicine and to enable the society to recognize in a tangible way excellent and thoughtful presentations. The topic of the essay may be any nontechnical aspect of medicine, including medical education, medical ethics, philosophy as related to medicine, reflections on illness, science, and the culture and history of medicine.

American Bureau for Medical Advancement in China

Open to fourth-year students. Several university teaching hospitals in Taiwan offer clinical clerkships to qualifying students. Electives of 2 months are optimal, although shorter ones will be considered. It is expected that students will be able to provide for their own transportation and room and board, but Warner-Lambert has provided a grant to accommodate several partial scholarships.

American College of Nutrition

Award based on original scientific work in Clinical Nutrition. Award: $500 plus transportation to meeting.

AMERICAN COLLEGE OF PREVENTIVE MEDICINE

$1,000 award for the best paper on preventive medicine–oriented topics; papers concerned with women's health issues encouraged.

National Council on Aging—Geriatric Fellowship

Sponsored by Travelers Insurance Aging, Inc., this program is designed to increase students' technical knowledge of geriatrics and to help sensitize them to social and personal problems facing older people. A fellowship of $3,000 will be provided.

Joseph and Rose Kennedy Institute of Ethics National Humanities in Medicine Seminar

This seminar was established to achieve three purposes: to provide selected medical students with an intensive experience in research and writing in the history of medicine, or philosophy of medicine, or literature and medicine; to encourage these students to develop programs of research and writing in a discipline of the humanities, which they will carry out during subsequent years of professional education and training and during careers as clinicians and humanists; and to link these students with other humanists in medicine across generational and disciplinary boundaries. Each student will receive a stipend of $1,200 to cover room and board. Students will be reimbursed for round-trip airfares to and from their school or home.

ACP-ASIM MEDICAL STUDENT ABSTRACT COMPETITION

Wanted: Students involved in research projects through their medical schools or community service programs they want to share with others, or who have come across as interesting case during an internal medicine rotation or through an internal medicine preceptorship program. If you are a medical student member of the ACP-ASIM, you are invited to submit an abstract to the annual Medical Student Abstract Competition. Ten winners will be awarded an expense-paid trip to the annual session. Abstracts may be submitted electronically using our online form at *www.acp.org*.

Medical Student Membership in the American College of Physicians–American Society of Internal Medicine

ACP-ASIM membership entitles you to special discounts on various college products, free attendance at ACP-ASIM annual session (the annual scientific meeting) and local chapter meetings, and a subscription to IMpact, the medical student newsletter.

AMA Political Action Committee (AMPAC)

AMPAC is a bipartisan group that serves to advance the interest of medicine within Congress, specifically by supporting candidates for office that are friendly to medicine. They also provide numerous programs to educate physicians, medical students, and their families on political activism. The board directs the programs and activities of this extremely important political action committee. Adding medical students to the leadership of this group will provide for better medical student representation within the group, as well as greater student involvement in this important process. Terms are for 2 years. Contact the American Medical Association for more information.

AMA FOUNDATION LEADERSHIP AWARD PROGRAM

This award is an exciting opportunity to advance your leadership skills within organized medicine. Medical students who have demonstrated strong nonclinical leadership skills in medicine or community affairs and have an interest in further developing these skills within organized medicine are eligible. The objective of the award program is to encourage involvement in organized medicine and continue leadership development among the country's brightest and most energetic medical students and residents. Twenty-five medical students will be selected. Travel expenses for award winners, including airfare and 3 nights' lodging, will be paid for directly by the AMA Foundation to attend the 2001 AMA National Leadership Development Conference. For applications, call 1-800-AMA-3211, ext. 4751 or 4746.

GENERAL AWARDS

American Medical Student Association (AMSA)

International Health Opportunities; *www.amsa.org/global/ih/ihopps.cfm.*

AMA-MSS Councils

The medical student section of the AMA (AMA-MSS) has several councils for which it seeks medical students. Application involves a current curriculum vitae, an essay on why you want to be a member of an AMA Council, which council(s) you prefer, what you consider to be your major strengths and qualifications for the position, and what benefits you feel are likely to result from your participation.

- Council on Constitution and Bylaws
- Council on Ethical and Judicial Affairs
- Council on Legislation
- Council on Long-Range Planning and Development
- Council on Medical Education
- Council on Medical Service
- Council on Scientific Affairs

EDITORIAL POSITIONS WITH MEDICAL STUDENT JAMA

MS/JAMA is the 7- to 8-page medical student section of the *Journal of the American Medical Association* (JAMA) that appears in the first JAMA of every month, September through May, and is also produced each month on the MS/JAMA web site. As a regular section of a major medical journal, produced by and for medical students, MS/JAMA represents a unique opportunity to train to become journal editors, writers, and contributors. The MS/JAMA web site is located at *www.ama-assn.org/msjama.*

AMA-MSS Committee Application

Medical students are sought to serve on the following AMA-MSS committees:

- Committee on Computers and Technology (formerly Computer Projects Committee)
- Committee on Long-Range Planning
- Legislative Affairs Committee
- Minority Issues Committee
- Ad Hoc Committee on Community Service and Advocacy
- Ad Hoc Committee on Membership Recruitment and Retention
- Ad Hoc Committee on MSS Programs and Activities
- Ad Hoc Committee on Scientific Issues Committee (CSI)
- Ad Hoc Committee on International Health and Policy

All applications must be completed and submitted with a CV to: American Medical Association, Department of Medical Student Services, 515 North State Street, Chicago, IL 60610. Fax: 312-464-5845.

RESEARCH AWARDS

National Tay-Sachs & Allied Disease Foundation

The primary objective of these awards is to stimulate interest in the field of lysosomal storage diseases. The research may be basic, applied, or clinical and should be performed under the direction of an investigator experienced in the field. Stipend: $1,500.

NEW YORK ACADEMY OF MEDICINE: THE GLORNEY-RAISBECK MEDICAL STUDENT GRANTS IN CARDIOVASCULAR RESEARCH PROGRAM

Three grants of $3,000 will be provided to support projects in either clinical or basic research initiated during the summer. Competition is open to MD candidates in a metropolitan area medical school in New York City, Long Island, Westchester County, or New Jersey. The award will be paid directly to the sponsoring medical school for distribution to the recipient. The deadline for submission of applications is March. *Contact:* Fellowship Program Coordinator, New York

Academy of Medicine, 1216 Fifth Avenue, Room 612, New York, NY 10029. Phone: 212-822-7204; fax: 212-996-7826.

New York Academy of Medicine: The Louis L. Seaman Medical Student Research Grants in Microbiology

Four grants of $2,500 will be provided to support summer research projects in the field of microbiology. Competition is open to MD students in a metropolitan area medical school in New York City, Long Island, Westchester County, or New Jersey. The award will be paid directly to the student, but is contingent on the submission of a written report on the project. *Contact:* Fellowship Program Coordinator, New York Academy of Medicine, 1216 Fifth Avenue, Room 612, New York, NY 10029. Phone: 212-822-7204; fax: 212-996-7826.

American Medical Association Education and Research Foundation Seed Research Grants

Up to $2,500 support for medical students for small research projects or, in some instances, to provide interim funding prior to large grant approvals from other sources. Grants will be awarded in two cycles during the school year: (1) September through November and (2) January through March. *Contact:* American Medical Association Education and Research Foundation, 515 North State Street, Chicago, IL 60610. Phone: 312-464-5357; fax: 312-464-5973; *www.ama-assn.org/medsci/erf/toc.htm.*

WEIS CENTER FOR RESEARCH GEISINGER CLINIC

Three-month program designed to expose medical students to career opportunities in research. Primary emphasis is at the cellular/molecular level of cardiovascular function. Stipend: $800/month.

John A. Hartford/AFAR Medical Student Geriatric Scholars Program

To encourage medical students, particularly budding researchers, to consider geriatrics as a career, the Medical Student Geriatric Scholars Program awards short-term scholarships through a national competition. The program provides an opportunity for these students to train at an acclaimed center of excellence in geriatrics. Each scholar receives a $3,000 stipend. Students in the New York metropolitan area can apply for funding through the Farr Fox and Leslie R. Samuels Foundation/AFAR Medical Student Geriatric Scholars Program. Contact American Federation for Aging Research (AFAR), 1414 Avenue of the Americas, 18th Floor, New York, NY 10019. Phone: 212-752-2327; fax: 212-832-2298; e-mail: *amfedaging@aol.com.*

Glenn Foundation/AFAR Scholarships for Research in the Biology of Aging

Inaugurated in 1994, this scholarship program was designed to attract potential scientists and clinicians to aging research. Provides PhD and MD students the opportunity to conduct a 3-month research project. Students will work in an area of biomedical research in aging under the auspices of a mentor. Each scholarship carries an award of $5,000. *Contact:* American Federation for Aging Research (AFAR), 1414 Avenue of the Americas, 18th Floor, New York, NY 10019. Phone: 212-752-2327; fax: 212-832-2298; e-mail: *amfedaging@aol.com.*

MERCK/AFAR RESEARCH SCHOLARSHIPS IN GERIATRIC PHARMACOLOGY FOR MEDICAL STUDENTS

To develop a corps of physicians with an understanding of medication use in the elderly, the Merck Company Foundation and AFAR created the Merck/AFAR Research Scholarships in Geriatric Pharmacology. Medical students will have the opportunity to undertake a 2- to 3-month full-time research project in geriatric pharmacology. Up to nine $4,000 scholarships will be awarded in 2001. *Contact:* American Federation for Aging Research (AFAR), 1414 Avenue of the Americas, 18th Floor, New York, NY 10019. Phone: 212-752-2327; fax: 212-832-2298; e-mail: *amfedaging@aol.com.*

American Oil Chemists' Society

Graduate students in any area of science dealing with fats and lipids who are doing research toward an advanced degree, and who are interested in the area of science and technology fostered by this Society, are eligible. Must be a graduate student who has not yet received his or her degree or begun employment prior to the AOCS meeting he/she is to attend. The award will provide funds equal to travel costs, hotel accommodations, and stipend to permit attendance at the national meeting of the AOCS held in the spring.

Biomedical Synergistics Institute—Ninth International Conference

Award for those individuals in training who submit the best original paper dealing with the Institute enhancement of human functioning. Papers published previously are not eligible for awards. Four student award categories with each receiving a prize of $250. The All Functioning Categories winner will receive a $1,000 prize.

AAA PRESLEY–CARL ZEISS YOUNG INVESTIGATOR AWARD

Recognizes excellence in research using light and/or electron microscopy. Must be a graduate student, medical student, postdoc (within 5 years of receiving PhD), or medical resident. $500 prize and certificate. Contact the Advisory Committee of Young Anatomists (ACYA) at 301-571-8314 or *exec@anatomy.org.*

AAA Zeiss Student Research Award

Recognizes excellence in research using state-of-the-art imaging methods, such as confocal and/or electron microscopy. Must be a graduate student or medical student. $500 prize and certificate. Contact the Advisory Committee of Young Anatomists (ACYA) at 301-571-8314 or *exec@anatomy.org.*

AAA/Genentech Student Research Award

Recognizes excellence in research using molecular biological techniques in the study of morphological changes at the cellular and/or whole animal level. Must be a graduate student, medical student, postdoc (within 5 years of receiving PhD), or medical resident. $500 prize and certificate. Contact the Advisory Committee of Young Anatomists (ACYA) at 301-571-8314 or *exec@anatomy.org.*

ALPHA OMEGA ALPHA RESEARCH FELLOWSHIPS

The purpose of the fellowships is to stimulate interest in research among medical students. Areas of research may include clinical investigation, basic research, epidemiology, and the social sciences, as related to medicine. The program is designed to stimulate students who have not had prior research experience. Fellowship is for $2,000.

American Medical Association Education and Research Foundation

Open to third- and fourth-year medical students who have completed the required clerkships in medicine, surgery, and pediatrics. The program consists of 4- to 6-week clerkships in general, pediatric, and surgical nutrition. Scholarships are only for students who do not have clinical nutrition clerkships available at their own schools. Students accepted into the program will receive a $700 award to defray living and traveling costs.

American College of Sports Medicine National Student Research Award

The National Student Research Award recognizes the most outstanding research project of the year at the graduate/professional student level. An important consideration for the award is the extent of the student's participation in the project. Each applicant must be enrolled in a graduate or professional program in the areas of clinical or basic exercise science or sports medicine at an accredited university, be principal author of a submitted and accepted abstract for presentation at the ACSM annual meeting, and be a member of ACSM or one of its regional chapters at the time of application and at the time the award is presented. The New Investigator and National Student Research awards provide support for the recipients to attend the annual meeting and present their research. Registration fees, travel expenses, lodging, banquet tickets, and framed certificates (presented at the annual awards banquet) are awarded to the recipients. *Contact*: American College of Sports Medicine, Graduate Scholarships for Minorities and Women, 401 W. Michigan St., Indianapolis, IN 46202-3233. Phone: 317-637-9200; fax: 317-634-7817; *www.acsm.org/*.

AMERICAN ACADEMY OF ALLERGY ASTHMA AND IMMUNOLOGY SUMMER FELLOWSHIP GRANT

Summer fellowship grants of $2,000 will be awarded to outstanding medical students who wish to pursue research in the following areas: physiology of allergic diseases, pharmacology of allergy and inflammation, basic cellular and molecular immunology, AIDS, and other topics pertinent to the understanding of allergic and immune mechanisms of disease. Eligibility: Full-time medical students residing in the United States or Canada who have successfully completed at least 8 months of medical school by the time the fellowship starts. Past Summer Fellowship Grant recipients are not eligible. *Contact*: American Academy of Allergy Asthma and Immunology, 611 East Wells Street, Milwaukee, WI 53202-3889. Phone: 414-272-6071; fax: 414-272-6070; *www.aaaai.org/*.

SUMMER EXTERNSHIPS

National Institute of Health Summer Research Award

www.training.nih.gov/.

Africa with Crossroads

Sponsoring agency: Operation Crossroads Africa

For senior medical school students who would like to work on a 5- to 7-week project in Africa that might focus on one of the following themes: (1) the community health approach, (2) diagnosis and treatment of tropical diseases, (3) preventive approaches to tropical diseases, and (4) the use of paramedics. Each project will also involve some labor. No stipend. The sponsoring agency will assist students in finding funds for transportation.

AMERICAN LIVER FOUNDATION STUDENT RESEARCH FELLOWSHIPS

To gain exposure in the research laboratory and possibly consider liver research a career option. Award is $2,500 per month for 3 months. *Contact:* American Liver Foundation, 1425 Pompton Avenue, Cedar Grove, NJ 07009. Phone: 201-857-2626; *www.liverfoundation.org/*.

Mucopolysaccharidosis Society Summer Fellowship

Eight-week summer fellowship for study of mucopolysaccharide diseases. Stipend: $1,500.

Utica College of Syracuse Summer Clerkships

Both of the following programs offer students clinical experience augment their classroom university instruction, reinforce clinical skills, and create interest in their future choice of both medical specialty and geographic area of practice: The summer clerkships (2–8 weeks) are designed for students who have completed either 1 or 2 years of training. Preference is given to second-year students. Stipend is $250/2 weeks. The clinical electives are credit courses offered on a year-round basis in 22 specialties for third- and fourth-year medical students.

MEMORIAL SLOAN-KETTERING CANCER CENTER SUMMER FELLOWSHIP

Sponsored by National Cancer Institute and Eugene W. Kettering Education Fund.

Eight-week summer fellowship offered to medical students in

their first 2 years. Objective of program is the educational enrichment of medical students by offering experience in research and clinical oncology and enhancement of their knowledge of cancer and promotion of future interest in the field. *Contact*: Chuck Ferrero, Box 187, Memorial Sloan-Kettering Cancer Center, 1275 York Ave., NY 10012 (212) 639-8457; *www.mskcc.org/mskcc/html/2637.cfm.*

Simon Kramer Externship in Radiation Oncology

Sponsored by the Thomas Jefferson Hospital, Philadelphia, this fellowship provides a unique opportunity for the medical student to obtain a 6-week experience in the Department of Radiation Therapy and Nuclear Medicine at Jefferson. Flexible beginning date; stipend of $1,200.

New York State Legislative Fellow

Fellows work as regular legislative staff members of the offices to which they are assigned. The work is full time, demanding, and is intended to use and develop the expertise of Fellows while offering an exclusive view of legislative procedures.

EDUCATION AND RESEARCH FOUNDATION OF THE SOCIETY OF NUCLEAR MEDICINE AWARDS

The purpose of the Student Fellowship Program is to provide financial support for students wishing to spend time in clinical or basic research activities in a nuclear medicine division for a 3-month period with a stipend of $3,000.

Student Fellowship Award Foundation of the Society of Nuclear Medicine

This fellowship provides financial support for students to spend elective quarters and/or summers in departments of nuclear medicine assisting in clinical and basic research activities.

Roswell Park Memorial Research Institute (Buffalo, NY) Summer Oncology Program

Provides direct support for students in the health professions engaged in research during the summer. Fellowships are awarded for an 8-week period. Research is restricted to topics in oncology. Participation in this program is limited to students completing their first or second year of study.

RUTGERS UNIVERSITY SUMMER SCHOLARSHIPS

Ten scholarships are available for this year's Summer School of Alcohol Studies to medical students. Award covers university fees, tuition, room, and meals ($975); weekend meals and travel are not included. However, a $200 stipend for related expenses will also be given to each scholarship recipient.

New York Academy of Medicine HIV Professional Development Project

Two-month internship in HIV-focused health care and social service settings. 35 hours/week, $10/hr.

Case Western Reserve University—Pathology

For those who have completed their sophomore year in medical school. This is a 12-month fellowship with a $12,000 stipend. The time will be divided between diagnostic pathology on the autopsy service and research related to the immunological and biochemical characterization of human cancer.

CLENDENING, LOGAN TRAVELING FELLOWSHIP

Sponsoring agency: University of Kansas Medical Center

This fellowship is open to registered medical students of any recognized medical school in the United States or Canada. The fellowship is of the value of $1,500. Applicants may elect to travel anywhere in the world for the purpose of studying any aspect of medical history of interest to them.

Costep of the U.S. Public Health Service

U.S. Public Health Service offers opportunities in Indian Health Services, Health Resources, and Services Administration, NIH, Food and Drug

Administration, CDC, Alcohol, Drug Abuse and Mental Health Administration, etc. U.S. citizenship and at least one year of medical school required. Positions are available all year round. $2,000/month plus travel costs. Information is available in Student Affairs; for application, call 1-800-279-1605 or 301-594-2633.

Cystic Fibrosis Foundation Student Traineeships

The Cystic Fibrosis Foundation announces student traineeships which are offered to introduce students to research related to CF. Applicants must be students in or about to enter a doctoral program (MD, PhD, or MD/PhD). Each applicant must work with a faculty sponsor on a research project related to CF. The award is $1,500, of which $1,200 is designated as a stipend for the trainee, and the remaining $300 may be used for laboratory expenses. For an application, write to: Office of Grants Management, Cystic Fibrosis Foundation, 6931 Arlington Road, Bethesda, MD 20814, or call 1-800-FLIGHT CF.

AMA-MSS GOVERNMENT RELATIONS INTERSHIP PROGRAM APPLICATION

The Department of Medical Student Services, in conjunction with the Washington office of the American Medical Association, is pleased to offer assistance to students seeking to increase their involvement and education in national health policy and in the national legislative activities of organized medicine.

Through the Government Relations Internship Program, stipends of $2,500 are available to assist selected students who are completing health policy internships in the Washington, DC, area. To be eligible for the program, students must be AMA members who have secured a policy internship in the Washington, DC, area. Through the program, students may also apply for an internship at the AMA's Washington office (two positions available), or at the Health Care Financing Administration in Baltimore, Maryland (one position available). Students participating in the program generally arrange their internships with congressional offices, specialty societies, or federal agencies in the DC area. A list of possible internship contacts is available.

The Betty Ford Center Summer Institute for Medical Students

Provides experiential education in chemical dependency and its treatment, primarily by student participation in the patient and family rehabilitation process. Five groups of 12 students will participate in the 5-day summer school program. Each session four Family Program participants follow the weekly schedule of family members, and eight students selected for the Inpatient Program are assigned to one of four inpatient treatment units. Program activities include lectures, meals, group therapy sessions, peer groups, exercise sessions, meditation, medallion ceremonies, and Alcoholics and Narcotics Anonymous meetings. Students are asked to maintain a focused journal. A basic set of books and a reference manual is provided to each student. Scholarships to this very special program include the cost of all materials, lodging, and meals. A travel stipend is also included. A total of 60 scholarships will be awarded. Students may apply to attend one of four summer sessions. For application information, write: Betty Ford Center Training Department, 39000 Bob Hope Drive, Rancho Mirage, CA 92270. Phone: 619-773-4108; toll free: 1-800 854-9211, ext. 4108; fax: 619-773-1697.

The Albert Schweitzer Fellowship

Provides complete funding for medical students who will work in Lambaréné, Gabon, as junior physicians, supervised by Schweitzer Hospital medical staff. Prior completion of clerkships in medicine, pediatrics, and surgery are required; some background or coursework in tropical medicine or parasitology is important but not a prerequisite. Because all patient encounters occur in French, a working knowledge of that language is absolutely essential. For more information, contact: The Albert Schweitzer Foundation, 330 Brookline Avenue, Boston, MA 02215.

HOWARD HUGHES MEDICAL INSTITUTE RESEARCH SCHOLARS TRAINING

Students in good standing in a medical school in the United States who have completed the second year but have not yet received the MD are eligible. The program is for at least 9 months and usually 1 year at NIH. Salary program $16,800, and other benefits are included. *Contact:* 1-800-424-9924.

American Diabetes Association, Inc. Medical Scholars Program Awards

The goal of the program is to produce new leaders in diabetes research by supplying physicians-in-training the opportunity to contribute to the process of discovery in basic or clinical research laboratories. Award is $30,000 for 1 year. Eligibility: Students must have completed at least 2 years of medical school. *Contact*: American Diabetes Association, Inc. Research Department, 1701 North Beauregard Street, Alexandria, VA 22311. Phone: 703-549-1500, ext. 2376; fax: 703-549-1715; *www.diabetes.org/research/.*

Pew Charitable Trust/ Rockefeller University Fellowships in Human Nutrition

One-year program designed to give hands-on laboratory experience and mastering of new methods in biomedical science for application to problems in human nutrition. Students should have completed their third year by July 1. Stipend: $14,700. Pierce, Chester Research Symposium.

UNIVERSITY OF PITTSBURGH PATHOLOGY FELLOWSHIP

One-year fellowship for medical students who have completed their second year and wish to spend an additional year of in-depth study of pathology in research (pathology, molecular biology, genetics, etc.) and practice before going on to the third year. The stipend is $11,000, and a scholarship for the next year of medical school (up to the state tuition rate at Pittsburgh) will be provided.

Association of Pathology Chairman Student Fellowship

Year-long full-time fellowship in participating schools for students after the second year of medical school. Intended to give students an in-depth research and/or clinical experience in pathology between the basic science and clinical years. Support varies by school, as do openings for students not from that school.

New York City Health Research Training Program

This is a practicum in public health research. The student participates in a project under the direct supervision of a preceptor. The projects are submitted by preceptors from within the Health Department or from outside agencies such as hospitals, medical schools, or other health-related institutions. A seminar series is part of the program. Work-study students are preferred. However, some alternative support is available for those not eligible for work-study. Full time in summer, part time during school year.

NEW YORK CITY URBAN FELLOWS PROGRAM

Year-long program offering the opportunity and challenge of an intensive field experience in urban government. Fellows work closely with city officials on long- and short-term projects and attend weekly seminars to gain an academic perspective on the workings and problems of local government. $17,000 stipend and insurance.

National Institutes of Health Summer Research Fellowship

With the guidance of a preceptor from one of the Institutes, students conduct research in a selected area of laboratory investigation. Program offers practical experience in research procedures and lectures and seminars designed to enhance education and investigative skills. Program runs a minimum of 8 weeks.

National Institutes of Health Clinical Electives Program

Medical students are invited to apply for clinical electives of 8 weeks with opportunities research and clinical experience with physician-scientists in Bethesda.

OSLER LIBRARY FELLOWSHIP PROGRAM

A fellowship program for historians, physicians, and students conducting research in the history of medicine. Intended to serve those who need to establish temporary residence in order to undertake research in the Osler Library.

Henry Luce Foundation Scholars Program

This program provides an intensive year-long experience in Asia designed to broaden the scholar's professional perspectives and to sharpen their perceptions of Asia, America, and themselves. The support consists of airfare, stipend, medical insurance, etc.

Echoing Green Foundation Fellowship

One-year fellowship providing entrepreneurial people with the opportunity to develop and implement an innovative public service project (health, environment, youth service, international development, etc.). Students must develop a proposal. Stipend is $25,000 per year.

HEALTH RESEARCH GROUP MEDICAL STUDENT FELLOWSHIP

One-year fellowship in Washington researching and monitoring federal health agencies, congressional lobbying, publication of consumer-oriented educational manuals, etc.

Rosalie B. Hite Cancer Center Research Fellowship

Sponsoring agency: University of Texas System

Fellowship open to graduate students or research workers in the area of cancer research. Selection of Fellows is on the basis of academic excellence of the candidate and applicability of the proposed program to the problems of cancer research. Graduate work is to be under the supervision of a faculty member of a component of the University of Texas at Houston, affiliated with the Graduate School of Biomedical Sciences Sciences degree-granting program.

Charles A. Dana Foundation Clinical Research Training Program

Sponsoring agency: University of Pennsylvania School of Medicine

Opportunity for medical students to participate in a year-long in-depth clinical research training experience under the guidance of selected faculty who are accomplished investigators in the fields of epidemiology, clinical research methodology, and the delivery of health care services. Training will be provided in clinical research methods, clinical epidemiology, biostatistics, and scientific communication. Stipend of $11,000 plus expenses.

CHARLES A. AND ANNE MORROW LINDBERGH FOUNDATION

A foundation dedicated to furthering Charles and Anne Morrow Lindbergh's shared vision of a balance between technological advancement and environmental preservation. Lindbergh grants are made in the following categories: agriculture; aviation/aerospace; conservation of natural resources—including animals, plants, water, and general conservation (land, air, energy, etc.); education—including humanities/education, the arts, and intercultural communication; exploration; health—including biomedical research, health and population sciences, and adaptive technology; and waste minimization and management. A Jonathan Lindbergh Brown Grant may be given to a project to support adaptive technology or biomedical research that seeks to redress imbalance between an individual and his or her human environment. Grants are made to individuals as well as educational and publication programs. *Contact: www.lindbergh-foundation.org.*

National Medical Fellowship—Commonwealth Fund

This program is designed to encourage academically gifted minority medical students to pursue careers in academic medicine and biomedical research. Open to those students who have completed their junior year. Duration is 8–12 weeks. Students have the option to participate in the summer or during the academic year. Fellowship award is for $5,000, with $2,000 earmarked for mentor to offset expenses during the research period.

National Institute of Arthritis and Musculoskeletal and Skin Diseases (NIAMS)

The Minority Travel Award Program provides travel funds for minority students and faculty members from minority institutions for attendance at national scientific meetings. *Contact: www.nih.gov/niams.*

NIH PREDOCTORAL FELLOWSHIP AWARDS FOR MINORITY STUDENTS

The National Research Service Award Predoctoral Fellowship for Minority Students will provide up to 5 years of support for research training leading to the PhD or equivalent research degree; the combined MD/PhD degree; or other combined professional degree and research doctoral degree in biomedical, behavioral sciences, or health services research. These fellowships are designed to enhance the racial and ethnic diversity of the biomedical, behavioral, and health services research labor force in the United States. Accordingly, academic institutions are encouraged to identify and recruit students from underrepresented racial and ethnic groups who can apply for this fellowship. Support is *not* available for individuals enrolled in medical or other professional schools *unless* they are also enrolled in a combined professional doctorate/PhD degree program in biomedical, behavioral, or health services research. *Contact: www.nih.gov.*

National Medical Fellowships, Inc.

NMF offers awards and fellowships to American Blacks, mainland Puerto Ricans, Mexican-Americans, and American Indians who are U.S. citizens enrolled in accredited schools of allopathic or osteopathic medicine in the United States. Funding is variable, yearly, and renewable. *Contact:* National Medical Fellowships, Inc., 254 West 31st Street, 7th Floor, New York, NY 10001. Phone: 212-714-1007.

Metropolitan Life Award Program for Academic Excellence in Medicine

This program recognizes and rewards third-year minority medical students for outstanding academic achievement and demonstrated leadership. $2,500 need-based awards to underrepresented minorities. Nominated by dean's office.

AMERICAN COLLEGE OF SPORTS MEDICINE MINORITY SCHOLARSHIP

The American College of Sports Medicine annually awards graduate scholarships for minorities and females of up to $1,500 each to be used to cover college or university tuition and/or fees. The purpose of these scholarships is to provide partial support toward the education of graduate and/or medical students with outstanding promise and a strong interest in research and scholarly activities as they pursue a career in sports medicine or exercise science. Scholarships are renewable for up to 4 years based on their research and professional activities and satisfactory academic progress in full-time study toward a graduate degree. Students who are not currently ACSM members are eligible to apply. Free student membership in the American College of Sports Medicine is also provided each year of an awardee's graduate scholarship. *Contact:* American College of Sports Medicine, Graduate Scholarships for Minorities and Women, 401 W. Michigan St., Indianapolis, IN 46202-3233. Phone: 317-637-9200; fax: 317-634-7817; *www.acsm.org/.*

Congressional Black Caucus Foundation, Inc. Scholarships

Offers grant money for doctoral study to minority students. *Con-*

tact: Congressional Black Caucus Foundation, Inc., 1004 Pennsylvania Avenue SE, Washington, DC 20003. Phone: 1-800-784-2577 or 202-675-6730; fax: 202-547-3806.

American Indian Graduate Center Grants

Grants of $250–$10,000 are available for American Indian students who are members of a federally recognized American Indian tribe or Alaska Native group, or possess one-fourth degree federally recognized Indian blood with financial need after exhausting available aid at their school financial aid office. *Contact:* American Indian Graduate Center, 4520 Montgomery Blvd. NE, Suite 1-B, Albuquerque, New Mexico 87109. Phone: 505-881-4584.

ETHNIC

DR. ANTHONY BAGATELOS MEMORIAL SCHOLARSHIP

Grant money available for Greek descent/Greek Orthodox faith with intentions to practice medicine within the nine-county area surrounding San Francisco Bay. Applications may be obtained by contacting: Annunciation Greek Orthodox Cathedral, 245 Valencia St., San Francisco CA 94103.

Chinese American Physicians Society (CAPS)

CAPS is offering 8 to 10 scholarships of $1,000–$2,000 each annually to two categories of medical students. The first is the Dr. Lester Chen Memorial Scholarships to students of Asian descent from the San Francisco Bay area. The other is the CAPS Scholarships to all medical students in need of financial aid regardless of their hometown, sex, race, or color. The applicants are judged according to their academic achievements, financial needs, community service records, and essays. Special credit is also given to those who are willing to serve the Chinese communities after their graduation. The deadline for submitting the completed application is usually the first Friday in October. Due to the huge number of requests for applications and our shortage of manpower, we can no longer send out the application by mail unless a self-addressed stamped envelope is enclosed with the request. Please obtain the applications from the student financial aid office of your medical school starting from April 1 each year. You can also print a copy of the published scholarship application from our web site. If you need more information about the scholarship program, please contact Chinese American Physicians Society, Lawrence M. Ng, MD, Executive Director, 345 Ninth Street, Suite 204, Oakland, CA 94607-4206. Phone: 510-895-5539 (voice and fax); e-mail: *scholarship@caps-ca.org*.

JAPANESE MEDICAL SOCIETY SCHOLARSHIP AWARD

$1,500–$5,000 grants to students of Japanese ancestry who are enrolled or accepted in a U.S. medical school. Applications may be obtained by contacting: Japanese Medical Society of America, Inc. Scholarship Committee, One Henry Street, Englewood Cliffs, NJ 07632.

JEWISH VOCATIONAL SERVICE ACADEMIC SCHOLARSHIP

For Jewish medical students living in Chicago. Applications are accepted December 1 through March 1. *Contact:* Jewish Vocational Service, One South Franklin Street, Chicago, Illinois 60606. Phone: 312-346-6700, ext. 2214.

Hellenic Medical Society Scholarship

Awards for medical students of Hellenic heritage from New York, New Jersey, Pennsylvania, Connecticut; must be a second-year student enrolled at an accredited U.S. school. *Contact:* Hellenic Medical Society of New York, 401 East 34th Street, New York NY 10016.

FOR WOMEN

AAUW Educational Foundation International Fellowship

This is a grant for foreign students to pursue graduate studies in the United States. *Contact:* American Association of University Women, 1111 Sixteenth St. NW, Washington, DC 20036. Phone: 1-800-326-AAUW; fax: 202-872-1425; e-mail: *info@aauw.org.*

AMWA CARROLL L. BIRCH AWARD

Sponsored by the Chicago Branch of the American Medical Women's Association, the award is presented for the best original research paper written by a Student Life Member of AMWA. Women must be enrolled in an accredited U.S. medical or osteopathic medical school to apply. The recipient of the award receives a cash prize of $500 and a plaque presented at AMWA's annual meeting. An article noting the award winner will appear in one of the Association's publications, and an abstract may be published in AMWA's journal. Contact your school's financial aid office for more info.

AMWA Bed and Breakfast Program

The program assists students who are traveling for a residency or job interview or physician members attending an out-of-town conference. Our members contact the national office with details of the trip. The national office responds by sending the traveler a listing of volunteers in the destination area. There is an administrative fee of $10 for students and $15 for physicians.

BPW Career Advancement Scholarship for Women

Grants of $500–$1,000 for women over 25 in their third or fourth year of studies with critical need for assistance. *Contact:* Scholarships/Loans Business and Professional Women's Foundation, 2012 Mass Ave. NW, Washington, DC 20036. Phone: 202-293-1200, ext. 169.

AWARDS AND LINKS TO MEDICAL SUBSPECIALTY SOCIETIES

American Society of Clinical Oncology Medical Student Rotation: *www.ascocancerfoundation.org/TACF/Awards/Award+Opportunities*

American College of Rheumatology Research and Education Foundation/Abbott Medical Student Clinical Preceptorship: *www.rheumatology.org/ref/awards/summerclinical.asp*

ACR Research and Education Foundation: *www.rheumatology.org/ref/awards/index.asp*

Agency for Healthcare Research and Quality: *www.ahrq.gov/fund/funding.htm*

Alliance for Lupus Research: *www.lupusresearch.org/grants_03.html*

American Autoimmune Related Diseases Association: *www.aarda.org/programs.html*

American Diabetes Association: *www.diabetes.org/main/professional/research/research.jsp*

Arthritis Foundation: *www.arthritis.org/research/default.asp*

Arthritis National Research Foundation: *www.curearthritis.org*

Crohn's and Colitis Foundation: *www.ccfa.org/science/research/*

Johnson & Johnson/Society for the Arts in Healthcare: *www.thesah.org*

Juvenile Diabetes Research Foundation: *www.jdrf.org/index.cfm?fuseaction=home.viewPage&page_id=8AC28525-1BC5-4E79-9A9079E0DE3C5739*

Lupus Research Institute: *www.lupusresearchinstitute.org/research_grants.jsp*

National Multiple Sclerosis Society: *www.nationalmssociety.org/research.asp*

National Psoriasis Foundation: *www.psoriasis.org/research/*

Robert Wood Johnson Foundation: *http://rwjfpfsp.stanford.edu/*

SLE Foundation, Inc.: *www.lupusny.org*

Scleroderma Foundation: *www.scleroderma.org/research/researchhome.htm*

Sjogren's Syndrome Foundation: *www.sjogrens.com/research/*

www.acponline.org/journals/ebm/ebmmenu.htm: Reviews the evidence for current medical practice.

www.ebem.org: Evidence-based emergency medicine home page.

cebm.jr2.ox.ac.uk: NHS Research and Development Centre of Evidence Based Medicine.

www.update-software.com/cochrane.htm: Web site for the Cochrane Library, the most well-known site for critically appraised topics or evidence-based reviews.

www.ebando.com: Bandolier: online publication on evidence-based health care.

www.shef.ac.uk/~scharr/ir/netting.html: Netting the evidence: A ScHARR introduction to evidence-based practice on the Internet.

www.ti.ubc.ca/pages/letter.html: Therapeutics Letter: Evidence-based review of pharmaceutical products.

www.ncbi.nlm.nih.gov/PubMed: Pub Med, a MEDLINE search engine through the National Library of Medicine.

igm.nlm.nih.gov: Grateful Med, a MEDLINE search engine through the National Library of Medicine.

www.cdc.gov: The Centers for Disease Control and Prevention: Contains full text issues of *Morbidity and Mortality Weekly Report.*

www.nejm.org: New England Journal of Medicine.

www.jwatch.org: Journal Watch.

www.bmj.com/index.shtml: British Medical Journal.

jama.ama-assm.org: Journal of the American Medical Association.

Index

H

M

N

O